EDUCATIONAL PSYCHOLOGY

Founded by C. K. Ogden

The International Library of Psychology

DEVELOPMENTAL PSYCHOLOGY
In 32 Volumes

EDUCATIONAL PSYCHOLOGY

Its Problems and Methods

CHARLES FOX

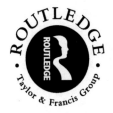

First published in 1925 by
Kegan Paul, Trench, Trubner & Co., Ltd.

Reprinted in 1999, 2001, 2002 by
Routledge
11 New Fetter Lane, London EC4P 4EE

Transferred to Digital Printing 2003

Routledge is an imprint of the Taylor & Francis Group

Printed and Bound in Great Britain by
Hobbs the Printers Ltd, Totton, Hants

British Library Cataloguing in Publication Data
A CIP catalogue record for this book
is available from the British Library

Educational Psychology
ISBN 0415-20988-9
Developmental Psychology: 32 Volumes
ISBN 0415-21128-X
The International Library of Psychology: 204 Volumes
ISBN 0415-19132-7

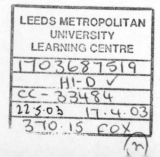

To
MY MOTHER

PREFACE

THE purpose of the present volume is to consider the contribution made by experimental psychology to the study of educational problems. In the last quarter of a century the volume of experimental work has expanded to such an extent that it is becoming well-nigh hopeless to get a conspectus of the position. Much of this work has reference direct or indirect to educational matters, and it is hoped that the survey here attempted may help the student of education to find his bearings in this territory. Enthusiastic experimenters are apt to forget that wisdom did not delay its entrance into the world until the reign of experimental psychology and that the experience of practical teachers gives them an insight into the mentality of youth obtainable in no other way. Nevertheless, the value of experimental observation cannot be gainsaid, and the science of education must take into account the evidence acquired by exact methods. The limitation to the experimental standpoint explains the omission of a full treatment of certain obvious topics which ought to find a place in educational psychology, but these are dealt with incidentally.

Wherever possible I have given historical details believing that some psychological problems cannot be adequately understood without historical treatment. This is more especially the case with the doctrine of mental discipline, the idea of which is very ancient whilst attacks on the notion are frequently directed against views which nobody has ever held.

Modern psychology gives a deservedly prominent

place to the study of instinctive tendencies or inherited impulses to activity, but the treatment is based on a very doubtful assumption. It is widely held that such tendencies are the only springs of conduct, the sole motive to action being in all cases some non-rational impulse. This belief was first formulated by Hume, who maintained as an ethical doctrine that reason could never of itself be a motive to conduct, but was confined in its operation to directing the conflict of such impulses. Recent writers, too, believe that only propelling and never attracting forces determine human conduct. As a corollary to this they are driven to assert that we can never acquire a new impulse to action but that all the energy is derived from inherited impulses or instincts. The doctrine has reached its predetermined psychological conclusion in Professor Freud's theory that all mental energy is derived from the sexual impulse. I have given reasons in the Chapter on habit-formation to show that there is no ground for the belief that acquired impulses are all derived from inherited tendencies to action.

It is a matter of considerable difficulty to separate the odd grain or two of educational doctrine from the great mass of psycho-analytic chaff. The exponents of psycho-analysis adopt the method of committing a violent assault upon the emotions. Harrowing or pitiable tales are told about mentally unstable people with a wealth of irrelevant and sometimes nauseating detail, the effect of which is to rob the reader of his sound judgment, when some obsolete psychological heresy is propounded and forthwith accepted on emotional grounds. The approach to the subject through the measurement of association times may aid in removing the bias, and releasing the reason. If 'cases' are avoided there is very little left to discuss.

In dealing with such questions as the nature of intelligence and mental fatigue I have tried to counter the doctrine that we have any need for a hypothetical central fund of mental energy, since although it is sometimes necessary to refer the unknown to the more unknown it is better not to do so if it can be avoided.

The treatment of mental tests is fast becoming a scandal. Testers have lost their mental balance and are confusing administrative with psychological procedure, so that devices invented for rapidly marking large numbers of answers have been erected into laws of the working of the mind. Hence we are offered tests in which the examinee no longer answers questions but merely selects a stupid answer forced on him by the examiner.

In many cases I have indicated where the next line of advance seems to me the most profitable, and the text contains several previously unpublished experiments. With the same object in view I have ventured as a stimulus to research to suggest a new view of mental imagery and a new theory of mental fatigue.

The method of placing all the references at the end of the book has been adopted in order to keep the student's attention fixed on the main line of argument. Only such references are included as deal with the matters directly discussed in the text and notes are frequently given chiefly by way of suggestion for reading.

I desire to thank the Editor of the *British Journal of Psychology* for permission to make liberal use of articles of mine in the Chapters on memory and observation ; and the Editor of the *Francis Galton Eugenics Laboratory Memoirs* to print the diagram in Chapter I.

CHARLES FOX.

WARKWORTH HOUSE,
CAMBRIDGE.
July 31st, 1925.

CONTENTS

xi

Chapter XI

Chapter XII

EDUCATIONAL PSYCHOLOGY
ITS PROBLEMS AND METHODS

CHAPTER I

MENTAL DEVELOPMENT

Theories of the Nature of Mind—(*a*) Compartment Theory—(*b*) Faculty
Theory—(*c*) Association Theory—(*d*) Structure Theory—(*e*) Gestalt
Theory—Mental Heredity—Terminology—Evidence for Mental
Heredity—Inheritance of Acquired Characters

THEORIES OF THE NATURE OF MIND

THE student of educational psychology will find his path
beset with insuperable difficulties unless he has clear ideas on
the nature of mental development. There is hardly a problem
in connection with the subject of our study which does not
assume some theory of development, and our first task must
be to examine the different views which have been accepted
in the past or are now current. It is the special danger of
workers in applied science to accept principles without
sufficient investigation and thereby to perpetuate age-long
errors. In the course of this book we shall have ample
opportunities of observing the confusion which has been
caused by accepting mistaken psychological theories as
though they were profound educational truths.

There are five theories of the nature and growth of mind
which need examination in this preliminary survey owing to
the fact that they are frequently employed consciously or

1

A

unconsciously in the application of psychology to educational
topics.   They will be referred to as

        (*a*) The Compartment Theory
        (*b*) The Faculty Theory
        (*c*) The Association Theory
        (*d*) The Structure Theory
        (*e*) The *Gestalt* Theory.

(a) *The Compartment Theory*

The compartment theory is so primitive that it seems
difficult to believe that such a view of the nature of mind
could have been resuscitated in a scientific age.   According
to this view the mind is regarded as a kind of receptacle
composed of different compartments, each of which is able to
store a definite amount of mental material of a particular
sort.   The nature of the material is not always clearly indicated but it is frequently supposed to consist of ideas, images,
affects and so on.   The various receptacles are assumed, in a
loose way, to have a more or less definite volume permitting
only a certain number of the contents to be stored in them.
If more are put in some must be squeezed out ; but sometimes
the images and ideas are regarded as being of a sort of gaseous
nature so that more can be forced in under pressure.   Mental
development consists of acquiring the mental elements and
arranging them into their proper compartments, after the
fashion of the files in an office, for convenience of reference.
Sometimes the compartments are dignified by the name of
systems but the underlying idea is the same.

Lest it should be imagined that nobody could conceivably
adopt this view I give a quotation from the exponent of the
most recent revival of the compartment idea.   " The unconscious system of the mind," says Professor Freud,[1] " may
be compared to a large ante-room in which the various mental

excitations are crowding upon one another, like individual beings. Adjoining this is a second, smaller apartment, a sort of reception-room, in which, too, consciousness resides. But on the threshold between the two there stands a personage with the office of door-keeper, who examines the various mental excitations, censors them, and denies them admittance to the reception-room when he disapproves of them. . . . The excitations in the unconscious, in the ante-chamber, are not visible to consciousness, which is, of course, in the other room, so to begin with they remain unconscious. . . . But even those excitations which are allowed over the threshold do not necessarily become conscious ; they can only become so if they succeed in attracting the eye of consciousness. This second chamber, therefore, may be suitably called the pre-conscious system." Although we are told that consciousness resides in the reception-room apparently the ideas and images (or excitations, which are queer things) do not awaken until, like the princess in the fairy tale, they have received the kiss of consciousness, rubbed their eyes and passed into a third compartment. What consciousness is apart from the contents of consciousness is a deep, not to say meaningless mystery. But this does not concern us at present.

This spatial notion of a series of compartments, owing to the ease with which it may be visualised, has captured the popular imagination ; and the fantastic theory of unconscious ideas which have all the characteristics of ideas as we know them except that of being conscious (which is the only constitutive property of an idea) has been accepted as sound psychology. In fact these crudities constitute the stock-in-trade of most of the exponents of psycho-analysis. The only person of this school who was not originally deceived by the theory was Professor Freud who states [2] that, " We may give free rein to our assumptions provided we at the same time preserve our cool judgment and do not take the scaffolding for the building." However he soon forgot this sound advice himself and his followers have never appreciated its significance. In dealing with functional diseases of the nervous system it is no doubt desirable for the practitioner to have a visual symbol in order to help in the analysis of the various complicated activities displayed in the psycho-neuroses. If the time relations of these activities can be conceived as split up into minor activities which exhibit a definite time sequence it is useful to symbolise the time relations by a spatial diagram. Thus if the origin of a certain phobia in an adult can be traced to some event occurring in his childhood it may be convenient, as a rough and ready mnemonic, to represent the original event as an idea persisting in an unconscious state for that will help to keep the cause in mind and will be useful for future reference. But, strictly speaking, there is no need whatever to assume a real spatial arrangement of the psychic system or to suppose that the mnemonics in any way resemble the structure of the living mind. In order not to be misled by the specious simplicity of all this spatial symbolism the student of educational psychology must remember that " these comparisons are designed only to assist us in our attempt to make clear the complication of the psychic activity by breaking up this activity and referring the simple activities to the single component parts of the apparatus." [3] In brief the various compartments are a device for representing spatially a series of time relations and should never be used for any other purpose. To build up a theory of mental processes on such a basis is like the attempt of the friends of an engaged couple to study the characteristics of their future children from a survey of the scaffolding of the house they are building.

(b) *The Faculty Theory*

Very little need be said about the theory of the nature of the mind as composed of a congeries of faculties, since no competent person now holds the view. It does however crop up from time to time and it is as well to see why it has been finally abandoned as a mode of explanation, though its terminology is often indispensable as a method of description. The criticism of Locke has never been bettered and therefore I quote from the Essay concerning Human Understanding.[4] " For, it being asked, what it was that digested the meat in our stomachs ? it was a ready and very satisfactory answer to say that it was the *digestive faculty*. And so in the mind, the *intellectual faculty* or the understanding, understood, and the *elective faculty* or the will, willed or commanded. This is in short, to say, that the ability to digest, digested ; and the ability to understand, understood. For faculty, ability and power, I think, are but different names of the same things ; which way of speaking, when put into more intelligible words, will, I think, amount to thus much ;—That digestion is performed by something that is able to digest . . . understanding by something able to understand. And, in truth, it would be very strange if it should be otherwise."

Since the faculties were intended to express the activity of the mind as shewn in the variety of functioning, if we abandon the use of them we must be prepared to attribute some power to the subject himself. Certain modern psychologists have, however, emptied the baby together with the water of the bath. Not only do they reject the complex faculties of memory imagination and the like, but they deny all power whatsoever to the mind, and fondly imagine that they can explain mental events without reference to mental activity. But this is ridiculous and no amount of talk about ideas acting, or images doing this or that, such as disappearing into the unconscious

and reappearing again like Jacks in the Box can dispense with
the notion of subjective activity.   As to the attempt to father
all the mental activity displayed by a living mind on to its
physiological substratum that is but an instance of the absurd
attempt to explain function by structure which we shall
consider later.   The nervous system is doubtless a necessary
condition of mental functioning but to regard it as the sole
sufficient condition is erroneous.   We shall see as we proceed
that many of the difficulties which educational psychology
is heir to originate in the denial of mental activity or the
attempt to substitute nervous activity in its place.

It has been recognised for some time that in order to
describe experience we require at least three ultimate descriptive terms.   From the days of Aristotle two aspects of experience had been recognised namely the cognitive and the
conative, but Rousseau forced attention to the third aspect
by insisting on the rights and importance of the life of feeling
in opposition to the view that feeling was a kind of obscure
thought or confused impulse.[5]   Since the time of Kant who
first applied the three descriptive terms consistently psychologists have recognised cognition, feeling and conation as
three attitudes which a person adopts in so far as he is mentally
alive.   But though these are analytically distinguishable, in
experience they are never found apart.   The suggestion has
been made that these should be called the ultimate faculties
of the mind but as this would imply a separation which, in
fact, never occurs it is more conformable with common
sense to regard them merely as descriptive terms with which
to describe the various subjective aspects of experience.

(c) *The Association Theory*

After running riot in Scottish psychology the faculties were
finally laid to rest by the association theory.   The history of

the " association of ideas " in psychology is a terribly long
and varied one.[6] Aristotle in a treatise on Memory had
noticed that " when we are recollecting we keep stimulating
certain earlier experiences until we have stimulated one
which the one in question is wont to succeed. And just so
we hunt through the sequence, thinking along from the
present or some other thing, and from similar or contrasted or
contiguous." Centuries elapsed and Descartes introduced
the notion that association was entirely a matter of brain
physiology. " The vestiges in the brain," said he, " render it
fit to move the soul in the same fashion as it was moved
before, and thus to make it remember something, even as
the folds which are in a piece of paper or a cloth make it
more fit to be folded as it was before." [7] This conception
has been accepted uncritically by most schools of psychology
especially those which pride themselves on being up to date.

When the association psychology was introduced into Great
Britain in the middle of the 18th century by Hartley in his
" Observations on Man " its ultimate result was to give the
quietus to the Scottish school which explained every conceivable mental act as due to a separate faculty. Thenceforward
in England until the last quarter of the 19th century theories
of philosophy, ethics, law and education were permeated by
the belief that all the most complex forms of mental life could
be adequately accounted for by the mechanical union of
simpler states. It is true that the doctrine of ' mental
chemistry ' by which the simpler states were supposed to be
combined in a manner analogous with the composition of
chemical elements in a compound eliminated some of the
more obvious failings. But neither this modification nor the
doctrine of evolution with which it was later combined, so
that the higher mental powers were regarded as evolved from
the simpler, made any real difference to the associationists ;
for no new principle except associationism was introduced

but the results of the association were merely supposed to be carried on from generation to generation. The wide extent of the principle may be gathered from a remark of J. S. Mill [8] commenting on the doctrines of his father, the classical English associationist. " In psychology his fundamental doctrine was the formation of all human character by circumstances, through the universal Principle of Association, and the consequent unlimited possibility of improving the moral and intellectual condition of mankind by education." For, if the mechanical association of ideas is the sole factor involved, it is clear that by providing the opportunities for making the correct associations we are doing all that we possibly can for intellectual and moral development, and we may make intelligence and character to order.

Although the doctrine of association of ideas as an explanatory principle was worked to death by the English school, Locke, who incidentally introduced the term dealt with it not to explain knowledge but to account for human error. According to him ideas, whether rationally related or not, may, by the force of habit, be so united in an individual mind that it is impossible to separate them. " They always keep in company, and the one no sooner at any time comes into the understanding, but its associate appears with it ; and if they are more than two which are thus united, the whole gang, always inseparable, shew themselves together." [9] Such connection which varies from person to person is dependent on inclinations, education and interest. He gave as an illustration the association of " goblins and sprites " with darkness : " Let but a foolish maid inculcate these often on the mind of a child, and raise them there together, possibly he shall never be able to separate them again so long as he lives."

As used by the classical English school association referred primarily to those sequences of presentations which occur in memory, imagination or thought, but was not confined to these. It was also used to cover the connection between sensations and movements or movements and ideas, and ultimately to explain the formation of habits. Thus Hartley illustrated the principle by shewing how the child learns to speak. He hears the word *mother* constantly when he sees her, consequently it was assumed that the visual sensation would stimulate the muscular movements of articulation ; or, later on, the mental image of his mother would be sufficient to set off the train of movements. In this simple way the whole structure of our memory and thought was supposed to be built up. What the associationists forgot, however, was that the child made the association because he had an innate impulse to speak and was interested in his mother as the source of all his joys ; so that not the bare conjunction of the " ideas " but the eagerness to satisfy an impulse was the real cause of the association.

Various forms of association have been enumerated such as association by contiguity, similarity, contrast, etc., but the only ultimate ' law of association ' is association by contiguity. The so-called association by similarity is a *result* observed by comparing the ideas *after* they have been recalled, and not therefore a cause of the revival ; as when the chimes of a clock remind me of the bells of Big Ben, which comparison I now make for the first time, i.e. after the association has been made. Contiguity, however, either in space or time is no real ground of association but simply provides the opportunity for the person to attend to the presentations in immediate succession, thus facilitating their recall.

It is very tempting to try to account for association wholly in terms of brain structure and theories of this kind spring up again and again. The most recent and thorough attempt is that of Professor Semon. He calls any enduring modification in living substance after it has been submitted to a stimulus a mnemic trace or engram and the process by which future stimuli touch off the engrams is known as ecphory. The principle of association is summed up in two ultimate mnemic laws. " All simultaneous excitations within an organism leave behind a connected engram-complex, constituting a coherent unity " and " The partial recurrence of the excitation-complex which left behind it a simultaneous engram-complex acts ecphorically on the latter whether the recurrence be in the form of original or mnemic excitations." Perhaps the meaning of the latter law may best be understood by an example. If I hear the phrase " all that glitters " I mentally supply its completion. Now the stimulus to the first word of the phrase " is not gold " is regarded as the auditory sensation of the preceding word, whilst the stimulus to the word *gold* is supposed to be the mnemic excitation set up in the engram-complex *is not gold*. This latter engram-complex has been ' left behind ' in my brain in accordance with the first law. So, to take a more primitive example, when a child simultaneously sees his nurse and receives food, both the optical stimulus and the taste stimuli produce their engraphic effects and the engrams are permanently associated. But all this leaves out the essential part of the process. Unless the child were interested both in the nurse and the food and more especially in the fact that these somehow go together the association would never be made. The attention to the combined stimuli which makes them parts of one interesting whole is the ultimate cause of the association. Thenceforward the sight of the nurse will act ecphorically to determine attention to the foretaste of the coming food.

The fundamental defect of the association theory lay in the denial, explicit or implicit, of mental activity or subjective selection amongst the ' ideas.' It was an attempt to account for the growth and development of mind on the ground of a marriage union between sensations, ideas, images, movements, etc., which act on their account, the person being passive in the process.   Thus Bain, one of the chief exponents, stated the law of Association by Contiguity which as we saw is the ultimate law of all mental association thus :— " Contiguity joins together things [he meant sensations, images, etc.] that occur together, or that are, by any circumstance, presented to the mind *at the same time.*" [10]   It was never explained what particular virtue resided in mere " Contiguity " which enabled it to do anything in the mental world.   How " ideas " could " associate " themselves remained and remains an inexplicable mystery.   Quite recently a new school of psychologists arose in America, the behaviourists, who dug up the corpse of associationism and thought that by substituting ' movements ' for ' ideas ' the remains could be revived and ' behave ' as though they breathed the breath of mental life.   But the carcase refused to function and simulate mental activity though it was provided for the purpose with explicit movements and, where these failed, with an illicit collection of implicit movements to do the work.[11]

(d) *The Structure Theory*

According to this view in its crudest form the mind is considered as a kind of structure having a form gradually built up in the course of experience.   Part of the plan of structure has already been laid down by the race before individual experience begins so that the subject does not start *de novo* but inherits a fabric which he proceeds to extend still further.   In order to realise how this idea arose it is necessary to refer to the hypothesis of *mental dispositions.* When a man is said to know mathematics, for instance, we do not mean that he is at that moment thinking of the subject, for he may be reading a novel.   What we mean is that he is capable of calling to mind certain mathematical propositions as he requires them and of forming correct judgments about mathematical ideas.   So, again, suppose I meet a man for the first time and then forget all about him ; on a future occasion I may recognise him although there may be nothing to shew in the interval that my mind is affected in any way. In both these and in all similar cases some psychologists as we saw assume that previous experience leaves behind some trace which determines subsequent mental processes, and such after-effects are called dispositions.   It is important clearly to realise that we have, so far, no independent means of knowing of the existence of the dispositions except by their effects. Or, rather, it would be better to say that the sole reason for assuming their existence is to enable us to give a connected instead of a piecemeal account of the facts of mental life. Hence to call them ' engrams ' or to refer to them by any other descriptive name such as ' unconscious mental modifications ' as is frequently done, is surreptitiously to assign to them certain hypothetical properties.

A man's present consciousness is determined by a set of conditions which are not completely enumerated when we have assigned all that is present at that moment to his mind. Thus if one tries to remember what one had for breakfast the possibility of recalling the various items of the meal with a sense of recognition is due mainly to what happened in the morning, and is only partially accounted for by the present situation and the effort to remember.   Hence the recollection is an instance of what has been happily called ' mnemic causality.'   To illustrate this, suppose " you smell peat-smoke and you recall some occasion when you smelt it before. The cause of your recollection, so far as hitherto observable phenomena are concerned, consists both of the peat-smoke (present stimulus) and of the former occasion (past experience).   The same stimulus will not produce the same recollection in another man who did not share your former experience.

. . . According to the maxim ' same cause, same effect,' we cannot therefore regard the peat-smoke alone as the cause of your recollection since it does not have the same effect in other cases.   The cause of your recollection must be both the peat-smoke and the past occurrence." [12] All habits are examples of such mnemic causality, and so is heredity, since it is possible to account for a present habitual act or an inherited ability by referring to the occasions on which it was practised in the past.

It would be possible by the help of the notion of mnemic causation to describe mental development without recourse to any permanently enduring latent mental traces.   However, our descriptions would be intolerably long, as we should be forced to include much of a person's past mental history in any attempt to explain his present activities, and for inherited abilities we should have to include the history of the race. To avoid this it is convenient to assume the existence of dispositions.   By doing this we are following in the wake of the physicists who suppose that energy which they attribute to steam owing to its capacity to do work must be caused by the heat which was used up in changing water into steam. The heat has disappeared but the steam can do work and to bridge the gap between heat and work the concept of energy is necessary.   For a precisely similar reason the concept of mental dispositions is helpful to psychologists.   So much may be conceded but all else that is implied in the structure theory is far-fetched hypothesis mingled with much error.

The ablest exposition of the structure theory is that given by Professor McDougall,[13] and since he shews more insight than others it will be as well to examine his account. According to him " The perfectly developed and organised mind would have a cognitive disposition for every individual object and for every species, genus, and class of objects ; and these would not be a mere unorganised crowd of dispositions,

but would be related in a perfectly definite treelike system."
This is a great refinement on any inorganic structure such as
we originally assumed and is so far to the good, for any sound
theory of the mind, since it is alive, must shew analogies with
living organisms. We learn further that the structure grows
" like a tree that puts out new twigs from the stem, forming
new growing points, which in turn divide ; until in the
developed human mind the structure is like a vast tree." It is
a pity that this suggestive figure was not left as it stands for
in the attempt to elaborate it much of its value is lost. The
final picture is painted thus : " The facts of mental structure
require for their diagrammatic representation a three-dimen-
sional diagram. As such a diagram we may take a bush
woven over by a multitude of spider's threads, stretching
from leaf to leaf, each leaf being directly connected with
many others by these threads. Such is the crude picture we
may form of the structure of the mind and of the way the
branches, twigs and leaves of the tree of logical knowledge
are woven together by the threads of historical association."
We must state that Professor McDougall attempts to vivify
the spider's webs by the help of a conative structure superadded
to the cognitive structure. But not all his disciples have seen
the necessity of introducing into the diagram the essential
mental activity without which it cannot work. One of his
followers apparently under the impression that the structure
of the mind is but another name for the structure of the nerves
has provided a complete set of engrams or neurograms in the
nervous system whereby every fact in the universe is mirrored
in a corresponding nervous tract.[14]

This is to confuse a principle of explanation with a visual
picture which enables us to grasp it more readily. Any
picture of mental processes must be erroneous and the figure
of a tree is only helpful provided that we never forget that all
the tissues are alive ; the essential thing is the function of

the parts and not the parts themselves. Psychological dispositions are functional not primarily structural and the sole reason for their assumption is to explain as far as may be the functioning of mind.   If we omit the function the structure is perfectly useless. What we require to explain memory, habit, heredity, etc., is not a set of dispositions fixed in a nervous structure, but subliminal functions ready to be called into play when certain opposing conditions are removed. " The naturalistic attempt to account for function by structure, though it is old as Lucretius, has hitherto always broken down." [15]

(e) *The Gestalt Theory*

Our preliminary survey demands an account of a view of the nature of mind that has received the name of the *Gestalt* theory. The German substantive *Gestalt* literally means form, shape or figure, but no English term exactly expresses what the theory conveys. We get nearer to the implication of the theory with the derivative word *Gestaltung* which means a conformation or configuration, but the closest approximation is provided by the compound word *Gestaltungs-fähigkeit*, i.e., plasticity. The notion that mental development can be explained by the building up of previously disconnected elements or factors tied by bonds of association the elements being sensations, ideas or what not crops up, as we said, again and again in educational psychology. It seems incredible that at this stage of psychological history Professor James' chief contribution to its study should be frequently overlooked. For in his famous chapter on the Stream of Consciousness he summed up his views in the witty observation [16] that " A permanently existing ' Idea ' which makes its appearance before the footlights of consciousness at periodic intervals is as mythological an entity as the Jack of Spades." Never-

theless such entities though frequently scotched still rear
their ungainly heads as we shall see when we come to study
mental imagery since much of what is written about such
images is a reversion to primitive mental atomism.   Images
are regarded as ' copies ' of former impressions, " which is
much like saying that the evening twilight is a faint *replica*
of the noonday glare as well as its parting gleam." It is
curious that the notion of function and development should
still be ignored by psychology.   Yet the idea of mental
development, like that of biological development, should
include within its connotation the three processes of differentiation, retentiveness and integration or assimilation, which may
together be described by the comprehensive term mental
plasticity.

If we hold fast to this idea of plasticity we must conceive
of mental phenomena, even the most primitive, as mutually
implicating each other.   Each mental phenomenon is what it
is only by virtue of its connection with all the others, that is
as a member of some configuration, just as the notes of a
melody are not isolated things but receive their colour and
value from the melody as a whole.   In fact the development
of a musical composition offers very good analogies with the
development of a mind, since it does not consist of independent
notes somehow strung together but of a continuous harmonious
whole.   The formation of a mental habit, for example, is
not the associative union of separate mental elements, nor the
formation of a mental structure, but consists in the attainment
of smooth functioning so that little effort is required to think
in accordance with the habit.   However, the growth of a
living organism offers better comparisons with mental development since the mind is alive and the segregation and
development of the fertilised ovum is the best figure, if we
must have a picture.

It is not necessary to give a more complete account of

the *gestalt* theory here, as owing to the new light it throws on important educational problems it will be explained in later chapters in some detail.[17]

Meanwhile it is interesting to note that the hypothesis of the *gestalt* psychology according to which all mental phenomena are figured or have a structure or pattern, frequently called a configuration is adequate to describe the law of association. No more than sensations come in isolation, but are always part of some larger background, do ' ideas ' occur divorced from others but are always part of some definite context by virtue of which alone they have a significance or meaning. This meaningful context we may describe as the configuration or pattern of the ideas. As Professor Stout puts it " In a continuous attention-process each successive presentation is apprehended in relation to the total object [the configuration] and the nature of this object is a most important factor in determining the flow of ideas." He might have said " the most important factor." [18] The problem of association is not to explain how ideas are associated for they never existed otherwise than as part of some configuration. When, by attention to the relations, the nature of the configuration has once been grasped the subsequent appearance of any part of the pattern serves to reinstate the whole. This simple formula is sufficiently comprehensive to include every distinct variety or mode of association. Thus ' association by contiguity,' as when the first line of a poem recalls the second, and so on, is an obvious case of completing a whole which is partially given. ' Association *by* similars,' as for instance the suggestion by a clear appearance of the sky of a frosty night because in my past experience this has often happened, is a further instance of a partial configuration suggesting its completion. And finally ' association *of* similars,' instanced by a present thunder-storm reminding me of a previous storm, is in the same way the completion of a configuration by virtue of some of its features being presented anew.

There is one problem of development which we have left aside in describing the variety of theories but which can no longer be ignored. The individual mind is not a *tabula rasa* at the outset of experience but has a fund of accumulated, but implicit experience at its disposal. How came it by this possession ?

MENTAL HEREDITY—THE TERMINOLOGY

The idea of organic inheritance is concerned with the attempt to distinguish what is due to Nature from what is due to Nurture. A considerable amount of experimental research has been devoted to the topic but an examination of the evidence leads to the conclusion that although a large array of biological and other facts have been accumulated very few generalisations have been attempted and all of them are debatable.[19] Amongst the host of difficulties encountered in the study of heredity not the least is that due to matters of terminology, and very little progress can be made until the meaning of terms is agreed upon. "Heredity," says Professor J. A. Thomson,[20] "is mainly a convenient term for the genetic *relation* between successive generations." Much popular and indeed scientific discourse obscures this idea by the belief that there is a mysterious form of energy or, at all events, a driving force of heredity. This is about as reasonable as the assumption that there must be a force of pupillarity urging students to a University because the relationship of the scholars towards their Alma Mater is expressed by the term *in statu pupillari*. Professor Thomson goes so far as to say that " All sociological talk that appeals to a ' principle,' ' law ' or force of heredity should be ruled out of court."

Biologists call the stuff of living material bioplasm and they distinguish two kinds, the germ-plasm of the reproductive cells and the soma-plasm of the rest of the body. Obviously it is only the germ-plasm which is handed on from parents to offspring, or perhaps it is better to say that the germ-plasm is at the outset the offspring. It was at one time held that when the fertilised ovum began to segregate or divide some of the cells remained apart, relatively undifferentiated, and gave rise to the reproductive organs. The germ-plasm, in other words, passed on from generation to generation relatively unchanged. It was also believed that the soma-plasm remained distinct from the germ-plasm during the course of the individual life, but this idea is now abandoned by all competent biologists; and in any case there is no necessary connection between the continuity of the germ-plasm between successive generations and its assumed independence.

The supposed separateness of germ-plasm and soma-plasm has served to perpetuate the notion that heredity is a *cause* or a *factor* producing certain results. But, as we have said, the term heredity simply refers to the fact of continuity and likeness between ascendants and descendants. Had there been no sexual reproduction this misapprehension never would have arisen.

If we consider, for example, the case of a strawberry plant, the notion of heredity becomes much clearer. The plant produces numerous runners and at intervals stalks appear above the soil with leaves and roots; and of course at this stage there is only one individual, since the bioplasm of the runners and the new shoots is continuous with that of the original clump. In the autumn the internodes of the runners die away and the clumps become independent, the process repeating itself continually, so that in each year new individuals are formed, which are descended from the first by continuity of

living substance. The formation of the new individuals is
not a new fact but merely a consequence of nutrition. Hence
it is manifest that heredity is merely a name for the relationship of continuity and resemblance between individuals
descended from each other. Continuity does not necessarily
imply similarity, for the individual does not necessarily
during growth always resemble himself exactly. This only
happens when the growth takes place in identical conditions.
If the climate, the soil, the food or all of them are changed
the individual becomes modified ; the farther the new shoot
springs up from the parent stock the more it is apt to differ.
Similarity then, gives place to unlikeness and we no longer
refer to heredity but to *variation*. When there are two
parents the fact of continuity is still evident but there is a
double likeness to be expected and consequently only a partial
resemblance to each parent. We may, therefore, say that
continuity with likeness constitutes the fact of heredity but
with the appearance of unlikeness we enter the domain of
variation. The similarity of the hereditary relation in the
lower organisms and man is suggested by the fact that such
properties as curliness of the hair, colour of the eyes, certain
facial characteristics, etc., in human beings seem to follow the
Mendelian rules of inheritance.

There is a fundamental distinction between physiological
and psychological inheritance which Professor Ward first
brought into prominence.[21] Unless this difference is carefully
attended to nothing but confusion can arise from the study
of mental heredity. In dealing with biological or physiological inheritance it is necessary to remember that we are
making a separation where none exists in reality ; for, as was
pointed out above, at the outset the organism and its inheritance
are one and the same. We can only consider them as two by
an effort of abstraction and the separation is attempted simply
as a matter of convenience. All those likenesses which can be

traced to the parents or other ascendants are considered apart (although of course they do not exist apart) and referred to as hereditary characters. Now this is very different from the use of the terms when we refer to hereditary property, for in this case no difficulty is found in separating the individual from his inheritance in thought or in reality. The proper use of the term mental heredity should resemble the latter of these meanings and not the former if we wish to be intelligible. In order to appreciate this, attention must be called to the varieties in the significance of the term *mind*, the meaning of which, like the spelling of Sam Weller's name is a matter of taste and fancy. Mind may mean the living subject, the *ego* or soul itself, and in this sense the continuity that we previously referred to as constituting the fact of heredity in the physiological sense of the term " so far from being an ascertained fact concerning this subject and any other subject, seems rather to be inconceivable even as a possibility." Fortunately we are not called upon as psychologists to give any account of the origin of souls or of their relation to each other. But the term *mind* may have a totally different meaning, a strictly psychological one with which the idea of mental heredity is bound up. It is highly probable that all heredity is ultimately psychological, and S. Butler in *Life and Habit* has given ample reasons for the belief that biological inheritance is a concept entirely devoid of significance unless we include in its connotation the idea of mental heredity. Use and habit were for him the key to the understanding of heredity, and since function determines structure, not *vice versa* it is clear that psychological factors take the precedence.

The second use of the term *mind* to which I have referred is that in which it is employed as equivalent to the *objective* side of experience, i.e. the *presentational continuum* of Professor Ward. Experience or behaviour has two sides, a subjective

activity and the objects attended to, namely, the presentations. With regard to such mental objects we find that " what
we call a presentation is still part of a large whole. It is not
separated from other presentations whether simultaneous or
successive, by something which is not of the nature of a
presentation, as one island is separated from another by the
intervening sea . . . we are led alike by particular facts and
general considerations to the conception of a *totum objectivum*
or objective continuum which is gradually differentiated."
The differentiation and growing complexity of this presentational continuum is what mainly concerns the psychologist
and is exemplified, let us say, in the overtones which the
musician distinguishes but which the non-musical person
does not hear. The musical person's note has parts and
relations which are absent from the other's. Now it is conformable with a good terminology to refer to this continuum
which the individual deals with as his mind. We may by
analogy with bioplasm call it the psychoplasm. " The
subject, on this view, is only called an heir because his ' mind '
or psychoplasm, like his body or bioplasm may shew, as it
develops, considerable resemblance to that of his parents."
In other words what is heritable psychologically is not the
psyche or soul but a psychoplasm which is continuous from
generation to generation being gradually modified as it is
handed on. Those modifications of the psychoplasm, by virtue
of which all individuals find themselves ready to face the world
with a set of reactions more or less adapted to certain situations
without previous experience of such situations, are called instincts. Other native endowments which may be referred to
the psychoplasm are untaught native abilities, untaught in the
sense that the person's interest in these directions requires no
prompting from others but compels him, as it were, to make himself efficient by practice in the direction of his talent as in the
case of Darwin who began to collect insects when a schoolboy.

There is a useful distinction frequently overlooked between the terms innate and inherited. The modifications in the psychoplasm which lead to certain responses are rightly called inherited. But there is no reason to think that genius though inborn is inherited; and whereas abilities can be native or acquired, genius being a matter of creativeness or originality can never be acquired. We ought however to speak of it as innate as all our knowledge goes to shew that it is inborn and must be the peculiar property of the subject or *ego* as opposed to the psychoplasm. It is not what he inherits which makes the genius but what he makes of his inheritance.

We have so far spoken of the individual without reference to his environment but this is to talk of an abstraction, for the terms are correlative implying each other. Rousseau blundered badly when he suggested that Émile should be educated apart from a social environment. There is no such thing as a human being apart from a social *milieu*. The relation between the two has been admirably expressed by Sigwart [22] who says: " If we call to mind how little on the average each of us acquires by himself alone and independently of others, how much of what he knows and believes is common property, one almost gets the impression that any distinctive individuality we possess really belongs only to our bodies not to our minds. As for the ideas and thoughts that animate us, they seem like the breath our lungs inhale, drawn from a common atmosphere and returned to it again." The environment alone will not account for human differences any more than the climate and soil of a region will wholly explain the diversities of the plants within it. Nevertheless the environment is of fundamental importance in heredity, for it may easily happen that an inherited characteristic fails to show itself owing to the absence of the proper environmental stimulus. Thus there is a wan newt called Proteus in the dark streams of Dalmatian caves that has no pigment in its skin, but we should err if we hastily concluded that the factor for pigmentation is absent. If Proteus is removed from the caves to daylight it first becomes spotty and then dark. If it produce young in the new environment they too are dark, and the eyes which are very degenerate in the cave attain to a greater degree of development. We may also call to mind that Plato's cave-dwellers could not attain to a knowledge of the good until they were dragged into the light of day. So, many a schoolboy acquires a reputation for incompetence because the environment or the teaching being unsatisfactory his native powers are dormant as there is no adequate stimulus to bring them into play.

EVIDENCE FOR MENTAL HEREDITY

Now that our terminological difficulties are partially solved it is time to consider the evidence that has accumulated bearing on the inheritance of ability. The first worker in this field was Sir Francis Galton who in 1869 published a book with the title *Hereditary Genius*. By the time he had corrected the edition of 1892 he had seen the error of his ways and explained that the original title was an obvious misnomer for the more modest *Hereditary Ability*, since he did not use the word genius in its usual sense, but merely as expressing an ability that was exceptionally high, and at the same time inborn. He pointed out that the distribution of faculties in a population could not possibly remain constant if, on the average, the children resembled their parents. If they did so, physical or mental giants would become more gigantic and dwarfs more diminutive in successive generations. Since this does not, as a matter of fact, occur it is manifest that the filial average is not the same as the parental, but nearer to mediocrity, i.e., it *regresses* towards the racial mean. In any stable community there is a typical centre from which individual variations occur in accordance with the ' normal ' curve of frequency. " The filial centre falls back further towards mediocrity in a constant proportion to the distance to which the parental centre has deviated from it." The technical term *variation* ought always to be used to express changes of this kind from the racial mean. As a result of his investigations Galton concluded that the hereditary relationship is similar both as regards biological and psychological characteristics, and also that it would be quite practicable to produce a highly-gifted race of men by judicious marriages during consecutive generations.

His method consisted in the careful examination of the relationships of over three hundred families containing between them about a thousand ' eminent ' men, regarding eminence as shown by high reputation as " a pretty accurate test of high ability." The eminent men were judges, statesmen, literary men, scientists, artists, etc. He found that there were enormous odds in favour of a near kinsman of an eminent man having ability of a high order as compared with one more remotely related. Eminent sons were more numerous than eminent brothers and there was a sudden dropping off at the second degree of kinship, namely grandfathers, grandsons, uncles, etc., whilst at the third degree of kinship there was a further dropping off. In this way he demonstrated an increase of ability in the generations that precede its culmination to eminence and a decrease in those that succeed.

Galton's work was taken up by Professor Karl Pearson [23] who likewise adopted the method of collecting family data. He elaborated and refined the statistical method of dealing with the facts and invented new modes for calculating degrees of resemblance. By the year 1904 he had collected nearly four thousand schedules referring to certain mental, moral and physical traits of brothers and sisters between the ages of 10 and 14 attending a large variety of schools all over the country from Aberdeen to Yeovil.   The physical characters were such things as stature, length of arm, cephalic index, eye-colour, etc., the mental characters were estimates of intelligence formed by the teachers on the basis of a sixfold graduated scale of ability, and the moral traits referred to such characteristics as vivacity, self-assertion, conscientiousness, good nature, temper, and so forth.   It ought to be remarked at this point that the statistical treatment of estimates of intelligence or moral qualities, however accurate, can never produce a finer scale than the rough one that we start with. That is we can never get more out of the figures than we put into them, and it is necessary to state this truism since some investigators perform the most elaborate calculations on the very roughest data.   It is absurd to calculate degrees of resemblance to three decimal places when the data are only quantitative, as it were, by courtesy.   For this reason in what follows I have not hesitated to eliminate the end figures freely.

Professor Pearson's argument is based on the following proposition : If fraternal resemblances for the mental and moral characters be greater than equal to or less than fraternal resemblances for the physical characters then parental inheritance for the former set of characters is greater than, equal to or less than that for the latter set.   An idea of the degree of resemblance may be obtained by considering the slope of the regression line.   For the physical characters, such as cephalic index, he found that the slope of the line of regression was about ·50, whereas the slope of the line for estimated intelligence or ability was ·47.

The following table shews the value of some of the correlations that were calculated from his data.

	Brothers.	Sisters.	Brother-Sister.
Head Length .	·50	·43	·46
Eye Colour . .	·54	·52	·53
Intelligence . .	·52	·50	·49

Further, it was estimated that the correlations between the siblings was approximately of the same value for physical characters as for qualities such as vivacity, conscientiousness, self-assertiveness, etc.   Hence, in accordance with the above stated proposition Professor Pearson inferred that " the physical and psychical characters in man are inherited within broad lines in the same manner and with the same intensity." But this statistical deduction was accompanied by the highly doubtful opinion that " the average home environment, the average parental influence is in itself part of the heritage of the stock and not an extraneous and additional factor emphasising the resemblance between children from the same home." However that may be, it would appear that, if these results are trustworthy, they suggest that whilst mental and moral qualities may be fostered by good environment in the home and the school they emanate from parental nature rather than nurture ; they are bred in the bone.

The investigations of Professor Pearson's pupils on adults have, on the whole, confirmed his results for school children.[24] By consulting the *Oxford Historical Register* it was possible to compare the classes in the B.A. degrees taken by all the men between the years 1830 and 1892 whose fathers had also been at Oxford.   It was found that the number of sons who took high honours fell off steadily according to the degree taken by the fathers.   If a father wants his son to take a good degree he had better do so himself, as the table shows.   Heredity is better than precept in the matter of degrees.

Degree taken by fathers.	Percentage of sons taking 1st and 2nd Class Honours.
1st and 2nd Class Honours . .	27
3rd Class Honours	15
Pass Degree	12
No Degree	9

The results are equally instructive if we take the sons' degrees as the standard and compare the relative percentages of fathers

who took high honours. The diagram printed on this page
shews that the percentage of fathers who obtained high honours
(1st and 2nd Class) diminish regularly, i.e. in a straight line,
as we pass through the various grades of sons.   On the basis
of all the figures it was shewn that, if unity is taken to represent perfect resemblance and zero complete lack of similarity,
" the degree of intellectual similarity between father and son,
as indicated by the degrees which each took is ·3." [25]   It is
very hazardous to indulge in speculations where statistics
and examination results are jointly concerned, but if we choose
to give rein to our fancy and assume that a student's mother
and father contribute equal amounts to his mental endowment, we may say that the psychoplasm which he inherits is
responsible for two-thirds of his ability.   When the degrees
of brothers were compared it appeared that of the first class
men, 45·5 per cent. had brothers who took high honours, of

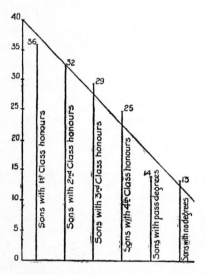

INHERITANCE OF ABILITY
(*After Schuster and
Elderton*)

Total number of Sons 2459

Date of Degrees of Sons
1860-1892

The heights of the vertical
lines shew in what per-
centage of cases the fathers
have taken either first or
second class honours.   The
diagram shews that the percentage of fathers who
obtained this degree of distinction diminishes with some
regularity, as one passes
downwards from the sons
with first class honours to
those with no degrees.

the second class 38 per cent. of brothers took high honours
and the percentage steadily diminished as one passed down
the scale of degrees.

Exception may be taken to all the results just considered on the ground that the estimation of ability by reputation or by examination results or by a crude scale is unsatisfactory. Since these researches there has grown up a new method of evaluating intelligence or ability by the use of mental tests. With the aid of the Binet-Stanford tests the intelligence quotient or mental ratio of over two hundred pairs of siblings in various orphanages in California was estimated. The coefficient of correlation between these brothers and sisters when corrected for age variation turned out to be ·54 which is in very close agreement with the results previously obtained. The same tests were given to siblings in two small schools in England. But the correlation coefficients were much lower in one school and the discrepancy was attributed to the paucity of the numbers and the influence of selection, whilst in the other school the results were very irregular. The method is a useful one and ought to be further extended in view of the fact that there is now available a great variety of standardised tests of ability. We have now considered the work which has any direct bearing on the problem of mental inheritance in human beings. It will be seen that the cogency of the conclusions depends very largely on the view that the resemblances which have been proved to exist are due to the hereditary relationship and cannot be the effect of the environment or nurture.

THE INHERITANCE OF ACQUIRED CHARACTERS

We must next consider briefly a problem of heredity which has given rise to infinite discussion and a large amount of experimental biology. Much of the discussion is vitiated by a loose use of terms as biologists are not skilled in dialectics and very little of the experimental work has any bearing on the problem of mental heredity which is the only side of the case that interests us. The question at issue is whether parents'

habits have any influence in making easier the formation of
similar habits in the offspring. Can parental nurture so
affect the psychoplasm that the children find themselves in
possession of a mental endowment varying in the same
direction ? Or to use Biblical phraseology ; when the fathers
have eaten sour grapes are the children's teeth set on
edge ? Lamarck believed that a new environment which an
animal encounters, requiring new modes of activity to secure
proper adaptation, leads to the modification of its organs ;
and if the activities are repeated for a sufficient length of time
modified organs will be transmitted to the descendants.
Weismann denied this possibility mainly on the erroneous
ground that the germ-plasm was physiologically distinct from
the soma-plasm and therefore he could not conceive how the
modification could be transmitted. But whatever is true of
biological heredity there is no doubt that Butler's view is
sound, namely, that habit in the individual life is the ground
of the hereditary relation in the racial life as far as mental
characteristics are concerned.

A large amount of biological evidence in favour of the
transmission of acquired characters has been accumulated,
but is chiefly concerned with changes in colour or in the form
of organs.[26] Thus if salamander *maculosa*, which has a black
colour spotted with patches of yellow, is allowed to pass its
life on a background of yellow loam the patches of yellow
increase in size. If the offspring are treated similarly the
whole surface of the skin becomes yellow with the exception
of a few streaks of black. Changes in the opposite direction
towards black can be produced by a black environment in a
couple of generations so that the offspring resemble in colour
a different species salamander *atra*. These results are of
value as shewing that there is no inherent impossibility in
the supposition that an induced change may give the offspring
a tilt in the new direction ; so that one may approach the

question of the mental heredity of acquired characters with an open mind. Evidence tending in the same direction has been obtained by examining the carefully kept records of English trotting horses which show a gradually improving time for the mile from generation to generation. But, of course, it is possible that the training has improved and that such influence of the environment acts separately on each successive generation.

Passing to human beings it is frequently stated that the Australians and the Americans have produced a new human type and that the descendants of the immigrants have lost their distinctive European characteristics. But such observations are largely subjective, and the so-called new types are probably due to the imitation of parents by the children and the continuous influence of a novel environment. There is little doubt that environmental influences may work profound changes in a relatively short time so that, without inheritance, what appears like a new type may be bred. The present head master of Christ's Hospital has assured me that within a couple of years at school the elementary scholarship boys are indistinguishable from the others in speech and manner, and that the rapidity of these acquirements varies directly as their intellectual ability. The environment in this particular case is especially favourable since the boys live in the country, far removed from disturbing parental factors and are all clothed in the same costume and live the same life. Again the Parsees of Bombay have lived in India for several centuries, and during the whole of this time have adopted the native Gujerati language, but their speech sounds still shew very decided phonetic resemblances with the Persian tongue, possibly owing to the fact that they congregate together and thus maintain an isolated social environment.

All such indirect evidence though highly suggestive can never produce complete conviction. Fortunately there is at our disposal a means of direct experimental investigation which we owe to the researches of the Russian physiologist, Professor I. P. Pavlov. His investigations are concerned with reflexes in the central nervous system and have a direct bearing on psychological heredity since they deal with the formation of acquired habits of response. Reflex activity, such as the blinking of the eyes, is a function of the lower centres of the central nervous system and such inborn racial reflexes are called unconditioned. But certain others may be acquired as the result of individual experience in which case they are called conditioned reflexes. The name is not particularly appropriate and it would be more descriptive to call the latter kind, reflexes due to a substituted stimulus. For if some novel external stimulus is made repeatedly to coincide with the action of an inborn reflex it acquires the power to produce the same reaction as the normally adequate stimulus. Thus, food is the adequate stimulus to produce a reflex secretion of saliva and gastric juices. When the feeding of an animal coincides frequently with a certain sound such as the ringing of a bell, this sound, previously indifferent, in the course of time evokes the same food reactions as the food itself. The intensity of the reaction has been measured by placing a tube in the salivary ducts and measuring the rate of flow of saliva, and it has been shown that the substituted stimulus of the ringing of the bell immediately produces a copious flow even in the absence of food. It is interesting to note that the conditioned reflex for salivary secretion has been demonstrated in man by placing a little suction disc connected to a tube over the parotid gland in the cheek, when the presentation of a substituted stimulus produced an increased flow of saliva.[27] A similar principle applies to the formation of conditioned reactions in the case of the instincts of self-preservation and sex ; normally indifferent stimuli may be substituted for the adequate stimulus in order to

evoke the instinct.   During the great war dogs were trained
for work in the front-line trenches by accustoming them to
the sound of the explosion of bombs whilst they were being
fed, and it was found that when they were sent to the front
line and a bombardment ensued, instead of bolting with
terror as their fear instinct prompted, they expected to be
fed, being no longer gun shy.   This is, in fact, the means by
which the individual man or animal gradually becomes master
of his instincts and adapts himself to the fluctuating circumstances of the outer world.   The unconditioned instincts
alone would not enable any animal to survive even for the
briefest period, and as for man the demands of the social
environment make it imperative that he should have the
power of controlling his instinctive reactions by substituted
stimuli.

Professor Pavlov established the conditioned food reflex
in white mice, i.e., he trained them to respond by certain
reactions to the sound of an electric bell in the same manner
that they normally responded to food.[28]   He caused the mice,
that is, to acquire a habit.   With the first set of wild white
mice it was necessary to repeat the combination of ringing
the bell and feeding 300 times in order to form a well established habit of response.   The next generation formed the
same habit after 100 repetitions only, the third generation
acquired it after 30 repetitions, the fourth needed only 10,
and the fifth found 5 sufficient.   The records of these startling
experiments have not yet been fully published, but it is quite
clear that the method of the conditioned reflex is a powerful
one and that a suitable beginning has been made in the
search for an answer to the vexed question of the inheritance
of acquired characteristics.   Moreover, similar experiments
are obviously possible on human beings and in fact they are
the nearest approach to a psychological method of solution of
the question.   It is not necessary, as Professor Pavlov seems

C

to think, to breed a generation that will respond without any repetitions in order to get a definite answer. For in the analogous case of learning to repeat a set of nonsense syllables (see the chapter on Habit), when they are apparently completely forgotten, a few repetitions may suffice for recovery, shewing that something may remain despite apparent oblivion. All that it is necessary to shew is that the children learn the habit with fewer repetitions than the parents.

The case for the inheritance of acquired characters is not, then, so desperate as some biologists suppose. Man is, in this respect, in a peculiarly favoured position, for even if it is not certain that changes in the individual psychoplasm are transmissible, yet he has an external heritage of tradition and convention, customs and institutions, literature and the sciences. Civilised society is itself a heritage of ideas and ideals which we inherit by being born into it. Changes in it are part of man's inheritance. Every pupil who enters a school with a good tone and long established traditions, or even new traditions if they are active, is in the position to inherit these. We may compare the *esprit de corps* of a given institution, such as a school, with the psychoplasm since it is the means by which tradition is handed on. When a great school master like Arnold or Thring promotes or induces variations in tradition these, in favourable circumstances, become the changed inheritance of many succeeding generations.

CHAPTER II

SENSORY DATA—VISION AND HEARING

Sense Training—Visual Acuity—Auditory Acuity—Legibility of Type—
Illumination—Psychology of Reading

SENSE TRAINING

MORE than any other single factor, the influence of Locke's sensationalistic psychology directed general attention to the importance of sense training in the education of children. Various educational reformers since the time of the Renaissance had pointed to the aid of the senses in acquiring knowledge ; thus, Mulcaster in his *Elementarie* stated : " The hand, the ear, the eye be the greatest instruments whereby the receiving and delivery of our learning is chiefly executed." But, as this quotation shews, they failed completely to grasp the fundamental idea that education of the senses is more than the means of acquiring knowledge ; that it is itself the earliest form of mental development. It remained for Rousseau basing himself upon Locke's ideas to stress the fundamental fact never thenceforward to be forgotten, that education must begin with sense training. Pestalozzi and Froebel contributed to the development of the idea and owed a debt in this respect to Rousseau. Nevertheless our exact knowledge concerning the part played by the senses in intellectual and moral development derives from a totally different source.[1]

The experimental investigation and practice of sense training began with J. R. Pereira (1715–80) who undertook the teaching of deaf-mutes, after having made a thorough study of anatomy and physiology.   He was the first to demonstrate the fundamental nature of the sense of touch and the possibility, as we may call it, of the substitution of one sense for another.   Deaf-mutes by practice improve their tactile sense, and by systematic graduated exercises based on the analysis of sounds Pereira was able to train his pupils to differentiate clearly the minute vibrations of the vocal cords. The pupils grasped the throat and mouth of their teacher, acquiring skill in the discrimination of the different vibrations. He also taught them carefully to observe by the sense of sight the position and movements of the throat, jaws, tongue, teeth and lips during sound production.   So delicate did their sense perception become that when under the influence of this training they began to talk themselves they reproduced their master's Gascon accent !   Not only did this education improve their senses but better social and moral development ensued.   More than a century later the blind deaf-mute Helen Keller, taught in a similar way, stated : " By placing my hand on another's throat and cheek I enjoy the changes of the voice.   I know when it is high or low, clear or muffled, sad or cheery.   The thin, quavering sensation of an old voice differs in my touch from the sensation of a young voice. . . . Sometimes the flow and ebb of a voice is so enchanting that my fingers quiver with exquisite pleasure."   Rousseau lived near Pereira, visited him, and saw his work, and probably the sections in *Émile* on sense training owe much to this source.

In order to appreciate the significance of sense training for moral and intellectual development it is necessary to turn to the observation of idiots. For normal children in their play and general activities, even without formal education, acquire control over their motility and sensibility. Not so idiots who exhibit inertia or merely spasmodic uncontrolled movements. Philosophers of the 18th century had a great predilection for the natural man unspoilt by the touch of civilisation. An opportunity of studying such a case occurred when a wild naked boy who had lived for seven years out of eleven or twelve in the woods in Aveyron was brought to Paris. Luckily he was not left to the philosophers, but entrusted to the care of Dr Itard (1775–1838). He turned out to be an idiot and the state of his sensibility may be judged from the fact that snuff did not make him sneeze or produce tears, loud shouts failed to attract his attention, he would seize hot coals or place his hands in boiling water. Pistol shots fired close to his head produced no effect, yet the cracking of a walnut of which he was very fond, immediately attracted his attention. Dr Itard succeeded after several years of patient effort by graded sense exercises in restoring some of his sensibility and though he failed to moralise him completely he did ultimately shew signs of moral qualities.

Dr Séguin (1812–80) carried on and improved the work of Pereira and Itard. With infinite patience and scientific insight he developed a complete system for training the motility and sensibility of mental defectives. He worked on the idea of the organic unity of body and mind in the educative process. By preparing a suitably simple environment with specially devised apparatus and carefully graduated exercises, he enabled the defectives to cope effectively with the simplest situations of social life. He demonstrated conclusively that by cultivating sensibility we achieve intellectual and moral progress. He also shewed that with these children the essential thing was to awaken wants, since it is only by spontaneous functioning that the senses are developed. Dr Montessori copied Séguin's methods and successfully applied the idea of a prepared environment and didactic sense apparatus to normal children. By her wonderful sympathy and affection for children she was able to inspire others with the ideas of her predecessors and make them widely accepted.

It is unnecessary to enter into details of the special methods employed in training the senses, since there is a large literature devoted to practical kindergarten work. However, it is desirable to call attention to an epistemological consideration the neglect of which may lead to educational mispractice. In the early stages of education a good deal of what the mind deals with is locked up in sense material or at all events needs the stimulus of sense-impression. The kindergarten teaches the discrimination of the various colours and shapes by practice with graded sense material and rightly teaches number in the same way by handling beads, sticks, etc. Hence it is easy to be misled into supposing that the knowledge of arithmetic like that of colour rests wholly on sense-data. But the similarity of the cases is only specious and the distinction has been most aptly pointed out by Mr Bertrand Russell who says, " a certain number of instances are needed to make us think of two abstractly, rather than of two coins or two books or two people or two of any other specified kind. But as soon as we are able to divest our thoughts of irrelevant particularity, we become able to *see* the general principle that two and two are four ; any one instance is seen to be *typical*, and the examination of other instances becomes unnecessary." [2]

It is a matter of insight for the teacher of the young to discern when the sense-training stage of the process is sufficiently complete, so as to relieve the mind from irrelevant particularity in order that the abstract may be freed from the mass of concretes. So, in teaching geometry, a practical course of measurements is highly desirable in the early stages in order to exemplify and suggest the general propositions underlying the science and to help the memory, but there is no other method than that of close reasoning by which the theorems can be really acquired. Yet when all is said, without the sensory basis the principles would not emerge, and general ideas are picked up largely by reading and the like sensory aids. Conformably to this there is some evidence in support of the view that lack of sensory acuity is responsible for reputed dullness and apparent stupidity in children. Hence we turn to the consideration of the sensory and environmental conditions without which education is likely to be ineffective.

VISUAL ACUITY

Measurements of sensory acuity are rough and ready, and yield figures which are comparative only for the readings taken by the same observer at one time. The standard acuteness of vision is taken as the power of the single eye to distinguish letters and characters which subtend an angle of five minutes on the retina, all the vertical and horizontal strokes which compose the letters and all the spaces between the strokes producing a retinal image of one minute. As the tangent of five minutes is ·00145 the size of the standard or test-type letters which are to be read by the " normal " eye at a distance of one metre is 1·45 mm. vertically and horizontally ; and proportionately greater, in a direct ratio, for longer distances. There are several factors which influence the measurements, such as variations in illumination, in blackness of the type, in the colour of the background, etc., so that it is difficult to compare the results of different observers. The fraction obtained by dividing the distance at which the letters of standard size can be read by the individual by the distance at which the ' normal ' eye can read them is taken as the measure of his acuity of vision.[8] The method is, at best, only approximate as much use is made of conscious and unconscious inference in reading the letters, and as we shall see later the legibility of type is dependent to a considerable extent on the forms of the letters. By a strange freak of typographical perversity the letters most frequently used, especially the vowels, are amongst the least legible of the letters. Some of these difficulties are countered by the use of single letters of the standard sizes such as a series composed of lines of E's, or with young children a series of squares with one side missing is employed and they are required to indicate, by pointing, which is the open side, or sometimes a series of small pictures of the standard sizes is used. It would be a great advantage for the comparative study of results if single straight lines of the standard size were uniformly used in all cases, and the persons tested were required simply to count the number of them. For more exact measures an international test is now used, consisting of a broken circle mounted on a rotating graduated dial. The observer indicates the direction in which the opening lies. The opening is turned in eight different directions and the observer must indicate five correctly. The size of the opening can be varied at will.

Sometimes visual acuity is measured by the greatest distance at which a particular kind and size of type can be read by the persons examined. In the anthropometrical survey of Cambridge students [4] in 1887, in which over two thousand men were examined, acuity was measured by the extreme distance at which ' diamond ' type could be read by each eye separately, the mean of both eyes being used as the index. The mean distance for all the students was 24·1 inches. They were next divided on the basis of general ability into three groups, A, B and C, comprising first-class honours men, other honours men, and those who read for an ordinary degree or who failed in honours. The mean index for each of the classes was A, 23·4, B, 24·1 and C, 24·4. There is thus a slight inferiority in respect of acuteness of vision amongst the most studious men ; and this defect was found to be largely due to the greater proportion of students in this group who could not read the type at any distance without glasses.   In other physical traits, such as height, weight, muscular strength, breathing capacity, etc., there was no difference between the groups, from which it was inferred that much reading tends to produce myopia.

The relation between close eye work and myopia is likewise suggested by the following figures obtained by examining over thirteen hundred boys and fifteen hundred girls in the rural schools of Cambridgeshire.[5] The inferiority of the girls is said by the medical officer responsible for the examination to be due to sewing, crochet and other fine work.   The table shews the percentage of children having " normal " vision :

				8 years	10 years	12 years
Boys	.	.	.	79·12	82·48	85·80
Girls	.	.	.	76·33	81·05	83·67

These figures indicate that the eyes only begin to reach their maturity as the age of puberty approaches.

The examination of over four thousand girls and boys in Middlesex, which is mainly an urban area verging on the rural, showed the following percentages of children whose visual acuity in one or both eyes was either $\frac{6}{12}$ or worse.

Ages				7-8 years	10-11 years	13 and over
Boys	.	.	.	14·1	12	15·7
Girls	.	.	.	16·1	13·9	16·8

Here, again, the errors of refraction are more common amongst the girls, and the medical officer attributes it to the fact that girls do needlework and more homework ; but he states as another reason the fact that girls are more prone to anæmia than boys, and as this condition affects the nutrition of all parts, it renders the eye less susceptible of withstanding strain.

A more extensive investigation of children in London schools yielded the following figures.   The number of children examined at the lower age was over 30,000 boys and an equivalent number of girls; and at the higher age more than 27,000 boys and about the same number of girls. All the numbers are percentages:

Ages	Acuity		$\frac{6}{6}$	$\frac{6}{9}$	$\frac{6}{12}$ or worse
8–9 years	Boys	. . . .	36·7	43·4	19·9
,, ,,	Girls	. . . .	32·2	46·1	21·7
12 years	Boys	. . . .	51·1	26·2	22·7
,, ,,	Girls	. . . .	43·8	30·5	25·7

The vision of the older children is more acute than the younger but the proportion of bad vision is greater in the older. That is, there is a gradual education of the physical and mental powers leading to an increase in the acuity of vision, and a deterioration due to pathological causes.

If these numbers are compared with those given above for rural schools it will be seen that the vision in rural areas is much better than that in urban areas.

The attempt to measure visual acuity in young children below the age of seven is subject to an interesting psychological difficulty.[6]

What do young children see when faced with a complicated visual object? It is usually said that they recognise the whole before the detail, the species before the individual; and this is no doubt true of the general course of development in the race. But it would be unsafe to draw conclusions as to the procedure of children without close and sympathetic observation. A couple of children between two and three years of age were closely observed as they looked at pictures in a magazine and made free comments. It turned out that they simply observed the juxtaposed details. There were no signs indicative of a general impression, but merely of an enumeration of haphazard particulars. Each detail was seized, then rejected, then another, and so on. When, however, the picture was limited to a single object there was an attempt to interpret it as a whole. It apparently makes no difference to the child whether the thing is known or unknown, for he assimilates it immediately to what he knows, e.g., a peacock is called a pigeon ; a swan, a pheasant, or even a giraffe or a camel is a cock and so on. The most characteristic procedure adopted by children is to pass from similar to similar. Anybody who looks carefully at the profile of the head of a cock with its characteristic line and curve can, if he fixes his attention solely on these, see the similarity between it and a giraffe. The caricaturist in taking advantage of these naïve similarities to produce startling effects helps us to realise the point of view of the child. The apparent absurdities of children's interpretations of pictures is due to the strong impression of a dominant trait promptly seized and held fast in the midst of an uncertain *ensemble*.

Owing to this difficulty of interpretation and the variability of children's answers but few data are available for the lower ages. Yet a careful investigation of London school children between the ages of 4 to 7 years yielded the following percentage results. They were taught to regard the tests as a game and were shewn a series of E's in different positions and they had to indicate, by pointing, which direction the open end of the letter faced. There were 410 girls and 393 boys between the ages named. The results were :

Acuity	Good $\frac{6}{6}$ ($_{least}^{at}$)	Fair $\frac{6}{9}$ to $\frac{6}{12}$	Bad $\frac{6}{18}$ or less	Other defects
Girls . . .	84	11	3	2
Boys . . .	86	10	3	1

The eyes of many of these children were hypermetropic, but by virtue of the extraordinary elasticity of the crystalline lens in the young they were able in these tests to overcome this defect. It is instructive to note that there is practically no difference between boys and girls between these ages, so that the suspicion is justified that the differences seen at later ages are due to environmental and functional influences.

If we compare the earlier ages with the period of adolescence we find a definite increase in myopia. Thus, as the result of the examination of a large number of Philadelphia school children, Risley found that whilst there was only a relatively slight change in the percentage of ' normal ' eyes there was a considerable increase in short-sight ; thus

Age	Myopia	Emmetropia	Hyperopia
8·5 yrs.	4·3%	7%	88%
17·5 yrs.	19·0%	12·3%	66·8%

At the age when school life begins the visual apparatus is immature, the refraction of the eyes is not yet fixed and the eye itself, its muscles and nerves have still to increase in size. As the figures shew there is a large amount of hyperopia, which means that the ideal condition in which the eyes see distant objects without any effort of accommodation is not yet reached. The visual deterioration in the direction of myopia becomes very evident at about the age of sixteen which coincides with the period when boys are about to take their matriculation examination.

There is a considerable conflict of opinion on the question of the inheritance of short-sight.[7] Myopia literally means to shut or blink the eye, which very short-sighted persons do in order to get rid of the diffusion circles of unclear vision ; for by closing the aperture of the eye a clearer outline is given to the blurred image. Now there are two main forms of myopia, either the axis of the eye is too long so that the principal focus falls in front of the retina or the same result is brought about by the excessive refractive index of the media of the eye ; and there are a large variety of conditions which can produce either form. In other words, myopia is not a mendelian ' unit character ' which can be easily traced from parents to offspring. Consequently attempts to discover whether myopia is inherited or acquired on the basis of statistics have yielded conflicting results. Professor Karl Pearson claims on statistical grounds that the complaint is inherited, but figures collected in Sweden about myopia in school children shewed a marked decrease with the hygienic improvement of the school conditions. Interesting confirmation of this view has recently been forthcoming from the Report for 1923 of the Chief Medical Officer of the Board of Education. He notes that the reports concerning myopia from all over the country point to the fact that visual acuity has steadily and continuously improved since school inspection began in 1908. The following table for all the children in London elementary schools substantiates this claim. It is based on the results of tests for visual acuity :

Year	Age—8 Years Boys		Girls		Age—12 Years Boys		Girls	
	Normal	Bad	Normal	Bad	Normal	Bad	Normal	Bad
1918	38·2	19·7	34·7	21·8	52·6	21·7	46·8	24·1
1919	39·7	20·1	35·6	21·6	51·6	21·6	47·8	22·7
1920	42·4	20·9	35·9	22·6	55·0	20·7	52·2	22·1
1921	47·1	19·4	43·7	21·2	56·9	20·3	52·0	22·1
1922	46·7	17·8	44·8	19·2	57·1	20·3	52·5	22·2

This improvement is attributed to the sight-saving campaign for improved hygienic conditions, and further, for the same reason, the disparity between boys and girls is diminishing, especially at the age of 12 years.

The weight of authority amongst ophthalmologists inclines to the view that whilst heredity cannot be excluded, environmental conditions are responsible for the increase of myopia during school life. Bending over one's work may produce congestion shewn by redness, watering and blinking, and injure the coats of the eye ; or the muscular strain of prolonged accommodation for near objects may bring on progressive myopia. Dr Edridge-Green regards certain infantile diseases such as measles and whooping-cough and especially the former as a chief exciting cause of myopia. But there may be a hereditary disposition towards functional myopia in which case unhygienic conditions causing undue strain will certainly operate to produce it, whilst good lighting, legible print and correct posture will aid in preventing its onset.

AUDITORY ACUITY

There are two methods employed to measure auditory acuity; both, as in the case of vision, yielding only comparative results. A sound is produced in a telephone receiver and its intensity diminished by means of electrical resistances until it can no longer be heard by the subject and the amount of resistance necessary to produce this result yields a measure of acuity. This method is only of service in cases where the ability to distinguish minute sounds of a specific nature amongst more intense noises, as in submarines, is required. For practical daily life the maximum distance at which the ticking of a watch can be heard when moved away from or towards the subject, or the distance at which the words said in a " forced whisper " can be heard are taken as measures of acuity of hearing. In using the whisper test it is advisable in order to secure a certain amount of uniformity in the results and prevent guessing to use a series of prearranged numbers instead of words; so that the percentage of the numbers correctly heard may be taken as the measure.

The whisper test more closely approximates to the kind of hearing which is required in schools, and fortunately it has been shown by a careful investigation that the measures yielded by it are more reliable than those of the watch test.[8] When both tests were repeated at intervals on the same group of subjects it was found that the results were not only more consistent in the case of the speech test, but the reliability as measured by the coefficient of correlation between the first and second applications of the same test was ·78 (p.e. ·04) for the whisper test, whilst for the watch test it was only ·61 (p.e. ·05). Now correlation coefficients of less than ·7 for the same capacity measured on different days lead us to suspect the accuracy of a single trial of such a test. Again different applications of the speech test shew almost no improvement since we have been practised in hearing speech all our lives, whilst, on the other hand, repeated trials by the watch test shew considerable and variable individual improvement. Bodily tone varies from day to day and this appears greatly to influence the watch test. It has been shewn that in closed rooms the intensity of sound does *not* vary inversely as the square of the distance, a fact which interferes more with the watch test than with the whisper test. Moreover, the sub-jective factors of fluctuations of attention and fatigue affect the watch test appreciably.

The following table shews the distribution of auditory acuity as measured by the forced whisper test for children in the rural schools in the county of Cambridge.

Age	*8 years*	*10 years*	*12–13 years*
No. tested	1027	605	1326
Distance :—			
20 ft. . . .	96%	95·9%	97·1%
10 ft. . . .	3·3%	3·5%	2·5%
5 ft. . . .	·4%	·6%	·6%

The same test applied to 100 boys and 100 girls in schools of the Lancashire County Council yielded the following results (the actual numbers are given) :

Number . .	171	8	11	11	11	5	5	5	2
Distance . .	20 ft.	20	20	10	10	5	5	less than 5	
Side . . .	R & L	R	L	R	L	R	L	R	L

M. Foucault examined all the children in two small French schools who were retarded for their age, namely 54, and found that 19 of these had auditory or visual acuity of a half the

normal or less.   He thinks that the retardation is the result of
their defective senses, but his observations of auditory acuity
were made by the watch test and cannot be accepted as final.[9]

LEGIBILITY OF PRINTING TYPES

Visual acuity should be distinguished from visual sensitiveness.   Every impression made on the retina must persist
for a certain time in order to excite a sensation and degrees of
sensitiveness have been measured by variations in the time
required to recognise the impression.   In order that a letter
of the alphabet may be read, the impression must persist for
more than a thousandth of a second.[10]   The shortest exposures
which suffice for the recognition of letters also admit of the
reading of short words ; in fact the time necessary for reading
words is shorter than that required for reading letters owing
to the greater facility in the recognition of a more extended
form.   Some letters as s, g, c, x are hard to see owing to their
form and others because they are apt to be confused with
each other, e.g., i, j, l, f, t.   Three times as many letters can
be grasped in one exposure when they make words and twice
as many words can be read in the same time when they
make sentences.   It is clear then that sensitiveness depends
not only on overcoming the inertia of the nervous system
but also on the facility of mental assimilation.   We respond,
that is, not to the bare impression received on the retina but
to the acquired meaning conveyed by it.

Attempts have been made and are still being made to
determine the relative legibility of the different letters of
the printed alphabet and of different ' faces ' of type.[11]   Two
methods have been employed for this purpose.   In the first
the letters are exposed for very brief intervals up to six-
thousandths of a second and the legibility is determined by
the mean percentage of correct answers for all the intervals,

account being taken of the nature of mistakes. A more satisfactory procedure is to display the letters for some time in
a dark room in an illuminated box, the observer assuming the
natural reading posture. The subject attempts to read the
letters at different distances, the box being moved nearer after
each attempt until all the letters are correctly read. The
average distance at which each letter can be read by various
people, together with misreadings and introspections are
recorded. In this way Miss Roethlein arranged the letters
of the alphabet in the following decreasing order of legibility
which corresponds approximately with the results obtained
by the time method

   m w d j l p f q y i h g b k v r t n c u o x a e z s.

Legibility also depends on the particular ' face ' of type which
is used, and some saving of eye-strain would be accomplished
if the more legible letters of each face were combined into a
single alphabet. But as this reform is not likely to be adopted
for æsthetic reasons, it would be an advantage if the internal
spaces within the letters of any one type were broadened, for
all authorities agree that this is of more importance to legibility than mere size of print.

The effect on the eye of different conditions of lighting
has been carefully examined under the auspices of the American
Medical Association.[12] By means of visual acuity tests,
records were made of the time that the eye could maintain a
certain standard of acuity and the time it fell below it during
a three minute test. The ratio of these times is regarded as
the measure of the ability of the eye to maintain its power of
clear seeing, and this ratio was calculated before and after
reading under different conditions of illumination. The effects
of evenness of illumination, diffuseness of light, the angle at

D

which the light falls on the object viewed, the evenness of surface brightness were all shewn to be important in maintaining visual efficiency. A field uniformly illuminated with light well diffused, and no extremes of surface brightness, such as is given by daylight, is the ideal condition for accurate and comfortable fixation and accommodation of the eyes. Systems of artificial lighting are classified as direct when the light is sent directly by a reflector to the plane of work, and indirect when the source is concealed from the eye and the light is thrown against the ceiling which reflects it diffusely. In semi-direct systems a part of the light is transmitted through a translucent reflector placed beneath the source and a part is reflected from the ceiling. The indirect systems and the semi-direct in which but a small portion of the light is directly transmitted were found to give the best results. In the indirect system the highest intensity of light may be used without discomfort to the eye. Unevenness of surface brightness in the field of vision brought about by direct illumination proved to be the most important cause of the eye's loss of efficiency, discomfort and fatigue.

Books used in schools should have paper without or with only a little gloss so as to avoid specular reflection producing differences of brightness which interferes with binocular vision. In order to secure greater legibility and less glare Babbage had tables of logarithms printed on paper of a primrose yellow tinge. Such a tint is very useful for all sorts of tabular work, especially in artificial light. Babbage selected this colour after tests of printing in various tints and finding out which his friends preferred; and he was of the opinion that different people might find different colours less fatiguing to the eye.[13] The French Government has adopted the plan in printing the official logarithm tables of the geographical survey for the army; and experience has shewn that this device does diminish the strain on the eye brought about by the intense contrast between white and black and irradiation effects in close work, so that those who are introduced to them prefer to use these tables to others. The colour is not meant for the ordinary reader for whom quality and texture of paper is much less significant for legibility than is usually supposed.

The loss of visual efficiency in an unfavourable illumination has been shewn to be muscular and not retinal. For the retinal loss in capacity (as tested by the power to discriminate colour and brightness, rate of exhaustion and recovery) was not greater in the above named investigation under one than another of the lighting systems employed, even after ten hours work.

Some of the muscular strain is the result of the effort of fixation and accommodation, but part of it is due to a cause first pointed out by Dr Javal in 1879. In reading, the eye proceeds by a succession of quick, short movements and pauses from left to right and then sweeps in one quick unbroken movement to the next line. The short jerks vary in extent and some of the pauses are longer than others. By photographic methods the extent and duration of the movements has been ascertained and it has been found that the movement spaces are irregular, a slight movement may be followed by one three to four times as great, the angular displacements being from 2° to 7°. The number of pauses for any person is, on the average, fairly constant for lines of the same length. With familiar matter there are fewer pauses, but the number is increased for foreign languages, detached words, lists, etc. Smaller type somewhat increases the number of pauses and movements. For fast readers the pauses are rather less than ·2 sec., but the variations are very great. Fast reading decreases the number of pauses and their duration but not the speed of the movements which is outside the person's control, so that fast readers perform less eye work. Children are found to make more frequent and longer pauses than adults, for it is the attention which is ahead as it were and pulls the eye along in reading.

Differences in the rate of reading depend largely, according to Professor Huey, on the ease with which a regular rhythmical movement of the eyes can be established and maintained. The swing from one end of the line backwards to the next has been happily compared with the motion of an oarsman's body between the strokes. The habit of swing is normally well established by the age of nine to eleven years, i.e., the necessary eye swing is then made without conscious effort and with considerable regularity. To accomplish this the length of the line in school books is important and uniformity is desirable. The small irregular movements are apt to be fatiguing to children and irregularity in the swing works to the same end.

THE PSYCHOLOGY OF READING

The actual reading range of the unmoved eye is restricted to a small area of a couple of centimetres radius round the fixation point.[14] Hence we must distinguish between what is actually ' seen ' by the eye and what is supplied mentally by suggestion or interpretation and unconscious inference. The interpretation is made so readily and the suggestion is so subtle that ordinarily a person thinks that the whole page is visible to him at once. The span of prehension is about five letters, i.e., the number of letters which can be grasped in one act of attention, as for instance by a momentary exposure, is limited to this small number. Yet, by practice, words have become united in unitary complexes, and sentences into larger complexes, which function as wholes so that by a single act of apprehension we can take in about thirty letters provided that they constitute a sentence. Anybody who reads characters in a foreign alphabet such as Greek or Hebrew can easily distinguish what is ' seen ' from what is supplied by the mind's store.

So, too, we are able at once to recognise the most complicated figures if they are presented in symmetrical form as a whole though the analysis into constituent lines may not be possible. A good deal of the æsthetic feeling accompanying symmetrical shapes is brought about by such facility in recognition. In a similar fashion, as has been often pointed out, we may find no difficulty in hearing the actors on an English stage, yet if we go to a foreign theatre we are at once struck, not so much by the effort to follow the language as by the physical difficulty of " hearing " the speech. Such an experience makes us vividly realise how slight are the ' cues ' which sensation supplies to our perceptions and how much interpretation is necessary in order to give them meaning. Words can be read at distances from the fixation point of the eye at which single letters are not recognisable. The length of the words and their characteristic general form as visual wholes are sufficient for recognition. For the same reason it has been demonstrated that words are recognisable when formed of letters not separately identifiable owing to their size or their distance from the eye. The whole word must consequently be taken in as a single unit in which certain forms are determinable and the rest indifferent. Only when the sequence of letters is unfamiliar is it necessary to be able to see the individual letters, as we find in twilight, when the power to read our own language may be unimpaired whilst a foreign language in which we are not very competent is only legible with increasing difficulty.

With greater familiarity the stimulus which determines the reading act becomes slighter and slighter. Fewer and more sketchy ' cues ' are necessary in order to touch off the act of recognition of word or phrase. A few dominating letters or shapes are a sufficient stimulus to enable us to supply the rest of the word in visual form.   There is much of what is known as preperception—the seeing in the light of what has been previously acquired, the completion of what is only partially given and the reading of meaning into symbols. The dominating, or characteristic form is filled out by the mind's eye into the complete visual form of the word or phrase.   The reader reacts not to the mere visual shape but to its acquired significance, or as Professor James says, " it is the total situation which is the ' object ' on which the reaction of the subject is made."   If he had substituted the term ' acquired meaning ' for ' total situation ' this statement would be an admirable summary of what the child does when reading.

The early reading of children is universally accompanied by lip movements and even though no sound is made the movements are accompanied by an inner speech.   Now this inner speech without noticeable movements of the organs of articulation is also common amongst adults.   Its elements are both auditory and motor, but it would be a mistake to suppose that it consists of the same elements as words when written or printed.   For it must be remembered that there is no phonetic basis for the division of a sentence into words, still less of words into syllables or letters.   In natural speech the sentence or phrase is an unbroken continuum which grammatical analysis has divided into words which are later separated artificially into letters, in much the same way as the separate pictures of a cinematographic film break up the continuity of movement into a series of static views.   The printed page gives an erroneous idea of the course of thought whilst reading or in inner speech, as it is not essential that the mind should grasp the details in order to understand the whole. For as Professor Stout has pointed out " it is certainly possible to think of a whole in its unity and distinctness without discerning all or even any of its component details," as when we think, e.g., of the meaning of such a term as ' wealth ' without having any picture of a bale of goods or a sack of gold. Generally, written or spoken words, and the same applies to inner speech, suggest simply their *meaning* which is apprehended at once without recourse to mental imagery. If, however, for any reason we are pulled up or stop to reflect or are baffled, then and then only does explicit inner speech tend to arise. Accordingly, it has been found experimentally that a characteristic correlate of slow reading is inner speech. Such awareness of the whole without discernment of the parts has been called implicit apprehension, the details becoming explicit as occasion arises. A few visual clues are adequate stimuli to arouse a whole wealth of meaning implicitly apprehended in internal speech. In learning to interpret the symbols of speech by reading, the child daily reproduces for us, as in a microcosm, the characteristics of the mental evolution of the race in its efforts to grasp the meaning of the macrocosm. So the best introduction to the study of educational psychology is to be found in an examination of the steps by which a child learns to read.

CHAPTER III

THE STUDY OF OBSERVATION

Preperception—Plan of Investigation—The Time Factor—Subjective
Activity—Quantitative Results—Qualitative Conclusions

PREPERCEPTION

THE examination of specimens, the study of pictures, charts
and diagrams, and so on, is an essential part of the technique
of teaching in most subjects. Apart from the appeal to the
senses, these devices are rightly supposed as we saw in the
preceding chapter to assist understanding. Every practical
teacher knows, however, that the mere looking at pictures or
objects or even the uncontrolled manipulation of them no
more assists comprehension than strolling round a picture
gallery develops appreciation of art. No understanding without insight. The educational value of sensory aids depends
on a training in observation, and it might be supposed that
experimental psychology would offer some aid in the study of
the process. The present chapter is the first contribution to
such a study and experimental details are given to assist
future investigation. There is an obstacle in the way of this
inquiry which we shall frequently encounter when dealing
with other matters. It is difficult to discover who placed the
obstacle there, but possibly Herbart with his doctrine of
apperception has the greatest responsibility.

According to his view all conative activity was denied to
the subject and transferred to the presentations for, said he,

" in the soul there are only presentations, out of which all
that is in consciousness must be constructed." He proceeded
forthwith to elaborate a dynamics of the presentations with
the appropriate differential equations in the place of subjective
forces. Such a parody of mental activity taken over into
educational psychology led, as might have been anticipated,
to a mechanical view of the educative process. But though
the doctrine died in the educational world frantic efforts are
made by the up-to-date psychologists to revivify it. There is
supposed to be, as we saw in the first chapter, an obscure compartment, the unconscious one, in which ideas and images
and affects crowd and jostle each other in their attempt to
get into freer compartments. They do all this by themselves
without any help from the conscious subject. All that he
has done is to shut them up and woe betide the man who does
so consciously or unwittingly for they are so anxious to get
out that they produce neurotic and other symptoms. The
unfortunate subject can only look on and wonder what the
pother is all about, for he never knows, and having no mental
activity of his own he is powerless. This theatrical show is
called dynamic or functional psychology apparently because
the subject has no function to perform.

If there were anything to be said for the theory it ought to
be possible by providing opportunities for the formation of a
set of images to exhibit their independent activity. Now the
experiment described in this chapter offered ideal conditions
for the establishment and arousal of visual images and their
subsequent use in the process of observation. The detailed
observations shew that there was no sign whatever of any
activity by the images themselves apart from the conscious
control of the subject. Previous activity exerted by the subject facilitated future activity and made observation easier
and more systematic. It is perhaps going too far to say that
images have no part to play in the process, but it is an inci-

dental or subordinate one. If it were desirable it would be quite possible to describe the whole of this process of observation by using the notion of mnemic causality without mentioning any images. Meanwhile it is safe to affirm that all attempts to dispense with the notion of subjective activity on the basis of experimental work have so far completely failed. We shall begin our study of observation with some account of the process of voluntary attention since on this effective observation depends.

In summarising the results of previous experimental investigations on perception in order to discover the nature of attention Professor James came to the conclusion that three factors were involved ; namely, the organic process of adjusting the sense organs, ideational preparation, and inhibition of irrelevant movements and ideas.[1] He considered that, in voluntary attention, the process of inhibition was merely an incidental feature and not an essential part of the process. It is evident also that conscious inhibition presupposes attention and, therefore, cannot, without circular reasoning, be used to account for it. The accommodation of the sense organs, although necessary for sensorial attention and probably always present in ideational activity, is a matter for physiology and need concern us no further. In any case, such adaptation is only a favourable condition of attention. We are left, then, with ideational preparation or preperception as the distinguishing feature of the attentive process. It is necessary, however, to avoid the doctrine of presentationism previously mentioned, according to which presentations are regarded as entities interacting amongst themselves ; and to do so we must keep clearly before us the fact that the interaction of presentations is always dependent ultimately on attention.[2] The mistake here alluded to is especially prevalent amongst experimentalists who are apt to confuse the conditions favourable to attention with the attentive

process itself.   Such process as we have affirmed involves the
conception of mental activity, which is evident whenever a
conscious state is the result of previous conscious process.

The term preperception was first used by G. H. Lewes.
He pointed out that the effect of previous experience was to
enlarge our present perceptions making us more and more
independent of the immediate stimulus, more and more
masters of the external world.   The present is largely the
resultant of the past revived as a present experience, " and
this revival makes *pre*perception a factor in perception."
In the same way a new idea " must be prepared for, *pre*-
conceived by the exhibition of its points of similarity and
attachment with familiar conceptions."   Both a new object
presented to sense and a new idea presented to thought must
be " soluble in old experiences " before either can be perceived or comprehended.   These phenomena have, of course,
been long recognised.   Thus, in the " Midsummer Night's
Dream " we read :

> " Such tricks hath strong imagination,
>   That, if it would but apprehend some joy,
>   It comprehends some bringer of the joy ;
>   Or in the night, imagining some fear,
>   How easy is a bush suppos'd a bear ! "

And Wordsworth wrote :

> " Of all the mighty world
> Of eye, and ear—both what they half create
> And what perceive."

Again in all ambiguous geometrical figures and patterns, a
strongly imagined effort to see one form rather than another
is usually successful in making us perceive the expected shape.

In his study of attention Professor James, following
Lewes, states the theory of preperception as follows : " *the
only things which we commonly see are those which we preperceive* and the only things which we preperceive are those

which have been labelled for us, and the labels stamped into our mind. If we lost our stock of labels we should be intellectually lost in the midst of the world." This doctrine, so vivaciously affirmed, consists of two distinct parts which, if true, are both of fundamental importance to educational theory. The first is that effective observation depends on preliminary knowledge of what we are about to observe ; and in some sense this must be true since the trained observer is more efficient in his own department than the untrained. The second statement is that language or an adequate terminology is essential to preperception. Both these positions are experimentally examined in this chapter so as to discover the precise difference made by previous knowledge and whether language is essential to the process of observation.

PLAN OF INVESTIGATION

Experiments with these aims in view were performed with over eighty University graduates, mostly honours men, taken in sets ranging from six to twelve in a group. The procedure employed with the last two groups is the most satisfactory and will be described in detail, but as the earlier experiments indicated by their results certain essential improvements in method they will be touched upon here. In general, the experiments were conducted on the following plan. Lantern slides were prepared, showing suits of armour, which were projected on to a screen in front of the subjects who were told to observe the picture as accurately as possible, as they would be asked to describe in writing all they had seen. After the first slide had been closely observed for about one minute it was withdrawn, and the subjects were told to note down immediately every detail they remembered in as concise a form as possible and also to state any general observations they had made. No time limit was imposed and each signed a declaration, before giving up his record, that he had tried but could not recall anything else. The set of subjects was now divided into two groups, one of which had a lecture in which the structure of a suit of armour was explained and illustrated by slides shewing drawings of each part, and the technical names of the parts were written up on the board. It was found that none of the subjects had any but the vaguest knowledge of armour, derived from hazy recollections of pictures or casual visits to museums, and the technical terms were almost absolutely unknown ; only three or four of the total number of students examined knew an odd term or two, but hardly knew exactly to which part it applied. When the lecture was over the two groups were again combined into one set and were shewn another slide of armour for one minute ; then they recorded their observations as before. Introspective records were also made. In this way it was possible to compare two groups ; one with, and the other without definite preperception. Marks were assigned on the following scale. Two were given for each part correctly noted (e.g., neck guard, wings on knee) ; one mark for each position correctly recorded (e.g., left foot advanced) ; and one mark for each correct description (e.g., arm guard chased ; solerets pointed). The same numbers with a negative sign were assigned for incorrect observations under these heads, i.e., marks were subtracted.

The first set of subjects examined consisted of twenty-three graduates of average age 26 years. When the first slide had been shewn and records of observations had been made they were divided into groups L and N consisting of eleven and twelve respectively. The lecture was given to group L and immediately afterwards both groups were combined and shewn the second slide, and then a third slide ; records of observations and introspections being made after each.

For group N the average marks for the three slides were

20, 22 and 25 (the medians being 21, 24, 20) ; for group L
the averages were 30, 38 and 38 (medians 30½, 37½ and 38½).
It will be seen that the groups were of unequal merit at the
beginning and that the group which had the lecture improved
relatively only slightly more, if at all, than the other group.
The outstanding feature of these marks is the surprisingly small
difference made by the lecture in the power of observation.
The introspective records make clear the reason for this ; for,
after the second slide, half the subjects in group L complained
that the endeavour to remember the technical terms confused
them and made observation more difficult.   Some of the introspections may be quoted as they illuminate different points.
Thus one subject said : " The technical terms were of use
only in so far as they broke the suit into pieces thus indicating
what parts to look for."   Another said : " The knowledge of
technical terms enabled me to work systematically," and this
was confirmed by several.   " The lecture aided the observation in that I used the sequence of the lecture and was able to
anticipate objects, e.g., I looked at once for the lance rest."
This may be compared with the following : " I would not have
seen the lance rest if I had not expected it.   I had to search for
it.   The lecture hindered observation because of the technical
terms.   If more time had been given after the lecture this
might not have happened.   The lecture, however, was of
direct assistance in that after it much less attention was paid
to such details as decoration which was immediately dismissed
as Milanaise, chasing, etc.   In *this* way technical terms helped."
The next two records indicate clearly why the lecture made so
little difference.   " The lecture aided me because (*a*) it prepared me to deal with the suit part by part instead of wondering where to begin ; (*b*) it was a guide to parts to look for.
The terms helped observation when they were thoroughly
known but hindered when I had a difficulty in remembering
them."   " The half-learnt terms obtruded when observation

was going on, tending to a mixture of two endeavours—to observe, and to fix on the right terms ; with the result that neither was properly accomplished. In the few cases where the name was recalled without effort, the observation was helped."

It is evident that the chief effect of preperception is to introduce order into the observation and that technical terminology is only of assistance provided that it is thoroughly well known.

THE TIME FACTOR

With the next set of sixteen subjects special care was taken to see that the technical terms were well known, for which purpose the lecture was repeated twice and the terms emphasised. Questions were also invited and answered. In order to secure a better comparison the subjects were divided into two groups of equal ability as measured by the marks obtained on the first slide. Two slides only were shewn this time. The results were puzzling since the group that had the lecture seemed to have profited by it astonishingly little compared with the other group, as the following figures indicate. The average marks of group N (the unlectured) for the first and second slide were 17½ and 31 (medians 15 and 29) ; for group L the averages were 17 and 34 (medians 19 and 33½). A further set of eighteen subjects gave the following averages for initially equivalent groups ; group N, 19½ and 37 (medians 20 and 35) ; group L, 19½ and 51 (medians 21 and 53). This last result is much more what might have been expected *à priori*. There were still baffling results obtained with other subjects owing to the eagerness of the groups who had the lecture to *concentrate on detail and to neglect general features*, which neglect caused a certain group of L subjects to score less than its equivalent N group in the second slide. Also several of the men required more practice to adjust themselves to the experimental conditions. The experiment was so interesting to nearly all the subjects that their eagerness militated against the calm which is essential to this kind of work ; especially when they were shewn the first slide. It was evident, also, that merely being familiar with the structure of armour and the terminology was not sufficient to display the full effects of ideational preparation. The subjects ought not only to learn their lesson but to have a sufficient period to digest it. Adequate time for mental assimilation of the knowledge given by the lecture turned out to be the kernel of the problem of observation. Attention is facilitated by preperception only when this condition is fulfilled. Time is of the very essence of the problem. During the interval there is an actual stamping in of the previous knowledge, a phenomenon to which Dr Ballard has given the name of Reminiscence. He says : " The belief that the change that takes place in the nervous system during conscious learning is to a certain extent continued when the learning has ceased is forced upon us when we consider those phenomena of reminiscence in which the physical basis is marked and manifest." He gives as instances the improvement of skill in swimming, skating, typewriting, etc., which occurs in the intervals when no practice is being taken ; and concludes that " an actual modification of brain structure, of the same nature as that which is supposed to occur during learning, gradually goes on during the interval." [3] The only objection to this view is that the changes are supposed to be purely nervous. There seems no sufficient reason to doubt that mental changes of a similar kind also take place during periods of inactivity. The results of the present series of experiments have convinced the author that mental changes, leading to better systematisation of facts and more adequate assimilation of terms, take place after the conscious learning has ceased.

SUBJECTIVE ACTIVITY

The final method of experiment adopted, which proved satisfactory in bringing to light the effects of preperception, may now be described. Sheets of paper were distributed to the subjects, divided into two columns with a subdivision for introspective remarks. The purpose of the experiment was announced as being the attempt to discover the difference made in observation by a preliminary knowledge of what one is about to observe ; and the subjects were also told that they would be asked to describe on their sheets everything they could remember. They were likewise informed that suits of armour would be projected from the lantern on to the screen. Slide (1) was then shewn on a screen in a darkened room for 1½ minutes. This time was discovered by several preliminary trials to be the optimum. All agreed that the time was sufficient for a complete observation, but when they were asked at the end of the whole experiment for how long they thought the slides had been shewn their answers varied from 1 minute to 5 minutes. If a longer time is given several subjects begin to get restless and are apt to let their attention wander ; with less time they feel hurried.

The slide was then withdrawn and immediately afterwards the subjects were asked to state in one column in brief cata-logue form every detail they could recall, and subsequently in the other column any general observations which could not conveniently be considered as detail. Any remarks they wished to make, not of an observational nature, were to be placed in the introspection column. As much time as was wanted was given to making these records, at the end of which the subjects wrote and signed the declaration " I have tried my best but cannot recall anything else." No sheet was accepted without this statement.

E

What the subjects were really trying to do was to read off from their memory image the details which they had noticed during their observation of the picture. It may be objected that a good visualiser will be able to decipher details which he has not observed, but, as it were, photographed and subsequently developed. But this view has been shewn to be a mistake. The best visualisers, who claim to have perfect imagery, are not capable of reading off details which they have not *definitely* attended to. It has been demonstrated, for instance, that such a person claiming to retain a complete mental picture of the front of a building (say) is unable to read off the number of pillars unless he has definitely counted them. Professor Woodworth, as the result of the study of his own imagery asserts that " it always consisted of facts previously noted." He goes on to say that " an actual situation presents an almost unlimited variety of facts or features, of which an observer notes a few, the rest remaining undiscriminated in the background. . . . Later he may ' remember ' the situation, but this is not to reinstate it in its original multiplicity or continuity. He recalls the features which he has observed, or some of them, but not the great mass of them which remained in the background. Lacking this setting or background, he is not in a position to make any fresh observation in recall." [4] Professor Woodworth's conclusions have been repeatedly confirmed in the course of the present investigation and also in some experiments undertaken by a totally different method by the present author. *In brief, we cannot study mental imagery without reference to mental activity and all that preperception can do is merely to facilitate such activity.* [5]

The next step in the method was to interchange the records amongst the subjects. The picture was again thrown on to the screen (this time in the lighted room) and they marked each other's papers in accordance with the scheme given above. Every doubtful point was referred to the author for his final decision and he subsequently examined the sheets. This method of marking has the great advantage that it forces the subjects to examine the picture in detail and stimulates interest and competition amongst the groups, which is necessary in this type of experiment. The method of evaluating the marks must take into account the fact that both groups have some practice in preperception; and this has been done in the calculations made below.

The whole process was repeated with a second slide (2) which was also shewn for $1\frac{1}{2}$ minutes and marked in the same way. The marks for the two performances were added together and, on the basis of the totals, all the subjects were divided into two groups of equal ability. For the particular set of fourteen subjects whose results will be considered in detail the combined marks for the two slides were 354 for group L (the lectured group) and 343 for group N (the non-lectured group). It was not possible to get closer totals, as one subject proved so considerably superior to the others. The advantage of combining two sets of readings lies in the fact previously noted that some habituation is required in order to allow several of the subjects to adjust themselves to the experimental conditions.

A lecture [6] on the structure of armour in which all the parts were named was now given to group L, the other group being dismissed. It was repeated twice and the various portions of a suit of armour were shewn on the screen, each technical term being written on the board. At the end of the lecture, slide (1) was again projected on to the screen and the parts indicated by name. Finally, the terms were copied into note-books by the subjects who were told to go over them during the following week until they were perfectly familiar with them. Questions were freely asked and answered during the lecture. In this manner the seven subjects of group L were enabled completely to assimilate all the terms and the details of the structure of armour, thus being placed in a most favourable attitude for preperception. All the subjects successfully learnt and could use all the terms freely. Exactly one week later both groups were recombined and two further slides (3 and 4) were exhibited, as before, the details of procedure being the same.

At the conclusion of the whole experiment, when the records had been marked and given up, the following questions were answered. Those who had the instruction stated whether and how their observation had been aided or hindered by the lecture and the technical terms ; those who did not have the lecture stated whether the absence of a terminology hindered observation and in what manner. They were expressly enjoined to give no theory but simply to describe their experience.

THE QUANTITATIVE RESULTS

The combined marks for each subject for slides (1) and (2) at the first sitting, and for slides (3) and (4) at the second sitting are given below :

Without preliminary knowledge (Slides 1 and 2)

Group L		Group N	
Subject	Marks	Subject	Marks
A	94	P	61
B	54	Q	60
C	53	R	53
D	51	S	57
E	42	T	42
F	39	U	41
G	21	V	29
Mean	50·6	Mean	49
m.d.	14·2	m.d.	10

Coefficient of variation,* 28   Coefficient of variation, 20·4

* i.e. $\dfrac{\text{m.d.}}{\text{Mean}} \times 100.$

A week after the lecture (Slides 3 and 4)

Group L		Group N	
Subject	Marks	Subject	Marks
A	153	P	85
B	114	Q	94
C	107	R	75
D	107	S	55
E	102	T	45
F	118	U	81
G	82	V	67
Mean	111·9	Mean	71·7
m.d.	14·1	m.d.	13·8

Coefficient of variation, 12·6   Coefficient of variation, 19

The effect of organised preperception can clearly be discerned in the differing variabilities of the groups. For the unlectured group N remains practically constant in this respect; whereas the group L displays a marked decrease in variability. It is important, for the theory of education, to realise that systematic training tends to produce greater uniformity within a group. Group N had, of course, some training in the observation of the first two slides and in marking them, but such training was undirected by precise knowledge, and unsystematic as compared with that of group L. Experiments of this nature may serve to differentiate the relative values of class instruction and individual work especially for weaker pupils; since the decreased variability, as the figures shew, is brought about by levelling up the less able whilst the trained group as a whole and individually shew better results.

If we desire to compare the trained group with the untrained from the point of view of the relative difference made by preperception, we must resort to the statistical device of using as our unit the standard deviation of the groups. For if one group yields more variable results than another this implies that variation in this group is easier than in the other. The crude figures in the above tables were converted into multiples of these units, yielding the following numbers when cleared of decimal points.

	Group L Marks (in terms of σ)			Group N Marks (in terms of σ)	
Subject	Slides 1 and 2	Slides 3 and 4	Subject	Slides 1 and 2	Slides 3 and 4
A	60	85	P	39	47
B	34	64	Q	38	53
C	34	60	R	34	42
D	32	60	S	36	31
E	27	57	T	27	25
F	25	66	U	26	45
G	13	46	V	18	37
Mean	32	63	Mean	31	40

As the figures are now comparable, we shall not be far out in assuming that if group L had no lecture they, too, would have risen to an average of 40 instead of 63. Consequently 23 marks is the gain due to preperception; and to find the percentage gain we must start not from their original average mark namely 32, but from 40. This is a gain of 57·5 per cent. To put it otherwise, these figures shew that as a result of preperception the trained group is able to observe somewhat over one and a half times as much as the untrained group; which implies, as pointed out previously, *that they are capable of so many more separate definite acts of attention.*

THE QUALITATIVE CONCLUSIONS

Having thus obtained a numerical estimate of the effects of preliminary knowledge in facilitating attention, it is time to consider the non-quantitative results which are, perhaps, of more significance. In dealing with these use will be made of the records of the whole of the eighty subjects and of their introspections.

One of the most important differences made by preperception is very difficult to describe, as it is so essentially subjective. The observer feels that his mental energy is being more effectively spent and this tends to make him feel more active. Such effective use of mental effort is accompanied by a distinct feeling of satisfaction, which seems to make the effort easier. Thus the person at one and the same time feels that he is more active with less effort. One of the N subjects put the matter in this way : " Lack of terms distinctly hindered my observation. I knew one technical term from reading Scott (tasset) and I always looked first to that part of the armour and had a *feeling of sureness* about this. Lack of terms hindered the mental separation of the armour into details ; I could only remember each detail as soon as it was separated."

After the lecture the subjects of the L groups took the initiative and went out on a voyage of active exploration to discover the definite parts named ; whereas previously the picture, as it were, had the initiative and the person was passively trying to remember what it offered to him. Or, to vary the figure, just as an animal expecting the appearance of its prey is ready to spring with all its muscles pre-adapted for that purpose, so the person expecting to see certain details in a picture has his mind prepared ready to pounce upon them. Owing to this difference of attitude it frequently happened that the elaborate decoration which was a feature of the last two slides confused or baffled those who had no lecture, so that they lost the wood for the trees ; but this never happened with the lectured group who were able to dismiss the decoration with a name, and subsequently to remember its nature. These experiments, therefore, yield confirmation of the view that recollection of an observed visual fact may be based on purely verbal imagery without any sensorial image of a visual nature being present.[7]

It will be remembered that the subjects were asked, at the end of the experiment, to say how the lecture and the knowledge of terms had helped their perception of the picture. The records shew that the greatest help is given in supplying a plan for the observation, i.e. in making it more systematic and definite. Recognition becomes more rapid as a result of preperception, and more certain—no subject ever complained that he could not *see* a detail after the lecture was given. The lecture makes the details stand out from the picture ; as one subject said, " The ordinary parts were emphasised because one knew where to look for them. Without the lecture it was the curious or outstanding parts that were noticed." The latter part of this statement is open to challenge. In the fourth slide the size of the ' lance rest,' when projected on to the screen, was about two inches in length and formed a conspicuous feature ; but it was hardly ever seen by a subject who did not know what it meant. In fact, it was this object which induced the writer, after the first set experiments, to insist on the declaration that everything that could be remembered had been recorded, as it was difficult to persuade a person otherwise that he had missed so conspicuous a feature. In one slide where the lance rest was inconspicuous owing to the ornamentation, it was never overlooked by those who knew what to look for. Finally, the absence of expected parts is immediately noticed ; several subjects declaring that they needed only to look for missing parts after the lecture in order to take in the picture. One subject of an N group who had considerable artistic skill pointed out a curious difficulty. He said that he failed to observe the picture accurately, in detail, because he could not separate constructional from decorative lines owing to lack of preliminary knowledge of the structure of armour.

With regard to terminology it became evident that its chief use was to facilitate description, i.e. to make it more concise, more ' telescoped.' But this is not all ; for frequently the mental image needed a word to fix it, that is to say, the terms formed ' pegs,' as one subject said, on which to ' hang ' the detailed observations as they were made. Closely connected with this is the aid given in discriminating parts by the use of words. Words make the dissection of the suit into parts much easier. For this purpose it is essential that the names should be perfectly familiar. The following introspective record illustrates this : " Terms did not help me because I thought of the armour in terms of my own making. My method was to consider the parts of the body covered and *then* the name. Breast plate was ' breast plate ' in my mind and ' cuirass ' only by an effort of memory. This does not apply to ' greaves,' since I happen to know this term as a literary one."

We can best, perhaps, see the utility of terms by noticing what the subjects who had no lecture reported. " With terms," said one, " I would have tabulated all the possible parts into a generalised suit of armour and I should have then gone through the given suit checking these off." In other words lack of terms prevents generalisation. Another subject stated that " Lack of knowledge of structure and terms hindered me owing to lack of definite starting points, and definite systematisation in classifying parts. Also by necessitating the use of roundabout phrases, which was apt to turn my concentration on the visual image to concentration on the terms expressing it." Several others pointed out the necessity of putting their observations into language, whilst the slide was shewn, in order to recall the detail later. Thus one particularly conscientious observer made the remark : " I could have mentioned several other points, but having no terms I was quite unable to express what I had noticed." He really meant that his memory image failed because he had no terms with which to retain it. Another remarked that he had a difficulty in retaining the relation of one part to another and he thought that terms would have helped him in this respect. Some few, however, denied all this and maintained that the absence of terms simply made their descriptions more clumsy. We are here probably dealing with ultimate differences in mental make-up.

CHAPTER IV

MENTAL IMAGERY

Primary and Secondary Presentations—Varieties of Imagery—Imagery
and Feeling—Meaning—Imagery and Learning

PRIMARY AND SECONDARY PRESENTATIONS

THE scientific investigation of mental imagery received its
initial impulse from Galton who attempted to study mental
contents by the comparative method.[1] He submitted a
questionnaire to certain selected individuals of high intellectual standing containing questions framed so as to help
their introspection. He asked them, for example, to state
definitely what was in their minds when they made an attempt
later in the day to recall the appearance of their breakfast-
table. His questions were chosen so as to secure replies based
on introspection with regard to clearness, vividness, stability,
etc., of the objects appearing in the effort to remember.
Galton started with the presupposition that visually evoked
objects were more likely to occur and more important than
others and consequently his questions were in the main about
visual things. Dr Betts considerably improved the *questionnaire* method by asking an equivalent number of questions
about objects belonging to the different sense modalities of
sight, hearing, taste, touch, etc., so as to counter any undue
emphasis on a particular sense.[2] His questions were more
carefully chosen so as to guide introspection to very definite
points and his subjects, who were University students and

teachers, were required to state whether the objects mentally recalled were as clear and distinct as their originals or only moderately distinct or whether, in fact, no object at all was present when the attempt at recall was made. A table of seven grades of vividness and distinctness was placed before the subjects, ranging from vividness which could not be distinguished from reality, to complete absence of vividness ; and they were asked with reference to each mental object recalled to assign a number representing its grade. It will be convenient to call mental contents which are aroused in the absence of the sense objects to which they refer by the name of secondary objects or presentations.

As a result of Galton's inquiries it had become the custom to classify persons as visiles, audiles, tactiles, motiles, etc., according to the kind of content or secondary objects with which they were endowed and which they employed naturally in the mental processes of remembering, imagining, reasoning and the like. Dr Betts' study of 47 men and 96 women led him to the conclusion that few, if any, were absolutely incapable of evoking secondary objects belonging to every sphere of sense. He found that the three highest grades of vividness and clearness were distributed amongst his subjects in the following proportions : visual, 68 per cent. ; auditory, 65 per cent. ; cutaneous, 61 per cent. ; gustatory, 58 per cent. ; kinæsthetic, 57 per cent. ; organic, 55 per cent. ; olfactory, 50 per cent. The author of this book has found a very similar distribution amongst various groups of University graduates. These figures, shewing the occurrence in roughly equal numbers of the different modalities, afford no ground for the classification into ear-minded, eye-minded, etc., if by these terms we mean to designate the native constitution of various people. On the contrary, they shew that clear examples of the various modes are to be found in different people in approximately the same proportions. The like results have been obtained for school children between the ages of seven and fourteen years, amongst whom an especially high correlation was found between the occurrence of visual and auditory secondary objects. The diagram printed on this page from data collected by the author shews the same thing by the similarity of the distribution for the three chief sorts of imagery.

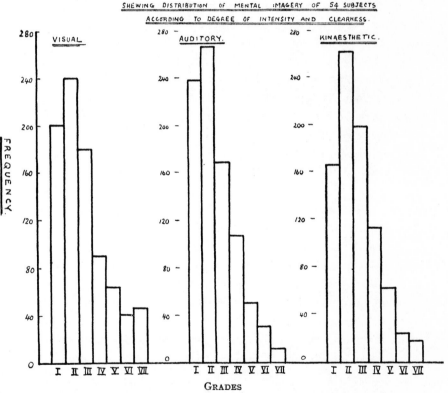

Explanation :—A *questionnaire* of 48 questions, 16 referring to each of the three kinds of imagery. Every subject, with a scale in front of him specifying the meaning to be attached to the grades, decided to which grade each image belonged. Grade I is the highest degree of vividness and clearness.

It must be borne in mind that in all the cases so far considered we have been dealing with images voluntarily evoked ;

but the ability to recall these objects by an act of will is not a necessary indication of their ordinary use. Although it would be erroneous to speak of visual, auditory or other types of mentality in the sense of differences in native constitution with regard to secondary objects, there is no doubt that individuals do select and prefer to use different categories ; and if we merely intend to refer to this preference in actual use there is no harm in speaking of differences of type. The so-called ' pure types ' are rare, if they exist at all ; and there is reason to believe that the various modalities could, by practice, be kept approximately at the same level if that were desirable. Thus Professor Titchener states : " my furniture of images is, perhaps, in better than average condition, because—fearing that, as one gets older, one tends also to become more and more verbal in type—I have made a point of renewing it by practice. I am now able, for instance, as I was able when I entered the class-room nearly twenty years ago, to lecture from any one of the three main cues. I can read off what I have to say from a memory manuscript ; or I can follow the lead of my voice ; or I can trust to the guidance of kinæsthesis, the anticipatory feel of the movements of articulation." [3]

This sort of evidence receives indirect support from the observation that the ability to evoke secondary objects belonging to any particular sphere of sense is not an influential factor in determining in what particular course of study a given individual will excel. Thus a person who can readily recall visual objects will not necessarily prefer geometry or drawing nor will an individual who can easily reproduce tones take to music. In fact it has been shewn statistically that there is an absence of correlation between the grades of voluntarily aroused secondary objects and success in college studies, either on the whole or in particular branches of learning.

By an obvious analogy secondary visual objects or presentations are called visual images and by an extension of this comparison secondary objects of all categories are known as images of the primary presentations or objects. This terminology is part and parcel of current discourse and psychologists freely talk of auditory images, tactile images and so on. The student should bear in mind that all analogies are apt to be misleading and this one in particular has doubtful implications. It is usually supposed that images differ from sense perceptions quantitatively only and not qualitatively and that this difference is mainly one of intensity. But it seems very difficult to believe that the image of sugar is merely a faint taste of sugar, for in that case a particularly strong image or a persistently repeated one would enable us to dispense with the real object, more especially in those cases where culinary art depends on the slightest suspicion of a flavour. Whoever derived satisfaction from an artificial rose by eking out its form with an image of its odour ? Or who can cloy the hungry edge of appetite by bare imagination of a feast ?

Unless the sense organ is stimulated there is a qualitative difference between a mental image and a sensation. In this respect visual imagery seems to differ from all other varieties of secondary presentations, for it has been asserted that the intense mental picturing of a secondary colour results in the sensation of the complementary colour, and also that the image of one colour may interfere with the after sensations of others ; which observations, if correct, would tend to shew that visual images exhaust the retina.

The total disparity between primary and secondary presentations is obvious to introspection, though the majority of psychologists seem unaware of the distinction. One very good observer has put the matter in an unimpeachable form. He says that to talk of reviving past mental experiences is not strictly correct, and gives as an instance his recollection of his morning's breakfast : " I have visual memory-images of the breakfast-room. . . . I have compound gustatory-tactile-thermal images of the taste of the porridge. . . . I have an olfactory image of the smell of the coffee and auditory images of the postman's knock. . . . Giving myself up to this memory experience, I *know* it is not exactly a reproduction, a renewal, a revival, a second edition of this morning's sense experience. If I close my eyes and shade them, my field of vision, after a little while, becomes quite dark, and with the exception of the *Eigenlicht* of the retina, I cannot discover anything. Peep I may as much as I like, into the darkness, not the faintest trace of the white of the table-cloth, or the gold rim of the cups and saucers can I discover, not a vestige of a visual sensation. Nevertheless, I ' see ' the breakfast-table quite plainly and vividly with the ' Mind's Eye,' as it is commonly expressed. That these memory-images are faint reproductions of the sensations, i.e. weak sensations, sensations of low intensity, is decidedly not true in my case, they are an experience, *sui generis*. I consider myself a good visualiser. . . . If, then, revival or reproduction is spoken of, these terms must not be understood literally." This sound introspection of a competent observer is in refreshing contrast with the confused nonsense talked by others about their mental imagery.[4]

The best psychological definition of a mental image, i.e. a definition in terms of experience, is that given by Professor Colvin, namely, " that activity of consciousness in which an object of sensation is experienced as not immediately present to the senses." [5] Unless the experience carries with it the feeling that the primary object is absent and only the secondary present, the psychosis is not properly described as a mental image. This distinguishes the image from all such mental objects as perceptions, illusions, hallucinations, dreams, etc., for all of these "are stamped with the quality which functions for immediate sensory presence of the object." What it is that we really experience when a mental image is said to be present will be considered later ; but meanwhile we may say that for all the modalities, except possibly vision and not certainly there, the use of the same terms for imagination and sensation, namely hearing, touching, etc., is unfortunate and only to be justified figuratively.   The inability to discriminate between hallucinations and normal mental imagery and the mental confusion thereby entailed is responsible for a psychological abortion called the ' eidetic image.'   To the Marburg school under the direction of Jaensch we owe the introduction of this monstrous confusion into child psychology. When the eyes are closed in a darkened room, and sometimes when they are open, hallucinatory visions are seen, brought about by pressure on the eyeballs, the slight stimulation due to lens adjustment, by changes in the convergence of the eyeball, etc.   Under emotional tension as in delirium it is easier by slight stimulation to produce these hallucinations. Now, the same sort of phenomena are evident sometimes when one stares at a dark surface in daylight.   If then a child is induced to look at a picture against a dark background and the picture is soon withdrawn he may be the victim of such hallucination so that he ' sees ' the picture after withdrawal. It is said that 60 per cent. of all children investigated, between the ages of ten to fifteen, produce these ' eidetic images.'   I have been present at such investigations and have been convinced that the whole operation is due to strong suggestion by the influence of the experimenter and the surrounding conditions, and the observations are worthless.

When Galton sent his *questionnaire* in the first place to distinguished men of science one of them made the following most pertinent reply.[6]   " It is only by a figure of speech that I can describe my recollection of a scene as a ' mental image ' which I can ' see ' with my mind's eye . . . I do not see it . . . any more than a man sees the thousand lines of Sophocles

F

which under due pressure he is ready to repeat." He received, to his great astonishment, the same sort of confession from several others, and it is difficult to see why he should have been surprised by such accurate observations. He also tried the experiment of suddenly accosting some person with the statement, "I want to tell you about a boat," and then inquiring what mental image was aroused by the word 'boat.' One of his victims, a young lady, apparently anxious to pay him back in his own coin, assured him, presumably without a smile, that " she immediately saw the image of a rather large boat pushing off from the shore, and that it was full of ladies and gentlemen, the ladies being dressed in white and blue." Another person, a philosopher this time, told him that the word 'boat' aroused no definite image as he had purposely held his mind in suspense. From these and a large number of similar observations Galton concluded that scientific men and other thinkers have feeble powers of visual representation, the faculty being starved by disuse. He appears to have been too ready to accept the introspections of the young lady and some schoolboys at their face value, whilst rejecting that of more competent observers. We shall see reason in the sequel to doubt the accuracy of the introspections of untrained observers. What makes one hesitate more than ever in accepting such statements is the repeated assertion of persons who claim to have very clear and vivid visual images that they could draw from them if only they knew how to draw ; whereas artists who *can* draw assert that their " imagery is so clear that if they had been unable to draw they would have un-hesitatingly said that they could draw from it." Much harm has been done to psychology by Galton's unwariness in dealing with his evidence about mental imagery and his mistakes have been handed on unthinkingly until they form the chief data of many a professed psychologist.

THE VARIETIES OF IMAGERY

Enough has been said to indicate that most of the primary objects of sense have their counterparts in the secondary presentations of imagination. Now, an integral feature of every primary presentation is some muscular movement ; thus in seeing the eyes are adjusted, in tasting the tongue is moved, in touch the muscles of the hand are brought into play, and so on with every sensory experience. In addition the muscular or kinæsthetic sense, due to strains and stresses in the muscles and tendons and pressures on the joint surfaces brought about by gross movements of the limbs, plays a predominant part in all our activities, adding their quota to the tale of secondary presentations.

Kinæsthetic or motor imagery has been widely investigated and it is convenient to have terms to distinguish its varieties. We shall use the word *somamotor* to designate the imagery of gross trunk, limb or head movements ; *manumotor* for those of the hand ; *oculomotor* for eye movements ; and *vocimotor* for images of the movements of the vocal organs. Although the majority of psychologists lay great stress on the importance of kinæsthetic imagery in mental processes there is a growing body of opinion that what are called motor images are, in reality, incipient motor sensations. Thus the attempt to recall words by vocimotor images is said to consist really of very slight movements of articulation definitely localised in the lips, tongue, larynx, etc. Again the effort to recall the movements of running or a stroke at tennis whilst sitting comfortably in one's chair may result in the feeble reinstatement of actual muscle, tendon and joint sensations instead of somamotor images. Whether this is the whole of what is meant by motor imagery or not there is little doubt that careful introspection does reveal slight resident sensations in the various organs when kinæsthetic imagery alone is said to occur.

Despite assertions to the contrary by those who maintain that they experience secondary presentations with the same fullness of detail as primary presentations there seems to be little doubt that all such recall is more or less sketchy and symbolic. Those features only are reinstated which are relevant to the particular moment of recall and the absence of the rest is usually not noticed because our attention is otherwise engaged. This is especially true of kinæsthetic imagery where a bare sketch of a movement is adequate for our purposes and even the sketch may be symbolic suggesting the movement rather than copying it.

The various modalities of imagery do not occur in isolation and it is a matter of some difficulty to distinguish between motor and visual imagery. Words may be recalled in voci-motor, visual or manumotor terms, and bodily movements as visual or somamotor images ; and it may be that in all cases all the varieties are mutually involved. Nevertheless, Professor Pear asserts that excellence in bodily skill may rest on a unique development of kinæsthetic imagery distinct from visual or all other types. Persons endowed with imagery of this sort would perceive and remember new movements, from the outset, in purely kinæsthetic terms. It is conceivable that if they could elaborate their particular talent in motor symbols that new concepts could arise and they could communicate their skill to others in motor terms. The vogue of gymnastics, dancing and eurhythmics in schools would thereby be facilitated and a new mimetic art might be evolved.[7]

All such views rest on an assumption which is palpably untrue, namely that secondary presentations can exist apart from their functioning or activity in much the same way that primary objects have an independent existence. Now images are not stored up ready to be recalled when required. I can produce the signature of my name at will, but it would be absurd to suppose that somewhere in my muscles the kinæsthetic images are kept ready waiting to make their appearance like actors in the wings of a stage. Yet this absurdity is countenanced by many psychologists. There is no kinæsthetic image apart from its use. When I say that I have such an image all I mean is that given the appropriate stimulus I can act in a particular way, i.e. write. Nothing further ought to be meant when I say I have a visual or auditory or any other sort of image. All these only come into being when some situation arises in which I must respond in a definite fashion either visually or otherwise. Thus if I am planning to lay out flower-beds in a garden I can do so easily if I walk about the garden or have a sketch of it in front of me ; failing this, a visual image of the garden is of service. It is as well to note, however, that I can do my planning equally well if I know the size of the garden and its shape in somamotor terms or in vocimotor imagery or even in words apart from any of these.

There is one variety of imagery not yet touched upon, namely organic, i.e. secondary presentations corresponding to organic sensations such as hunger, thirst and all other primary sensations dependent on particular bodily conditions. It is doubtful whether such so-called organic images are not in all cases real sensations of minimum intensity. The direction of the attention to any part of the body is likely to yield a sensation in that part, which may be interpreted to mean that sensations are continually occurring from all parts of the body but are usually ignored either because they are too faint or because of their unimportance. The mental importance of organic sensations lies in their relation to our emotional states which are among their most prominent causes ; and as we shall see later, a confusion is apt to arise between such states and what is erroneously regarded as imagery.

THE IMAGES OF CHILDREN

It is universally believed that the imagery of children is more vivid than that of adults, but after what has been said this can only mean that they make more use of their images. The only certain way of discovering a mental image is by introspection. All investigations which rely on indirect means, such as presenting material to be learnt by the eye or the ear alone and inferring the images from the correctness of the learning are, as the sequel will shew, erroneous. Binet's method [8] of getting direct introspection is the correct procedure, but it is a difficult and treacherous one where children are concerned and the results must be accepted with the greatest caution. As the result of a study of the introspection of school children between the ages of $7\frac{1}{2}$ to $14\frac{1}{2}$ years Dr Rusk [9] maintains that imagery between these ages is particularly rich and detailed, consisting of all varieties ; auditory, visual, tactual, kinæsthetic, organic, etc. In some cases the imagery was said to be so vivid as to obliterate whatever was in the field of perception, producing an abstracted look due to concentration on the secondary objects. It was also observed that the children themselves are frequently projected into their own imagery, so that they observe themselves doing things as though they were spectators of the scene, just as in a dream. This feature of self-projection was noticed in the children of all ages. Those of the most fertile imagery, however, were by no means those of the highest school intelligence. Other observers, too, have found that the correlations between vivid and clear visual and auditory imagery and school intelligence are low, or it may be negative. A pupil may have clear and correct images of the illustrations of a lesson, for instance, and yet have learnt very little if he fails to grasp the underlying meaning and relations. As far as school studies are concerned vivid mental imagery may be detrimental or rather it bears no relation to the effectiveness of the mental processes which it accompanies. Even in the lower mental processes such as sensory discrimination of colours, musical tones and pitch, shapes, etc., imagery is helpful only to a small degree ; less so in the case of auditory than visual images. The value of sense training in schools, rightly urged by educational reformers such as Rousseau and Pestalozzi in opposition to the reliance on words alone, rests on its intrinsic nature and its assistance in mental development, rather than on the cultivation of mental imagery. Without the sensory basis the thought processes could not begin to work, as was shewn in the case of the savage of Aveyron. But the ability to evoke images by an act of will is no index to the extent to which images are used in the various thought processes. It has been shewn, for instance, by taking records of the reaction-times, that many persons appreciate the meaning of a word or phrase in a shorter time than they take to recall the corresponding image.

There is evidence to prove that the vividness and clearness of imagery can be improved by practice. Whistler's master trained his pupils to note carefully the details of landscapes which they were subsequently to paint and the efficacy of the method was certified by a French Government Commission which shewed that as a result of the training the artists could remember and reproduce the complicated pattern and colour of a Persian rug in its absence after studying it carefully for a short time.

IMAGERY AND FEELING

The artists referred to reproduced the pattern so that, as the published colour reproductions demonstrate, it was difficult to believe that they were not painting from the primary object. But this is not to say that they were necessarily painting from a visual image. For it would be quite possible to reproduce the shape and colour of the rug by means of kinæsthetic and verbal imagery. If I remember that the colour of an object is bottle-green and its shape that of a lozenge I do not need a visual image in order to reproduce it.

Suppose ten straight lines of different lengths are drawn crossing at random so as to make a meaningless figure, and exposed for five seconds, and a person is asked to reproduce it afterwards. Professor Piéron [10] who devised this experiment found that, on the average, fifteen such exposures, each followed by an attempt at reproduction, were sufficient for correct recall, i.e. for recall of the direction, approximate length and angle of crossings of all the lines. Now a photographic visual image of the figure is quite out of the question for this implies that all parts of the figure are seen at once, but in actual fact only a small portion is focused and the rest is vague. The eye must actively explore and fixate the various portions before the whole is seen clearly, so that the sensory data for a considerable quantity of kinæsthetic imagery are present.

We should expect then that kinæsthetic imagery would play a considerable part in memorising the figure and this is what Piéron found. His subjects relied largely on motor imagery ; in calling up the angles for instance they had kinæsthetic impressions of different movements. He also noticed that there was a certain amount of intellectual reconstruction of the figure.

The author of this book has repeated the experiments on over twenty University graduates who had been trained to introspect and found that the average number of exposures for correct reproduction was thirteen. The subjects were, of course, left free to choose their own methods of memorising. In only one case was there a distinct visual image and all the subjects built up the figure piecemeal. Where an attempt was

made to get a visual picture of the whole it soon proved
ineffective and was abandoned in favour of a series of kinæsthetic efforts. At first sight the figure presents the appearance of a confused jumble of intersecting lines entirely devoid
of meaning. The instructive part of the experiment lies in
the discovery that the subjects, without exception, make
attempts, more or less successful to read meaning into the
chaos, to intellectualise it by the help of language or verbal
imagery. Visual images, even if they exist, which is very
rare, do not aid recall and the reproduction is only effected
when the figure is made significant. The real stimulus is not
the confusing appearance but a meaning which the subject
extracts from it, for the mind has an innate tendency to read
meanings into its presentations and the reaction is made to
these meanings and not to the bare stimuli. Such meanings
were almost entirely embodied in language. Thus one subject,
who after thirteen exposures was able to reproduce the figure
correctly an hour later, started with kinæsthetic images which
gradually disappeared and were replaced entirely by language.
He analysed the chaotic drawing into the following formula :
" Cross, telegraph pole, parallelism, point, parallelism, in-
equality," which being remembered *verbally* enabled him to
retain the figure.

Now the meaning of an impression can be retained in yet
another way which is of the first importance for the understanding of mental imagery. It is very questionable whether
olfactory images have any independent existence apart from
present sensations. Yet Shelley wrote

> Odours, when sweet violets sicken,
> Live within the sense they quicken.

The lyric in which these lines occur is suffused with delicate
feeling and what " vibrated in the memory " of Shelley was
doubtless the undying emotional tone with which his soul

responded to beautiful objects. Such emotional reawakening is frequently mistaken for imagery. The organic resonance which accompanies recollection, due to changed heart beat, disturbed respiration, intestinal movements, etc., is sufficient to account for the air of reality which memory yields giving a secondary presentation the tang of an object present to the senses. It takes very close introspective observation to distinguish emotional states and the organic response which is their expression from sensory imagery, so that the evidence of untrained persons with regard to their mental furniture is almost worthless. Such a careful observer as Professor Colvin [11] as the result of the study of his own imagery concluded that what passes for an auditory image is frequently a mixture of kinæsthetic and other sensations. He says that the chief factors of his own auditory images consist of " various accompanying sensory phenomena, in part those due to motor adjustment and in part those coming from bodily sensations in connection with the emotional accompaniments of tones."

A passing whiff of hay carried by the breeze will instantly reinstate scenes of our childhood or a pleasant summer vacation. The pleasure and intimacy of such recollection is almost wholly due to the revival of organic sensations and emotions which odours are peculiarly fitted to arouse. So the snows of yesteryear may live in our memory solely by reviving the feelings which they once accompanied and independently of any visual imagery. When, for any reason, the same emotional tone is aroused in us we are apt to get the feeling of living through the original sensory experience. The present author is frequently surprised to find himself imagining he is at sea when passing a kitchen door and is able to trace the illusion to the sickly odour of peeled potatoes which he endured on a voyage long ago. He is thus able to endorse Professor Piéron's acute observations on the precautions necessary to be made in studying images, which must be quoted in the original.[12] " Il peut même arriver qu'une évocation purement affective soit prise pour une évocation proprement visuelle ; ainsi, lorsqu'on évoque un objet sombre ou clair, on croit parfois y réussir alors qu'on éprouve des impressions, des sentiments, en rapport avec lui, sans qu'une image clair on sombre apparaisse le moins du monde. On doit prendre garde aux illusions d'introspection."

In the laudable attempt which is now being made to cultivate literary appreciation in schools much attention is paid to the stimulation of imagery. Lessons are given in which the pupils are asked to concentrate on the images whilst a poem is read to them. No doubt the enjoyment of the piece is thereby enhanced in literature where the meaning is contained in the imagery or forms a large part of it. But, on the other hand, concrete and distinct imagery may prove a hindrance when the images are not essential to the thought but merely enrich or develop it. Experience has shewn that poetry containing many pictures is not necessarily easier for a pupil to grasp than a piece devoid of images. Moreover, the enjoyment of literature and its appreciation come largely from the thoughts which call forth heightened feeling when expressed in appropriate rhythm ; and although a large amount of imagery may be present, it is usually only a subsidiary feature of æsthetic taste.[13]

MEANING

Much discussion has centred round the question of the occurrence of imageless thought. In one sense all thought is imageless for it is concerned with propositions or meanings and not with bare subjects or predicates. Images are simply part of the material supplying the data which thought manipulates. Just as written language consisted at first of pictures

becoming in the course of time more and more symbolic,
so thought in its early stages may need the support of sensory
images, gradually replaced by vocimotor imagery which in
its turn may yield place to meanings alone in which the
sensory basis is almost entirely swamped.   Similarly the child
in the kindergarten is guided to his number concept by means
of sticks and balls, whilst to the astronomer manipulating his
symbols the realities signified may be as remote from his
sensations as an undiscovered planet.   As soon as meanings
become clearly defined and ideas proceed smoothly images
tend to disappear from the focus of consciousness.   They
reappear again only when any impediment occurs obstructing
the free flow of thought so that as the author of this book has
shewn " any delay or conflict in consciousness is a favourable
condition for arousing a relevant mental image, that is one
that will in some way help towards a cessation of the
conflict." [14]

When images are present in thinking or other mental processes they function as symbols only.   For this reason it is by no
means necessary that they should be detailed copies of sensory
presentations and in fact too much detail would often be a
positive hindrance.   It frequently happens that when we think
we are able to recall a man's features, say, with great exactness,
we are astonished to find on being asked that we do not know
whether he has a moustache or not.   What is recalled in these
cases may be the barest symbolic indication of a face or a
typical expression.   In like manner too with auditory images ;
when we think we can recall a friend's voice we may find
that there are no defined vowels or consonants before us
but simply a suggestion of the quality of voice or enunciation.
Only these latter things interest us, unless we happen to be
phoneticians, and what is resuscitated is confined to what we
are mainly interested in.

Some people can recall the colour of an object without its

specific shape or even the gloss without either provided that they are interested in these alone. As was previously stated a person's confidence in his ability to evoke a mental image in all its concrete setting is due to the revival of certain emotional characters. Again, in al perception, in addition to the sensory experience involved there are certain specific conscious attitudes distinct from kinæsthetic sensations. Such attitudes add new content of a non-sensory kind to our perceptions and these non-sensory elements may be sufficient for recall of an imageless nature. In memory and imagination such attitudes and emotional experiences may form the tissue of our thinking, the sensory elements being subsidiary and irrelevant. Imageless thought in this sense is not only possible, but of frequent occurrence amongst those who, by careless introspection, confuse these experiences with sensory images.

It was said above that thought is concerned with meanings of which images are simply the vehicles or carriers. There is, however, a persistent attempt amongst psychologists to identify imagery and meaning. Whilst some urge that imagery is but the stimulus and meaning the response, or to put it in another way that image is the structure whilst meaning is the function, others maintain that the image is itself all that there is in what is meant by meaning. Nobody is more competent or has a greater claim to respect when introspective matters are at issue than Professor Titchener who goes so far as to state that the meaning of *meaning* is itself an image. Here are his introspective findings. " I see meaning as the blue-grey tip of a kind of scoop, which has a bit of yellow above it (probably a part of the handle), and which is just digging into a dark mass of what appears to be plastic material. I was educated on classical lines ; and it is conceivable that this picture is an echo of the oft-repeated admonition to ' dig out the meaning of some passage of Greek or Latin.' " [15] As Professor Titchener tells us that he takes great pains to keep his visual images up to the mark by constant practice, he will inevitably find these specks of the past brought to light by introspection. But to regard them as *meaning* is like the attempt to study the constitution of light by paying attention to the motes in the sunbeam which the rays make visible.

Driven from the stronghold of visual and auditory phenomena the sensationalists who regard meaning as exclusively sensory or imaginal in content may still take refuge in kinæsthetic images. This, in fact, is what is frequently done. The meaning of a physical object is said to be constituted by the motor adjustment made towards it. When a dog cringes at the sight of a whip or jumps and barks joyfully at the sound of his master's whistle, the cringing and the frisking adjustments are thought to be the whole of what is meant to the animal by the whip and the whistle ; nothing more. Meaning in short is movement and the more complex meanings involve simply finer and more delicate responses. The behaviourists assert indeed that the movements must be primary presentations overt or incipient so that the meaning of an equation, say, consists simply of the manumotor and vocimotor reactions which are suggested by it. No new element is involved when the reactions are taken to be not primary but secondary kinæsthetic imagery, for meaning is still said to be adjustment.

The enthusiastic advocates of handwork as an educational instrument have been only too ready to adopt the behaviouristic standpoint as their psychological theory instead of taking their stand on the intrinsic importance of an all round development of mind and body. Manual work does not need the support of erroneous doctrines, but may justify itself as an educational organon on the ground of its social and artistic significance satisfying urgent concrete needs which abstract scholastic traditions completely overlooked or suppressed.

Now a fatal objection to the theory which regards meaning as adjustment lies in the fact that we adjust ourselves to meaning and not to impressions. To use a witty illustration devised for a totally different purpose. Suppose a behaviourist confronted first by a bear in a modern zoological garden terrace and then by a bear at large ; to the former he offers a bun to the latter a clean pair of heels. Will he now undertake to explain in terms of behaviour alone his very different responses in the two cases ? Only by the knowledge that the free and the confined bear *mean* totally different things can the vastly different adjustments be explained, not *vice versa*. As the illustration shews it is to the meaning of a total situation that we react and not to detached portions of it whether sensations, images or what not. Meaning is prior and psychologically supreme. Experimental work on word associations has proved that the purpose to respond in a definite way is sufficient to produce specific reactions when the subject is totally unable to detect any image and when he is barely conscious of the stimulus word but only of its general meaning. Allowing for justifiable exaggeration as a counterblast to sensationalism we may adopt the position that mind deals only with meanings ; that " we always see meaning as we look, think of meaning when we act. Apparently we are never distinctly conscious of anything but meanings." [16]

The researches of Binet in France, Woodworth in America and the Austrian school of psychologists have given the deathblow to the crude sensationalism which regarded impressions whether primary or secondary as adequate to explain mental structure and function, and meaning as a mysterious and troublesome result of their interaction, to be explained away. On its structural side we previously called this view atomism since it conceived of mental life as a congeries of elements held together by associative bonds. Meaning was a new element superadded to the complex when it began to function.

But the whole notion of mental elements is artificial and invalid. Mental life is an organic unity and all parts are what they are by virtue of the living whole. Meaning is not a new element added to pre-existing elements, but permeates the whole structure which is steeped and dyed in it, or rather without which it has no vitality.[17] A good analogue of mental life is to be found in a living language where the play of meanings is the informing spirit of the whole, whilst sentences, parts of speech, words *et hoc genus omne* are the disarticulated parts of the skeleton separated by grammatical anatomists. We may as reasonably expect to construct à language with these dry bones as to exhibit mental life as an association of impressions plus meaning. The direct method of teaching modern languages in schools, apart from its infinitely greater effectiveness in practice, is founded on the sound psychological instinct that without life there can be no feeling and that *sprachgefühl* is of the very essence of language.

There are certain features of the mental life which the researches of the Austrian school have emphasised and which no account of meaning can afford to overlook. The method of investigation is remarkably simple.

A person is asked to perform a simple operation such as to decide on the heavier of two similar looking weights, or to write down the first half a dozen words that occur to him, or to react to a word that is shewn to him by some associated word either made ' freely ' or under some constraint such as that of whole to part (e.g. chair-leg), or to answer ' yes ' or ' no ' to some simple statement read to him, or to give his opinion on some doubtful point and so on. Immediately after the reaction is made or the opinion given, or in some cases during the course of making up his mind, the subject is asked to give as complete an introspective account as possible of what was in his mind during the experiment and aided his judgment or thinking.[18] The most highly trained introspective psychologists have been the subjects of these experiments. What they found was that in addition to sensations, images, ideas, volitions, etc., certain conscious attitudes or postures were present, distinct from all these. In describing such attitudes the observer has, of course, to explain them in terms of ideas, feelings, etc., but these are stated not to be present in the experience itself *as it is felt*. Examples of such attitudes of a cognitive and conative kind are doubt, certainty, hesitation, conviction, awareness of a relation, realisation of the task, etc., etc., all given in a flash of consciousness and felt as an undiscriminated whole. Sometimes the attitudes are affectively toned and at others they are neutral but in either case, as experienced, they are peculiar modifications of consciousness totally disparate with imaginal contents. Their intimate nature appears to suggest that they must be peculiarly subjective attitudes, which, like the elementary feelings are totally unanalysable.

IMAGERY AND LEARNING

At first sight it might appear that the mode of presentation would determine the particular kind of imagery used in recall. Thus material presented to a subject visually or aurally might be expected to be reproduced by visual or auditory imagery and so with the other varieties. This obvious assumption is frequently made by teachers in devising methods of presentation of their material in the belief that they are thus able to influence the mode of learning and remembering. In this respect teachers have been misled by psychologists who ignore or deny subjective preference or selection. Now a pupil is never the passive recipient of impressions but always exerts selective activity on what is presented to him. In particular, visual impressions are not registered passively as on a photographic plate but what is visually retained, is,

G

as we saw above, influenced by what the subject is interested in and definitely attends to. Professor Meumann and others have demonstrated that the images of reproduced words are primarily those which the subject prefers to use and are only secondarily influenced by the mode of presentation. When material is presented aurally to subjects whose preference is for visual imagery the reproduction is made in terms of the latter. The mistaken view here alluded to is widely prevalent not only amongst psychologists and teachers, but generally. Much literary criticism is vitiated by the assumption that it is possible to get an insight into an author's imagery and mode of composition by examining his written productions. Nothing could be wider of the mark. One of the chief delights of Heine's poetry is its haunting musical lilt which is quite unreproducible in any translation. Yet Heine himself denied that he relied on the sound of the words and insisted that it was the sight of the words and constructions which was his main help in composing. When he had become almost blind so that he was forced to dictate his poetry he complained of the difficulty, thus: "Our language is adapted to the eye; it is plastic, and as regards rhyme, not only the sound, but also the manner of writing has its influence. . . . The German must, in my opinion, see or have practically formed (plastisch) before him what he colloquially creates. Verses which one finishes in one's head are easier to dictate than prose, and yet I could not do that."[19]   If Heine could not rely on his auditory imagery in composing who can ?

G. H. Lewes reported, indeed, that Dickens told him that " every word uttered by his characters was distinctly *heard* by him before it was written down," and assuming the correctness of this he very rightly attributes it to hallucination. Forster, the biographer of Dickens, rejects with indignation the hallucinatory theory of his genius but admits that it might possibly have occurred during periods when he was over-

wrought and ill. When he was suffering under the severest
trial of his life he wrote to Forster that he thought " it was a
wonderful testimony to my being made for my art, that when,
in the midst of this trouble and pain, I sit down to my book,
some beneficent power shews it all to me, and tempts me to
be interested, and I don't invent it—really do not—*but see it*,
and write it down." [20] The well-known hypersentimentality
of Dickens and his extraordinary sympathy with all his
creations may possibly have provided the affective background
for most of what he " saw " ; he, like others, confusing feelings
with images, unless his jarred nerves produced true
hallucinations.

A similar doubt is suggested by the following account of
Whistler's method of studying his Nocturnes. [21] " We had
left the studio after dusk . . . when he suddenly stopped,
and pointed to a group of buildings in the distance . . .
shewing golden lights through the gathering twilight. . . .
After a long pause he turned and walked back a few yards ;
then, with his back to the scene at which I was looking, he
said, ' Now, see if I have learned it,' and repeated a full
description of the scene, even as one might repeat a poem one
had learned by heart." Who will be prepared to say after
this description whether Whistler relied on visual or verbal
imagery in painting ?

An investigation recently undertaken on the effect of the
mode of presentation upon the process of learning has confirmed
these views and extended their scope. [22] Lists of words and
meaningless syllables, presented in diverse ways, were learnt
by various students trained in introspection whose normal
imagery was of different kinds. The forms of presentations
were variously combined. In some cases, for instance, the
words were exposed visually and the subject repeated them
aloud, or he saw them and inhibited the tendency to repeat
whilst the experimenter said them aloud ; sometimes the

words were read to the subject who wrote them and saw his writing or wrote them with his eyes shut, and so on in various other ways. The introspections revealed the fact that for learning this sort of material it is difficult, if not impossible, to inhibit vocimotor imagery whatever the form of presentation, and the attempt to do so intensifies auditory imagery. With combined visual and aural stimuli the subject attends to one only not to both. When words are recalled which have been read aloud by the experimenter, if any auditory image is present, it is that of the subject's own voice not that of the experimenter. Subjects whose normal imagery was vocimotor used this type of image when the presentation was auditory or visual. In general the particular mode of presentation did not determine the modality of the imagery employed by the subject either in learning or recall. As far as imagery is concerned the learning process depends much more on the mental make-up of the learner than on the method by which he is taught. Where, however, there is a difficulty in remembering so that the words do not readily come the imagery corresponding to the mode of presentation may be aroused. A clearer instance of the importance of subjective activity in learning would be hard to find.

Combined with the specific images of the words, recall is often aided by a schema of a visual or kinæsthetic kind or sometimes by a rhythmic schema of a vocimotor nature in which no definite words need be present.

It is very instructive to learn that in no case either of learning or recall did a subject use a manumotor image. The motor sensation in the hand produced by writing is not a factor in the learning process, but any help which is given comes from the attention to the visual word as it appears slowly during the writing operation. There is no doubt that too much stress has been laid by teachers on the importance of written exercises in helping the memory. In the early stages of learning much more attention is now devoted to oral work both by teachers of arithmetic and of modern languages, which practice has ample psychological justification and may with advantage be further extended.

CHAPTER V

HABIT FORMATION

The Nature of Habit—The Rôle of Impulse—The Form of Progress—
Importance of Purpose—Improvement in Retentiveness—Neural
Basis of Habit—Imitation—Rate of Growth—Rate of Decay

THE NATURE OF HABIT

IN the realm of habit the effects of education, in the widest
sense, are enduring. Any persistent effort repeated over a
sufficiently prolonged period, with a definite purpose, will
produce permanent effects on the intellectual and bodily
activities of the individual. When, for example, a child is
learning to talk, he takes a keen delight in trying, repeatedly,
to produce the sounds which he hears, and in the course of
time reflects accurately the particular vowels and accent
current in his environment. No doubt, as he progresses, some
modification may be produced by subconscious assimilation,
without any apparent effort, but as the child is naturally
imitative of his elders he tries, with more or less persistence,
to repeat whatever he hears them say. An accent or any
trick of speech acquired in this way, is notoriously permanent,
and though it may be masked by subsequent education it is
always beneath the surface ready to spring into action when
for any reason self-control is weak. In a similar fashion, the
student of mathematics gets habituated to respond automatically to certain frequently occurring symbols and forms of
expression, and the student of biology to facts of organic life

with a train of evolutionary ideas which arise spontaneously. In all these instances it is obvious that, although the finished reactions are effortless, or nearly so, the actual progress to this desired end was marked by a succession of trials and failures; and only by holding fast to the correct modes of acting and thinking was the final achievement possible. The method of trial and error, by itself, however, is incapable of giving rise to any habitual mode of conduct, as the facts adduced later will abundantly shew.

In forming a habit the individual, as it were, saves future effort by accumulating acts of volition in the form of a permanent investment, on the interest of which he may live for the rest of his days. This characteristic feature of habit by virtue of which the effort ceases when its purpose has been finally accomplished, is the foundation both of the utility and danger of habit-formation. Unless the effects of practice were to make our conduct and thinking more facile in certain directions, progress along such paths would be ruled out. It has been said that we rise on stepping-stones of our dead selves, but though this belief may have a certain ethical significance, it is nevertheless a psychological blunder. When a man is trying to solve a problem in mathematics, for instance, he will not be able to proceed far unless he is so grounded in all the elementary processes that he can safely trust to his habits, unless, that is, they are so much alive that they need no present effort on his part to make them active; and so he is able to devote all his attention to the problem itself.

But there is another side to the picture; for extreme habituation is often a bar to progress, especially where ideas are limited. The constant repetition of the same thoughts in the same grooves makes it difficult to diverge from them and strike out into new directions. So much is this the case, that in the great majority of persons escape is impossible, for they are incapable of making the strong and persistent effort

which is necessary.   Only the fortunate few can break through
the hard crust of custom.   Of others it may be said

> The moving finger writes and having writ
> Moves on, nor all your piety nor wit
> Can lure it back to cancel half a line
> Nor all your tears wash out a word of it.

In addition to habits of thought and of action there are
also so-called habits of will, by which is meant the ready
carrying out in practice of a resolution or purpose when once
it has been firmly implanted; such as the habit of punctuality.
Closely allied with the last-named are such virtues as honesty,
veracity, etc., for the virtuous man has so habituated himself
by steady purpose that action in opposition to the virtue
gets no lodgment in his life.   In so far as moral training is
effective, moral action becomes action in the line of least
resistance.   Plato correctly believed that all virtues except
wisdom could be acquired habitually ; for, he said, " the
other so-called virtues seem to be akin to bodily qualities, for
even when they are not originally innate they can be implanted
by habit and exercise." [1]

A considerable amount of experimental work has been
performed in order to study the growth of habits and, as
might be expected, most of this has been devoted to the
study of habits of action as these are most easily observed.
It should be borne in mind, however, that much of what
is said in this chapter about bodily habits applies *mutatis
mutandis* to the other categories of habit.

THE RÔLE OF IMPULSE

A bodily habit is the expression in terms of muscular
movements of the improvement, acquired by practice, in the
facility of adapting oneself to similarly recurring conditions.
Thus, in learning to swim, or to write, or to act in any other
way, the diffuse, unco-ordinated and awkward motions of the

tyro are gradually replaced by the restricted, co-ordinated and facile movements of the adept, carried out nearly automatically as a response to similar circumstances. The unerring mechanical precision of such acts is evident from the fact that a rubber stamp is often used as a substitute for a man's signature ; and as far as the outline is concerned there is nothing to choose between them. In fact a close consideration will shew that in other respects they are similar, for whether a man stamps or signs his name, he uses a tool to carry out his purpose ; only in the one case the tool is made of rubber, in the other of muscle and nerve. Fully fledged bodily and intellectual habits thus tend ultimately to become the mechanisms or tools by means of which our wider aims are accomplished with dexterity and celerity.

Is then, the study of habit-formation to be considered merely as a branch of physiological mechanics ? This question raises the important issue as to whether a habit is to be regarded as an acquired impulse to activity ; whether in brief education in skilled activities can create new springs of conduct. Now an impulse is the driving force or prompting to vital activity and it is necessary to see whether such a ' drive ' can be acquired by experience or whether experience is limited to giving new directions to pre-existing impulses.

The overwhelming urgency of vital impulses is best discerned in those cases where for any reason their free expression is thwarted or hindered. Human beings, together with the higher animals, have an instinct to communicate with their fellows by vocal sounds, and this impulse normally finds satisfaction so readily that its overbearing force is seldom realised. Prior to her education the blind deaf-mute Helen Keller had no means of expressing this instinct except by a very limited number of artificial signs which she had herself invented. " Meanwhile," she writes,[2] " the desire to express myself grew. The few signs I used became less and less adequate, and my failures to make myself understood were invariably followed by outbursts of passion. I felt as if invisible hands were holding me, and I made frantic efforts to free myself. I struggled—not that struggling helped matters, but the spirit of resistance was strong within me ; I generally broke down in tears and physical exhaustion. . . . After awhile the need of some means of communication became so urgent that these outbursts occurred daily, sometimes hourly." The urgency of the instinctive impulse was obstructed in this case by lack of sensation, but the interference with any innate impulse by any method will produce similar results.

A couple of instances may be given to shew the impossibility of suppressing an innate tendency, or to divert it into other than its proper channels. Handel's father, a surgeon, regarded music as a degrading pursuit, or, at best an idle amusement ; and " he strove to stifle in every way the alarming symptoms of musical genius which appeared in his son almost in infancy, while he refused even to send the child to school lest there, among other things, he should also learn his notes." [3] Nevertheless, the boy managed to get possession of a small spinet in which the strings were bound with strips of cloth to deaden the sound ; and, having it concealed in a garret, he taught himself to play without being discovered. When he was seven years old his father set out on a journey to visit a notable person who kept a private chapel with an organ and Handel begged to be allowed to accompany him ; but, his request being refused, so strong was his persistency of purpose that he followed the carriage on foot for a considerable distance, until he got his way, and finally managed to get permission to use the organ.

Benvenuto Cellini was destined by his father to be a musician and strenuous efforts were made to cultivate this talent from his early years when he was taught to sing and play the flute. " And though I was of very tender years when little children are wont to be pleased with a whistle and such-like playthings, I had a particular dislike to it." All through his childhood he had a strong passion for drawing and nothing would induce him, despite his father's strong desire, to adopt the career of a musician. At the age of fifteen he apprenticed himself, against his father's wish, to a goldsmith craftsman so that " I might be free to draw as much as ever I liked. . . . My desire to excel in this art was great, or rather, I might say, my love for it ; but, indeed, both were strong in me." [4] It is not surprising after this to learn that in a few months he became noted for his workmanship and design, and thenceforward his genius carried him to distinction in his chosen art.

The direction of many impulses is relatively indeterminate, but, as in the instances just given, it may be quite specific. Moreover it sometimes happens that the purpose is quite unknown to the subject himself, who experiences a vague restlessness, as we see, for example, at the onset of puberty. Others have a definite tendency which is clearly known to the person concerned. In so far as the urgency of an impulse is consciously experienced it is called a conation. There are, however, great differences to be found in the consciousness of the direction of the impulse.

Some impulses exhibit a tendency to subside after a period of activity unless they subserve a conscious purpose or desire which is valued by the subject or is useful to the race. A good example of this tendency to fade away after a period of activity is furnished by the grasping reflex, which is present in all children at birth, so that they are able to support their weight, with either hand, up to about the hundred and twentieth day, after which the impulse subsides. Some instincts shew a similar tendency. Thus, Professor Stanley Hall [5] quotes a study of the collecting instinct in which over twelve hundred boys and girls were examined, the strength of the impulse being measured by the number of things collected. It reached its greatest intensity at ten years of age and then declined, although with considerable persistence, through the teens. Two hundred and fourteen kinds of collection for each sex were observed, with strongly marked differences between the sexes at adolescence. From the age of twelve the interest appeared to pass from the things themselves to their relations, classifications, etc. Girls were found to be more prone to receive and boys to hunt or trade for their collections.

It is clear from the last example that there is an innate conative impulse to acquisition, the urgency of which is very widely if not universally experienced. The *élan vital* has been differentiated in the course of evolution into this mode of activity, whilst the nature of the objects collected is a matter of the environment. Contrast this with the habitual act of putting on one's neck-tie. There appears at first sight to be no impulse to perform this activity *per se*, but rather it is carried out in order to subserve some pre-existing motive, such as the tendency to imitate or the desire to adorn oneself. Here the relation of habit to impulse is analogous to that of the executive and directive functions of a social organism. Some habits, then, are the ministers of innate impulses, their executive agents ; but just as it would be rash to assume that no agent has energy of his own, so it need not be supposed that all the energy spent in carrying out a habitual act is derived from pre-existing impulses.

Professor McDougall, however, takes the view that no habit can ever yield any impulsive energy or be a motive for conduct.[6] He denies that any motor habit, such as repeating the alphabet, which he strangely regards as his 'most practised habit,' or playing the piano, can in any circumstances become an impulse ; and asks : " Does any such habit, no matter how perfected and how much repeated, become in itself a drive ? . . . Does it generate, or is it sustained by, an appetite ? Is it *in itself* a source of purposive activity ? To all these questions the answer is clearly—No." He contrasts these cases with the impulse to strike an angry blow when hurt or insulted. Now it may be admitted at once that the occasions on which one is impelled to repeat the alphabet are rare, except perhaps to replace the blow by those persons whose careful bringing-up has taught them to count numbers or repeat the alphabet instead of giving way to anger. The efficacy of this method of response has been attested since classical times, for Athenodorus, the tutor of Augustus, bid him repeat the letters of the alphabet before acting on an angry impulse. Seeing that such reactions as this are commonly acquired as a response to situations which normally call forth the angry impulse, it is odd to refuse to call the alphabet reaction an acquired impulse. Anyhow, the reaction *is* sometimes effective as a substitute for the native impulse of anger and it would seem that such a powerful spring of conduct could only be checked by something which has itself the energy of an impulse. Religion can mould human nature in opposition to the most powerful of native impulses and a whole nation may acquire new characteristics by this means. The Professor of Chinese at Cambridge believes that the mildness of the Chinese people is due to their religion. " One result of this is that the Chinese hate war and violence, as may be noted in their street quarrels, which provide an unlimited amount of abuse, especially of ancestors, on both sides, but rarely come to blows."

He who doubts whether an impulse can be acquired need only consult those students who work at definite hours and in habitual ways, and he will soon find out that they experience a curious restlessness if anything interferes with their normal routine ; and only rarely do they feel any desire to work at other periods. Or, take the case of the hardened swimmers who have acquired the habit of indulging in an early morning plunge, the strength of whose impulse may be gauged by the intense discomfort they are willing to endure to get it. That only their acquired habit can satisfy the acquired impulse is shewn by the fact that they do not derive satisfaction from a mere cold bath, however cold and uninviting. As to the query whether any habit can give rise to, or be sustained by, an appetite, the answer surely is in the affirmative. Everybody who has indulged the habit of smoking over a long period feels a strong craving which cannot be allayed in any other way ; and the appetite is so specific that if he has cultivated the pipe habit neither cigarettes nor even strong cigars will satisfy the longing. The impulse is so accurately adjusted to the habit, from which it is derived, that one who is accustomed to smoke at definite hours, say after dinner, experiences the ' drive ' only at those periods.

We may safely conclude that habitual actions are, on the whole, the expressions of acquired impulses. What gives the contrary view a certain plausibility is the failure to distinguish impulses, whose ends are clearly felt by the subject, i.e. conative impulses, from those whose purpose is not a matter of conscious experience. A good case may be made out for believing that all our primitive impulses are, at the outset, unconscious in the sense that their ends are not foreseen by us and that we only come to know what we want by wanting it. This phenomenon is, in fact, not peculiar to our innate impulses but pervades our whole mental life. In the preface to a widely read sociological work the author [7] says : " Now that the book is finished, I can see, more clearly than I could while I was writing it, what it is about." The Freudians maintain that our desires start by being fully conscious and then become suppressed ; but it is equally plausible to hold that they were all more or less unconscious in the above sense from the beginning and only became conscious in the process of being satisfied. " Desire for flowers comes after actual enjoyment of flowers. But it comes before the work that

makes the desert blossom." [8]   So that the problem for educational psychology is not to discover the mechanisms by which
our desires and wishes become submerged, but the course of
education by which we come to realise their meaning, and the
methods most suitable for directing them into the proper
channels.   The education of the will by forming stable habits
of action in new directions is a creative act in that it implants
in the individual life new sources of energetic impulse.

THE FORM OF PROGRESS

In the practical study of the formation of habits the rate
of growth and decay of habitual activities are investigated
and recorded as curves of progress or evanescence.   The
records may represent the time required for a set performance ;
or the amount of performance, such as the number of letters
recorded correctly in a stated period ; or the number of errors
made in performing a definite amount of work.   Such graphic
records are called time, attainment and error curves respectively.   Other forms of curve have been plotted, such as the
attainment in certain units which can be reached without
error, or with a given number of attempts, and so on.

Most habit curves display features which are worthy of
careful study ; they fall in the case of time or error curves or
rise in attainment curves very rapidly at the initial stages of
practice, and at later periods they may become flat, exhibiting
what are called ' plateaus ' from which there may be a subsequent *sudden* rise or fall.   The plateau is well shewn in the
accompanying diagram.[3]   The rapid rise or fall in the initial
stages is usually explained as shewing very great relative
progress in the early stages of practice.

It should be remembered that every habit is composed,
not of a single series of movements, but of several such series ;
forming a sort of hierarchy in order of difficulty, or compre-

hensiveness, or both. Just as, in recording a naval battle the official reports of the individual captains reduce the

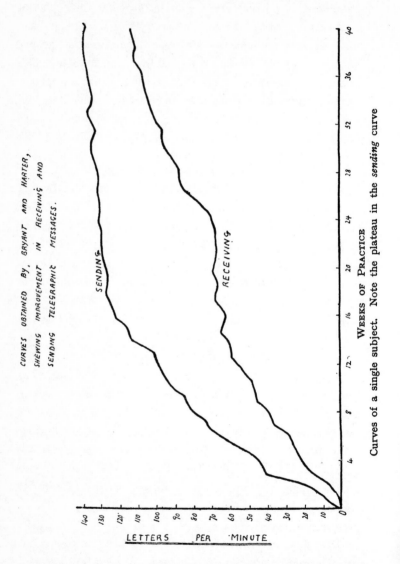

CURVES OBTAINED BY, BRYANT AND HARTER, SHEWING IMPROVEMENT IN RECEIVING AND SENDING TELEGRAPHIC MESSAGES.

SENDING

RECEIVING

LETTERS PER MINUTE

WEEKS OF PRACTICE

Curves of a single subject. Note the plateau in the *sending* curve

observations of a number of individuals into one story, and the despatches of admirals are an attempt to telescope the reports

of individual captains ; whilst the Admiralty report attempts
to reduce them all to a single focus. Some of the lower orders
of movements in the hierarchy consist of series of actions,
the working plan of which is either instinctive or habitual
and which therefore require little or no practice ; consequently there is apparently great initial progress. No doubt
also the zest of work is greater in the initial stages which may
help to explain the rapid improvement. The higher or co-
ordinating series of movements in the hierarchy are relatively
novel and must be slowly built up. It is only when all the
lower series have been made automatic, and fused
together, as it were, that the higher order habits can function
easily on the basis of the lower. Thus to write or speak
fluently in a foreign tongue, for example, it is essential to make
the vocabulary and grammatical forms mechanically perfect
before the higher language habits connected with the combination of words into connected discourse can display themselves
freely. There is consequently a plateau period followed by a
sudden further improvement which resembles the rapid progress in the initial stages. The receiving and sending curves of
Messrs Bryan and Harter may be taken as typical of the growth,
i.e. of the varying rates of progress in learning a task such as
a language. Careful study of these figures shews that the
progress in the earlier stages is represented by an S-shaped
curve and this has been observed in many other cases. It
should be noticed that the curves would present the same
general form if the units of time had been hours or days, etc.,
instead of weeks.[9]

Professor Thorndike has given another explanation of the
form of these curves. He thinks that all mental development
consists in forming associations between indeterminate
impulses and movements, an error which we considered in an
earlier chapter If all bonds of association were equally
easy to form and once formed were not forgotten, the habit

H

curve would rise as a straight line until the physiological limit of improvement, when the plateau would begin. But after each bond is formed it tends to decay, and requires practice to keep it at full strength ; so that part of the work done goes to preserve old bonds of association instead of being used to form new ones. There is thus a negative acceleration as the result of the expenditure of the work required to keep the bonds already formed in an efficient state. The result of this is a diminished rate of progress with the same amount of practice, when the plateau is near.

It has been suggested by Professor J. Peterson [10] that some of the peculiarities of habit curves are due to the method of plotting the results and not to variations in the rate of learning. The initial rapid rise or fall in the curves may be partly explained by this cause. For it is clear that the units are not strictly constant, an error for instance being different at different parts of the scale ; nor are equal practice intervals or the performance of the same objective work homogeneous units during the whole period. The curves in the diagram on the next page represent the same data plotted in different ways and it is seen that whilst the error curve displays the initial rapid fall the attainment curve does not shew the rapid initial progress, but on the contrary, uniform progress at first with acceleration at the end of the period. Plateaus, also, may be magnified or obscured owing to the same causes, but as is pointed out in the notes at the end of the book the curves are not fairly constructed.

Numerous experiments have been carried out on the rate of verbal learning, for which Professor Ebbinghaus devised nonsense-syllable material [11] in order to eliminate meaning as far as possible. Such researches are usually called investigations into memory, but in reality they are mainly concerned with the formation of vocal habits. Evidence in support of this view is supplied by investigations on snails, which

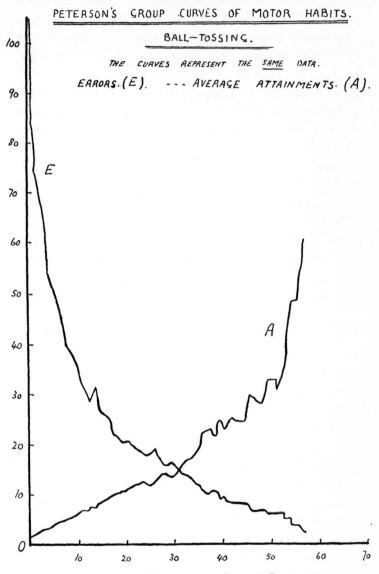

PETERSON'S GROUP CURVES OF MOTOR HABITS.

BALL—TOSSING.

THE CURVES REPRESENT THE SAME DATA.

ERRORS. (E). --- AVERAGE ATTAINMENTS. (A).

PRACTICE PERIODS. 200 CATCHES EACH
Combined Curve of 25 subjects

react to a diminution of light or to a shadow by withdrawing into their shells.   Professor H. Piéron shewed that
these gastero-pods cease to withdraw after a certain number
of obscurations ; then, after a period of rest, they react again
to shadows, but cease after a smaller number of stimuli, and
so on after repeated trials.   The animals, in fact, form a
habit of movement : and the law which best summarises the
rate of the decline of the inhibitory effect is the same
as the law of forgetting nonsense-syllables after varying
intervals.

Just as there is an optimum interval for giving small
impacts to a heavy pendulum in order to get a long regular
swing so it has been shewn that there is an optimum interval
between the separate repeated acts necessary to form a habit.
This interval is a measure of the period required for maturing
or fixing the impression and is different for different acts.
The succeeding impression in order to be maximally effective
should come at the end of the optimum interval, otherwise
work is lost.   After this interval there is a period of evanescence.   It has been suggested that such gradual maturing
of impressions may be one of the factors producing the plateau.

THE IMPORTANCE OF PURPOSE

The only way in which an impulse can be detected by an
outside observer is by watching the actions carried out in
order to satisfy it.   We may call the temporal order, co-ordination, and localisation of the movements involved in carrying
out a specific action the " working plan " of the act.   If this
plan is inherited the action is usually called instinctive, as in
the case of walking.   The distinction between inherited and
acquired is not absolute, for whilst walking is an acquired
art the child would be prompted by his locomotor impulse to

perform the movements at a certain stage of his growth owing to mere maturation, even if not encouraged by others. When on the other hand the working plan is largely acquired by the individual in the course of his experience, the action is called habitual as in learning a language in obedience to the impulse to communicate with others.

Habits are formed by repeated purposive acts, which create new bodily functions, facilitating future action of a similar kind. Psychologically, then, function determines structure; the conative impulse creates the instrument by means of which it may issue in action. Much psychological theory, as we saw earlier, is vitiated by the adoption of the physiological standpoint which inverts this relation between function and structure. As the organ becomes increasingly more perfect it becomes more automatic, and the conscious direction of the movements tends to become subconscious. When creating a new habit it is possible by careful introspection to watch the gradual disappearance of effort and attention as one increases in facility. In deeply ingrained habits, such as writing, the strokes of the pen are made quasi-mechanically; there is the intention to write but no specific purpose to make the pen strokes, which go on almost of themselves. Owing to this feature of perfectly acquired habits it is erroneously inferred that the bare mechanical repetition of an action is sufficient to form a habit. But this is to confuse the end-product with the means necessary to bring about its formation. Now the stimuli which set a habit going are not exactly the same on any two occasions. Vital activity is distinguished from purely mechanical response by the power to adapt itself to considerable change of circumstances. Beneath the apparent stereotypy of habit there is always some variation which the subject, when acting, usually ignores because he has other and, it may be, more important purposes in hand. Yet it has been well said that if a habit is to have " sufficient generality to adapt itself to variations in its external stimuli, it must be combined with and supported by some organised body of ideas." [12]

The rôle of purpose in habit-formation has been subjected to experimental research, and it has been shewn that mere repetition without consciously directed effort is almost useless to establish a habit.

Messrs Bryan and Harter found, in the case of telegraph operators who were learning to send messages, that the rise from the plateau in the attainment curve only took place when there was a deliberate attempt to improve on the part of the subject owing to some strong incentive, such as the desire to secure extra pay.   It is the intense effort which results in effective learning.   Similar results have been obtained by Miss M. Smith and Professor McDougall in learning to reproduce series of nonsense-syllables.   They shewed that the greater the passivity of the subject the more numerous were the repetitions required to learn a series by heart.   In other words, when reliance is placed on mechanical repetition, learning is slower and more difficult.   Thus, on one occasion 13 and 9 repetitions were sufficient for these subjects, on the average, to learn a series of twelve nonsense-syllables when they each made a maximum effort.   When, however, they adopted a passive attitude an average of 89 repetitions was necessary for one subject and 100 for the other.   It may be thought that the vastly increased number of repetitions would secure better retention of the material learnt.   But this was shewn to be fallacious.   For on attempting, after an interval of some days, to relearn certain sets of series, which had been originally learnt either actively or passively it was found that a greater number of repetitions were required in the latter case.   In fact most of what had been learnt passively was forgotten after about one week.[13]   The will to learn plays a real part in habit formation.

Habit is, thus, not mere mechanisation, but demands the co-operation of set purpose, at the very least, the purpose to learn. For as Professor Dewey [14] says: " How delicate, prompt, sure and varied are the movements of a violin player or an engraver. How unerringly they phrase every shade of emotion and every turn of idea. Mechanism is indispensable. If each act has to be consciously searched for at the moment and intentionally performed execution is painful and the product is clumsy and halting." The difference between the artist and the mere technician lies in the fact that the latter is the slave of mechanism ; it is mere routine. So, in intellectual matters progress and skill rest on the formation of habits of thought, but whilst intelligence needs such habits, which are the condition of its guidance along definite channels of expression, the rôle of the artist is always an integral part of the performance.

IMPROVEMENT IN RETENTIVENESS

It is a matter of common observation, repeatedly confirmed by experiment, that individuals improve by practice in the facility of accomplishing habitual tasks. Thus a person, who sets out to learn a number of series of nonsense-syllables of the same length by heart, finds that he can within limits learn each series with a less number of repetitions as time goes on. Moreover, the number of repetitions required to relearn a series after an interval also diminishes with practice. The question arises as to whether the improvement shewn in relearning such series is due to an increased power of retention or whether it is due to greater facility in learning. Some interesting experiments have been carried out by Miss M. Smith and Professor McDougall to decide this point.[13]

Five subjects had almost daily practice for six months

and one subject for twelve months in learning series of syllables; on one day a series was learnt and a day later it was relearnt and so on. Now it is clear that any improvement due to better methods of learning will operate equally in the relearning process. Consequently if evidence of increased retentiveness is desired it must be looked for in a greater relative improvement in the relearning process as compared with that of learning. The table below gives the results obtained:

Subjects	Average of 8 expts. giving no. of repetitions for learning at beginning	Average of 8 expts. giving no. of repetitions for learning 6 months after	Gain	Average no. of repetitions to relearn at beginning	Average no. of repetitions to relearn 6 months after	Gain
A	14	8	43%	7	4	43%
B	16	9·6	40	5·6	3	47
C	8	7	—	3	3	—
D	9	5·6	38	2·8	1·2	57
E	13	11	15	9	6	33⅓
F*	12	8	33⅓	6	4	33⅓

* Interval of 12 months.

It will be seen that B, D and E shew a greater relative improvement in relearning. For these subjects, therefore, it seems as though the practice has resulted in increased power of retentiveness. The other subjects either shew no improvement or equal improvement in both processes. It would be hazardous to base any conclusions on these experiments until they are confirmed by more extensive investigations. The method is sound and the topic is well worth more extended research, for owing very largely to the influence of Professor James [15] there is a widespread belief that a person's native retentiveness is a physiological property of his nervous system which he can no more change than he can by taking thought add a cubit to his stature.

THE NEURAL BASIS OF HABIT

The classical accounts of habit-formation regard it as completely a physiological affair, a series of reflex-arcs somehow established in the nervous system. A reflex system in its simplest form is composed of a chain of anatomically distinct nerve units or neurones functionally connected in a sensori-motor arc. Consider, for example, the movements of fixation-accommodation of the eye, i.e. the automatic movements made by the eye, when stimulated by light, which serve to bring it into such a position that the image of the fixated object falls on the retina in the place of clearest vision, namely the *fovea centralis*. This involves two relatively distinct sets of movements, namely movements of the eyeball secured by contraction of the muscles attached to the eye bringing the *fovea* into the correct position, and variations in the degree of curvature of the lens to ensure proper focusing as a result of the contraction of the ciliary muscle. For the sake of simplicity let us confine our attention to the eyeball movements alone, though it must be remembered that these are complicated by movements of the head also, and, it may be, of the whole trunk.

Now the reflex-arc is usually described as composed of three distinct parts ; an afferent portion, the receptor or so-called sensory part which receives the stimulus ; an efferent portion, the effector or motor part which brings about the movement ; and finally an inter-central portion which serves to connect up the anatomically distinct sensory organ with the motor organ. Corresponding to these parts there are afferent, central and efferent neurones, and in the simplest ideal case a chain of three neurones would suffice. When the sensory neurone is stimulated, say, by light falling on the periphery of the retina, energy already stored up in the nerve is released, which in its turn fires off the stored energy in the central neurone, and this liberates the energy in the motor neurone leading to a muscular contraction which brings the *fovea* to bear on the luminous object, thus completing the sensori-motor arc. Nothing could well be simpler or more beautifully arranged for a mechanical explanation, as in the case we are considering the ' pathway ' of discharge is already laid down in the nervous system, though it is said to be made smoother by maturation and experience.

In accordance with this view it is maintained that the most complex habits can be explained as a combination of such reflexes,[16] being " nothing but concatenated discharges in the nerve-centres, due to the presence there of systems of reflex paths, so organised as to wake each other up successively— the impression produced by one muscular contraction serving as a stimulus to provoke the next, until a final impression inhibits the process and closes the chain." The only difficulty in this explanation, according to its author, is to account for the original formation of the ' pathway,' since when a wave of energy has once traversed a sensori-motor arc nothing is easier than to imagine that it should travel along it more readily the second time.

In considering this explanation the student must be warned carefully to discriminate between the facts of observation and theoretical deductions therefrom. Otherwise, he may be inclined to suppose that physiologists have discovered central connections between sensory and motor processes which the psychologist is at liberty to use, whereas the direct contrary is the case, and the nervous connections are merely hypothetical connections prayed in aid by psychologists in order to explain the observed facts. The fact to be explained is the apparent mechanisation of habit by repetition and the fixed inter-central pathways are pure theory.

Let us, however, test the theory by trying to apply it to our original example of a reflex act. The actual movement of

the eye in order to fixate a definite point in space depends
not only on the particular part of the retina stimulated, for
which it is possible that a definite (though an uncomfortably
large number) of central connections are provided, but also
on the original position of the eye with respect to its orbit
and likewise on the initial position of the head. All this
presupposes that each retinal point must be connected with
an indefinitely large number of central neurones. But the
microscopic size of nerve cells and their numerous dendrites
provide the psychologist, who hankers after a neural basis
of explanation, with such enormous numbers of possible
central pathways that he need not be disturbed by mere
magnitude.

Experimental observation introduces a new difficulty in
the way of the theory. Marina, experimenting on apes,
performed an operation on the eye and interchanged the
superior rectus muscle for the lateral rectus, i.e. the muscle
moving the eye outwards was eliminated and its place taken
by the muscle which normally lifts the eye upwards. After
the wound was healed the animal ought to have made the most
surprisingly awkward eye-movements in the endeavour to
fixate points in the field of vision and to save the theory of
neurone connections from disaster. Instead of which, when
he got over it, he calmly carried out both voluntary and
automatic lateral movements properly ; and Marina concluded
that " the anatomical association-pathways from the centres
to the muscles are not fixed." If then we cannot rely on the
fixed pathways in the nervous system to account for reflexes,
the theory of the neural basis of habit which rests on it
becomes very shaky indeed.

These, and the like difficulties, which are usually glossed
over or ignored by psychologists, not only make it difficult to
believe that habits are due to a concatenation of reflexes but
also lead to doubt as to the existence of fixed nervous con-

nections between the sensory and motor sides of habitual actions. Habits do indeed tend to become quasi-mechanical with repetition, but it is too readily assumed that this implies that they become stereotyped; whereas we saw earlier in the chapter that such a view is untenable. Take, as an instance, the act of signing one's name, which is about as mechanical a habit as a man can acquire. Sometimes the paper is to the right, sometimes to the left, sometimes forward and again near, on occasions level with the edge of the desk and on others tilted at an angle; and in every position a more or less different set of movements is necessary. Again, one may write with a pen on paper or with chalk on a blackboard, and in the latter case a very different group of muscles is employed, for instead of moving the fingers and the wrist the whole arm is involved. Yet every time the same form of signature is produced. What, then, becomes of the fixed chain of inter-central neurones; or are there several chains each appropriate to a different set of circumstances? The difficulty is accentuated when it is remembered that if I write simultaneously and unreflectingly with both hands the left hand produces a mirror image of the right hand movements. Are we to suppose that the establishment of the right hand set of intra-central neurone paths led originally to the formation of an equivalent series for the left hand? Anyone, who is still sceptical, may easily convince himself by the experiment of sitting on a chair with one leg pointed straight forward, and he will be able with little difficulty to trace his usual form of signature in the air with his big toe. As he has, presumably, never done this before, there can be no central pathway in the nervous system to account for the movements.

It is much more in consonance with the actual facts to turn aside from the fixed pathways and to describe the matter in psychological terms only. We say then, and all the facts of observation support the description, that what a person is trying to do on each occasion when he signs his name is to adapt his movements to a somewhat similar sensory configuration or pattern. The partial movements constituting the act of writing are reflexes but, even so, the whole act is something other than the sum of these movements, just as a melody is a different thing from the mere collection of notes contained in it. And as a melody can be played in different keys so, we have seen, can a habitual act be reproduced in a variety of forms. The musical analogy has been deliberately chosen, since it gives a truer conception of the growth of habit than the hypothesis of tracts or pathways in the nervous system uniting the sensory and motor sides of the process.

At one time it was the fashion, owing to the prevalence of the association theory, to explain all mental growth in terms of bonds of association between isolated mental data, and the theory of habit which we are challenging is nothing but the doctrine of associationism applied to bodily movements. Instead of starting with a chaos of disconnected movements, sensations, ideas or other ' mental atoms ' subsequently reduced to order by the magical virtue of association we believe that a certain arrangement dominates conscious life from the very beginning. If movements were originally independent of the sensory or ideational processes it is difficult to explain how they ever became associated together. The doctrine of associationism is no more intelligible when the assumed elements are reflexes than when they are ' ideas ' ; it simply will not work. From the very outset a child's experiences are comparable to the discrimination of notes within a chord, the rest of the chord consisting as yet of an undifferentiated volume of sound to be subsequently analysed. The chord is the primary experience and it is the psychologist's task to explain how the separate tones come into experience, if indeed they ever do so. The fatal blunder of mental atomism or associationism was to start from the most developed experience, the separate tones, and as might be expected it failed completely to shew how the experience of a chord could ever be derived from the sensations of separate notes. The modern *gestalt* theory rightly insists that form, order and arrangement dominate mental life from first to last. There is no such thing as a ' mental factor ' isolated from others, but all mental life is figured or has a structure or pattern *ab initio*. We do not require any theory to account for the structure since that is our datum, but rather we should call for an explanation of isolated units if they were ever found. So, it is reasonable to demand an explanation of the psycho-analytic ' complexes ' since these are said to be cut off from the rest of conscious life. The main reason for assuming fixed inter-central pathways or tracts was to account for the so-called bonds of association between sensations and movements. But as these are not separate but parts of a figured whole such bonds no longer interest us, since we do not require hypothetical neural connections to account for the union of elements which were never sundered.

To revert to our previous analogy, a musical person hears an opera differently from an unmusical, but neither of them hears separate tones, they both listen to melodies. The musical person has however a greater insight into the structure or configuration of the melodies. Just as intellectual growth may be considered as consisting of greater insight into the harmonies which the world offers for our appreciation ; so habit-formation is the reproduction in terms of movements of the configurations presented to the senses. In forming a habit the person is persistently trying to translate the meaning of sensory impressions into motor language. Why, then, it may be asked is repetition necessary to form a habit, unless we are blazing a trail through a forest of neurones in order to establish a permanent pathway ? The answer to this question has already been given, for we saw that mere repetition of movements is useless. The attempt to learn a series of nonsense-syllables by passive repetition is wellnigh hopeless. It is only successful, if at all, because it is impossible to keep the mind perfectly passive. If success is attained the series is rapidly and completely forgotten for as we stated there is little difference between the number of repetitions required for re-learning what has once been learnt passively and the number of repetitions required to learn for the first time.[17] When on the other hand, such a series is learnt with determination it is never completely forgotten. On the assumption of the linking up of a chain of neurones such a difference is inexplicable ; for as far as the nervous connections and muscular movements are concerned it is immaterial whether we repeat the series with or without the desire to learn. The function of repetition in habit-formation is, therefore, not to establish paths of low resistance but to attune the muscular system to the appropriate configuration, just as a violin only yields the best tune after prolonged use by a master-musician.

To form a habit is, in short, to compose a movement-melody, and the act of composition cannot be carried out passively since the structure or form of the melody must be kept steadily in view. The situation pipes a relational tune and the person dances in the appropriate rhythm. It is necessary to repeat the actions again and again in order to reconstruct the proper rhythm. As soon as the suitable configuration has been realised, but not before, further repetition makes the behaviour steadier and more facile. This is doubtless part of the explanation for the sudden rise from the plateau in habit curves as the result of practice ; for as long as the configuration remains unclear progress is very gradual, but once it is clearly discerned improvement is made with a bound. A steady continued purpose to understand and act on the situation is an essential feature in habit-formation. Mere repetition without such insight into the pattern of the situation will never produce increased facility. Thus we

see that the motor neurones respond to the sensory because
together they form a unitary physiological organ in which
the parts function in harmony.   It should not be difficult in
these days of ' wireless ' instruments to conceive how a trans-
mitter and a receiver can function together without a fixed
pathway of connection.   All that is necessary is that the one
should be attuned to the other.   Future research must discover the physiological mechanism on which such attuning
in the animal body depends before a satisfactory theory of
the neural basis of habit can be formulated.[18]

IMITATION

If we take a wide survey of human conduct it is evident
that many of our important habitual actions owe their origin
to the copying of the same activities in others.   Everybody
is influenced in his modes of thinking, feeling, and willing by
the particular social milieu in which his life is passed.   As our
habits are acquired in a social atmosphere the problem of
imitation is an essential part of the study of habit-formation,
as may be seen from the fact that our fundamental habitual
acts, such as speaking or writing, could never arise without the
aid of models to imitate, despite the fact that both are
ultimately based on the imperative native impulse to communicate with our fellows.   The rapid spread of a new fashion
or a new game may serve to illustrate how potent is the
influence of imitation in forming habits of conduct.   As
fashions usually spread from the ranks of people occupying a
higher position in the social scale we may surmise that a
certain degree of prestige is necessary in order that a habit of
action may diffuse throughout a community.   This view is
confirmed by the historical observation that, with the spread
of Roman conquest, Roman civilisation was adopted by the
subject peoples.   But although the Greeks were subdued they

did not imitate the Romans but rather were imitated by them, so great was the prestige of Greek culture and civilisation. We see the same cause in operation daily, for when a new idea or theory comes with the prestige of a great name or a great institution it is immediately adopted, whether intelligible or not, by the generality of mankind. It is difficult to say in what prestige consists, but anything which is or is thought to be authoritative has some of this quality, and a newspaper with a large circulation may use such authority to change not only the habits of political thought of its readers, but also their modes of living and the very food they eat.

Imitation is often described as being either imitation of the movements required to bring about certain ends or imitation of the ends themselves. But it is hard to find unimpeachable natural examples of the former kind of imitation. The closest approximations to the imitation of movements are seen in drill, the object of which is to secure as uniform a habit as possible. Being entirely artificial in nature drill has no educational significance. Anyone who contrasts the rigidity and uniformity of a drilled troop with the flexibility and variety of a performance, say, in eurhythmics will easily realise that imitation of movements is at once artificial and sterile. The soulless imitation characteristic of an earlier generation in teaching the rudiments of learning to young children, whereby they were forced to uniform repetition until they fitted the Procrustean pedagogical bed is a warning against artificial imitation of movements and is happily almost completely given up. In this respect teachers are in their current practice far in advance of psychologists in their theories. For psychology still follows in the wake of popular tales and attempts to construct a theory of imitation based on physiological connections in order to bolster up incorrect observations. Thus one writer says that,[19] in its more strict sense, the term imitation is applicable only to the

I

" copying by one individual of the actions, the bodily movements, of another."

Apes are popularly believed, by those who observe them
through the bars of a cage, to be imitative animals *par excellence*,
and educational psychology follows suit with wonderful
tales of the imitation of every movement by young children.
Now Professor Köhler has spent several years in the careful
and acute observation of chimpanzees, taking the precaution
of getting at very close quarters with them and providing
them with tasks well within the limits of their capacity.
He entirely rejects the explanation of their behaviour which
assumes that habit and imitation are due to the formation and
persistence of nervous pathways of low resistance. The
' same ' movements, he rightly insists, never recur ' as practically none is performed twice over in the same way.' He
makes the following pregnant remarks in summarising his
observations which ought to give the *coup de grâce* to any
theory of imitation which relies on neural connections between
perception and movements. " No observer, even with the
best of efforts, can say ' the animal contracts such and such a
muscle, carries out this or that impulse.' *This would be to
accentuate an inessential side-issue, which may change from
one case to another* (italics his). . . . Which muscles carry
out which actions is entirely immaterial." [20]   If there are no
permanently fixed movements involved in carrying out a task
how can there be fixed nervous pathways ?   Professor Köhler's
prolonged observations and experiments led him to the conclusion that apes do not imitate as readily as popular belief
supposes.   They never imitate movements, but only the ends
to which the movements are adapted.   But, and this is the
important point, whenever they do imitate it is always some
action that they are already familiar with and which they
understand fully ;   for " none of the observations give the
slightest ground for thinking that animals could ' simply '

and *quite without insight* have imitated important parts of their performances. The chimpanzee cannot do this." [21] Nor, it may be added, can anybody else. Whenever an intelligent ape learns anything by imitation the problem is always of such an order of difficulty as to lie well within the bounds of what he could do by himself unaided. For the same reason a man who really has insight into the game of chess can readily reproduce a game of several moves which he has watched. Not so the man who does not understand, however good his imagery may be. Professor Stout had an inkling of this when he wrote that ' Imitation may develop and improve a power which already exists, but it cannot create it.'

It is evident that learning by imitation is not a copying by summation of part activities, but of an articulately figured whole, and improvement in the process consists of a better insight into the relations of the configuration. When I pull out my watch because another person has pulled out his, what I imitate is *seeing the time,* for my watch may be in a different pocket from my neighbour's and unattached to a chain ; in fact, I am not interested in his movements at all, but simply in the configurative whole which is presented by his action. Thus an act of imitation is never a photographic copy but always a reproduction of a movement configuration, just as one may be said to ' imitate ' a melody on a violin which has been heard on a piano. Similarly when a child runs because his playmate does what he imitates is the *running* configuration and by no means the leg and trunk movements of his fellow. On rare occasions the child does, in a spirit of fun, try to imitate movements, as when he tries to copy the motions of a corpulent uncle whose walk appears to him a comic performance, and then he only caricatures the waddle since he is attempting an impossible task.

In short, we may say that imitation consists of the reproduction of the rhythm of sensory patterns or configurations by means of corresponding motor rhythms, leading to a similar result. What is copied or aimed at is the purpose, which is attained by a repetition of the underlying melody-figure. Now such configurations or patterns may be already part of the individual's psychoplasm, inherited or acquired, and in that case the mere perception of the imitated act is sufficient to start off the appropriate rhythms. Or, it may be, that the pattern is a new one, as in learning a new game, and here constant repetition is necessary for effective imitation. By the help of this conception borrowed from the *gestalt* theory it is possible to give an explanation of imitation in purely psychological terms. We have no need for the assumption of innumerable afferent nervous paths each appropriated to a specific perception to be copied, nor for central neurones somehow connected with these and leading to the imitated movements. Our account has shewn that every item of this explanation is riddled with insuperable difficulties. The desperate situation to which a physiological view of imitation is committed is shewn when it is necessary to conjure up separate sensori-motor arcs for everything which can be imitated spontaneously. " It may be," says an exponent of the view,[22] " that every child inherits a considerable number of such rudimentary instincts, and that they play a considerable part in facilitating the acquisition of new movements, especially perhaps of speech movements." But the child does not copy speech movements, he imitates *speech ;* and what an amazing number of afferent inlets would be required to account for all the nuances of consonant and vowel sounds of a language in all their living complexity ! Only the trained phonetician gets within measurable distance of copying the speech movements of another, for which he requires the help of instruments and diagrams, and even then experts fail to agree on the copy. Yet the amazingly clever child does it all in a very few years without adventitious aids ; so potent is the influence of

home education. There must be something wrong with the
physiology which leads to such results. How much simpler
the whole problem becomes when placed on the psychological
plane.

Association by imilars, as when I expect the clock to
strike as soon as I hea r the chime, [23] is a well established psychological law and can do the work demanded of it in this connection. If a perceptual configuration or pattern has a similar
rhythm with a movement configuration then all the essential
data are present for a reproduction of the movement. It is
no doubt astonishing that a configuration of a sensory sort
should call up a similar one in a totally different set of terms ;
but the law of association is indeed remarkable. We are so
familiar with the phenomenon that it never occurs to us to
wonder, for instance, at the reproduction in a dance of the
rhythm of the music. Classical psychology tells us that the
common element is sufficient to account for such reproduction
which is neither more nor less remarkable than that the chimes
of my clock recall the city of Bruges. " It is to be clearly
understood," says Professor Stout, [24] " that the revival of
similars by similars does not at all depend on the similarity
having been previously noticed. . . . But if an entirely new
acquaintance reminds me of an old friend because they are
like each other this is a pure case of the revival of similars."
What is true of the reproduction *of* similars is equally valid
for revival *by* similars ; and it is not necessary, therefore, to
assume that the child, whilst imitating, is definitely conscious
of the similarity which he reproduces.

We are thus led back by a different path to the conclusion
reached in the preceding section where we discussed the neural
basis of habit. There is an immediate psychological connection between the sensory and motor processes resting on
similar configurations in both. Such a connection, in the case
of learning to speak, is immensely aided by the hereditary

impulse to communicate, which is the ground of the remarkable aptitude which the child displays and the rapid progress he makes in such a complicated performance. When the hereditary stimulus is lacking, as it is in most of the things we imitate later in life on the basis of our acquired impulses, learning becomes more of a task ; which gives point to the remark that man never learns so much in the same period of time as he does when a child.

RATE OF GROWTH

The experimental investigations into habit formation, in so far as they consist of objectively measured results, are the records of physiological acts and it is possible, therefore, to treat them mathematically.[25] Various attempts have been made to find an empirical formula of interpolation to express the curve of progress. After trying several different equations Professor Thurstone [26] came to the conclusion that one form of the hyperbola best satisfied the observed results for *attainment* curves. In its ideal form, where there are no previous effects of practice, his formula reduces to

$$y = \frac{an}{n+b}$$

where y represents the amount of attainment in terms of the number of successful acts per unit of time, n the number of practice acts since the beginning of practice, a the physiological limit in terms of units of attainment ; b is stated to represent the rate of learning (an obvious error since the rate is only constant when the curve is a straight line), but really is dependent on the subject's capacity for the task. This formula has little to recommend it but is given here to stimulate inquiry.

The author of this book has devised the following method for arriving at the formula of the *time* curve. Several persons working together are given a simple fixed task to perform, such as pricking holes in a regular order through a disc which is seen in a mirror. The operation is performed fifty times by every subject, and the time of each separate performance for each person is recorded. The median times of the whole group are found for the separate performances and plotted on a graph as ordinates, the abscissæ being the number of the performance. In some experiments instead of the median the upper quartile, or the reading which divides off the top third of the series has been taken. This procedure eliminates times of excessive duration which are often due to preventible causes. A smooth curve which best fits the readings so obtained is drawn and its form is determined. The formula obtained on several occasions with different subjects by this method was

$$t = \frac{K}{(n+p)^c} + T$$

In this expression t represents the time necessary to perform the

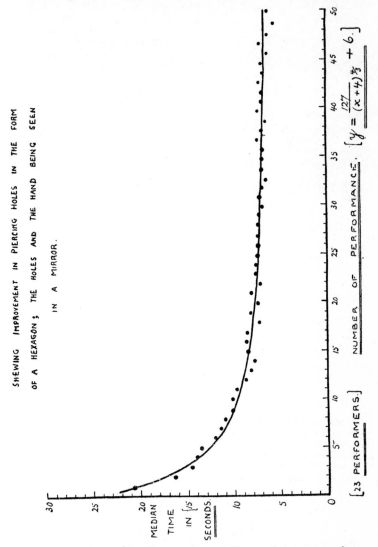

SHEWING IMPROVEMENT IN PIERCING HOLES IN THE FORM OF A HEXAGON; THE HOLES AND THE HAND BEING SEEN IN A MIRROR.

$\left[y = \frac{127}{(x+4)^{\frac{2}{3}}} + 6. \right]$

NUMBER OF PERFORMANCE.

[23 PERFORMERS.]

MEDIAN TIME IN 1/5 SECONDS.

single operation, n is the number of the performance, c is a small number greater than unity, and K, p and T are constants.

K depends on the nature of the test and the subject's capacity, p represents the fact that in no skilled movement does the subject really start from the zero point for he has used the same movements in other operations though not in the same way,[27] T represents the time necessary for the operation when the subject is on the plateau.

Recently, another attempt has been made to determine the equation of the learning function for time curves. By making the assumption that the function of the time varies first at an ever increasing rate, later, after passing through an inflection point, at an ever decreasing rate Messrs Meyer and Eppright [28] derive the equation

$$t = \frac{(L-1)T}{\pi} \text{ arc. cot } (n+p) + T$$

where t is the time for a complete operation, n the number of such operations which have preceded any definite task (e.g., when t is the duration of the third test, n is 2), p is the equivalent of a certain number of practice units which our previous experience has contributed to the particular task, T is the time when the final plateau is reached, and L is the individual's " learning ability " due to his native endowment which would presumably have the same value whatever the task. The derivation of the equation on theoretical grounds, though ingenious, is hardly justified in our present state of ignorance, but will stimulate further investigation.

RATE OF DECAY

Having obtained some idea of the rate of progress in the acquirement of a habit it is desirable to inquire into the rate of evanescence. Ebbinghaus [29] was the pioneer in this field of work. His procedure was to find out the average time required to learn by heart a definite number of nonsense-syllables ; after which he allowed varying intervals to elapse, and relearnt them, taking note of the time saved on the second occasion and thereby finding the amount he had retained and forgotten in each interval. He found that one hour after the original learning one-half was remembered, after eight hours one-third, after six days one-quarter, and one-fifth was retained after a month.

In an investigation by the present author a group of persons were required to reproduce a diagram composed of ten straight lines of varying length, intersecting at random, and exposed for five seconds at a time. After each exposure an attempt at reproduction was made. The average number of exposures for correct reproduction was fourteen. After half an hour's interval the average number of exposures necessary for relearning shewed that one-eighth was forgotten, and after a lapse of fifty days one-third was lost. Swift found that, after forty-eight hours' practice on a typewriter followed by a two years' interval, only ten hours' practice was required to recover the same speed.

It is evident that the rate of decay is very rapid at first and then slows down with the lapse of time until it becomes negligible.[30] The numerical results of his experiments led Ebbinghaus to formulate the law that the ratio of the amount retained to the amount forgotten is inversely proportional to the logarithm of the time calculated in minutes from the end of the learning.

Expressed in symbols the law of decay reads as follows:

$$m = \frac{K}{(\log t)^c}$$

where m is the above-named ratio, K and c are constants, and t is the time in minutes since the end of learning. The formula has been tested by the present author on a number of students, who were divided into groups of equal ability as measured by the number of repetitions needed by each to learn series of 15 nonsense-syllables. When the division into equal groups had been effected all the subjects learned a new series of 15 syllables, by saying them at a prescribed rate, until they could repeat them correctly. At varying intervals afterwards the number of repetitions required by each to relearn the new series was ascertained, which yielded a measure of the average amount forgotten by each group. It was now possible to deduce the constants and it was found, approximately, that

$$m = \frac{9}{(\log t)^3}$$

the values of c varying from 2·96 to 2·87.

Professor Piéron has also tested the formula with certain subjects who learned groups of digits and were tested at intervals from 7 to 120 days. He then proceeded to calculate the percentage economy (M) in the number of repetitions required to relearn each group and came to the conclusion that the formula of interpolation which best fitted his results was somewhat more complicated, namely

$$M = \frac{K(\log t)^a}{t^b}$$

where t is expressed in days ; the values of a and b were in his experiments respectively 2 and 1·25. This formula, according to Piéron, gives more consistent results than that of Ebbinghaus.

For practical purposes he suggests a simpler formula still, namely

$$M = \frac{K}{\sqrt[n]{t}},$$

where n is greater than unity and in some of his experiments had the value 2.

It must be carefully remembered that as we are not in a position to interpret these empirical formulæ it is a matter of convenience which shall be used. All that can be said at present is that the rate of decay is not as rapid as would be indicated by a hyperbola asymptotic to the line of time, but evidently presents a hyperbolic inclination.

CHAPTER VI

MEMORY

The Meaning of Memory—Reminiscence—The Effect of Distribution—
Memory and Interest—Can Memory be Trained ?

THE MEANING OF MEMORY

DESPITE the large volume of experimental research devoted
to the elucidation of the problem of memory very few generalisations of unimpeachable significance have been achieved.
As with many other topics in psychology the difficulty arises
from the loose use of terms. Experimentalists following in
the wake of theoretical writers on the subject have equated
memory with a universal function of organised living matter,
namely *retentiveness*.[1] In this wide use of the term a new-
born baby who exhibits the grasping reflex by supporting
his weight with his hands, since he is assumed to repeat
an action which was once useful to his ancestors in climbing trees, is said to remember the act. Nay, further, a
daisy kept alive in a pot in the dark which closes its petals
at dusk and reopens them at dawn is said to reproduce in
memory its previous activities in the field. If we believe as
Samuel Butler did that all such physiological retention is
ultimately the outward expression of some life purpose, and
there is a good deal to be said in favour of such a view, it
illuminates the situation to call the above cases expressions
of habit. But only confusion ensues if they are denominated
by the name memory as this leads to the belief that what is

true of them applies equally to memory proper. We shall have occasion to see in the sequel that this belief is erroneous. The term memory should be restricted to revival in idea in so far as such revival consciously reproduces a previous experience without transforming it. Such a state of affairs is an unrealisable ideal, as the witness in the law court who is expected to reinstate the past, the whole past, and nothing but the past experience very soon realises. Nevertheless this is what the experimental psychology of memory ought to aim at investigating, and it should especially distinguish the phenomena of habit from those of memory proper.

An illustration will make the situation clear. Suppose a boy is asked whether he remembers the binomial theorem, he will probably repeat the formula $(a+b)^n$, etc. And it may be that the whole thing is incomprehensible to him. Assume, however, that he has recently followed the proof of the theorem for the first time and has been lucky enough to grasp it and that he is now asked whether he remembers it. After some hesitation he may recall the various steps as he followed them, each suggesting the next and possibly the order in which they were presented, or he may have forgotten this and yet reproduce the logical sequence. Recalling the formula is psychologically very similar to the reproduction of a series of meaningless symbols, for schoolmasters know perfectly well to their cost that it is a mechanical habit ; whereas the recollection of the proof is a different phenomenon involving habit, no doubt, but being in the main an act of true memory.

Now every concrete act of memory contains these two relatively distinct processes mingled in various proportions. The habit process which is the predominant one in all instances of learning by rote was studied at some length in the preceding chapter. There we saw that in such learning the various repetitions were consolidated into a single quasi-mechanical set of movements, and during recall the movements were repeated in the order in which they were learnt.   True memory has different characteristics ; it involves self-consciousness and the recall has a definite date, place and setting, i.e., its individuality is not merged, at first, into other similar activities. In course of time, with repetition, the personal aspect may fall into the background and we get almost impersonal memory where the distinguishing marks of date and setting tend to disappear, as when the student at college reproduces the proof of the binomial theorem, having begun to forget when, where and how he learnt it.

Professor Bergson, who first called attention to the distinction named the two processes, habit-memory and image-memory respectively.[2]   The former he acutely observes is not so much a part of the subject's past as of his present and future activity, whilst the latter is re-presented in its setting and unlike the former which must be reproduced piecemeal, it may be revived as a whole in a single act of intuition.   But, as we said above, no useful purpose is served by calling the former memory, though it may be descriptively designated as ' habit enlightened by memory ' or physiological memory. For Bergson's true-memory the name image-memory is objectionable as being too restricted, since it would exclude the possibility of imageless remembrance, or the memory of meanings without recognisable images.   To distinguish it from the other we may conveniently call it psychological memory, though as previously indicated the two forms are never found apart in human experience.   It is a trite remark, but well worthy of emphasis, that there is no such thing as a memory ; there are only persons remembering.   Were it not that it would lead to intolerable circumlocutions it would be as well in any discussion of the subject to write about persons instead of memories when many difficulties, such as those concerned with memory training, would be avoided.

Interesting experimental verification of the distinction

between habit and memory has been forthcoming,[3] and similar experiments ought to be repeated with other material. Various tests involving the capacity of retention were given to about forty persons and marks were assigned for correct performance. Since both habit and memory involve retentiveness the tests were of two kinds, some requiring the reproduction of unique experiences in which habit could therefore play no part, others, such as the learning of nonsense-syllables demanded the reproduction of movements learnt by repetition. The correlation coefficients of the marks for the former tests were ·61 and for the latter ·53, whilst the marks for tests taken from different groups shewed, on the contrary, no correlation. Success in one set of tests did not necessarily carry with it success in the other. An additional test consisted in reproducing the substance of a prose passage read to the subjects, which is typical of the kind of memory demanded in scholastic work. This test shewed affinities with those of both groups yielding an average correlation coefficient of ·24 with the members of the first group, and ·41 with the latter. It is evident that such a test comprises both processes, for several phrases are already well known and will be reproduced verbatim as verbal habits, but if the subject-matter of the passage is previously unknown, its reproduction calls for an effort of pure memory.

Experiments on the rate of evanescence also point in the same direction. When the material to be learnt consists of meaningless syllables it has been shewn that the popular view is correct, namely, that, other things being equal, what is learnt more slowly is also retained longer, and that quick acquisition means quick forgetting. In other words there is a negative correlation between quickness of acquiring a habit and its retention. When we pass to such a task as the learning of German-English vocabularies where there is more admixture of psychological and physiological memory the relation begins to be reversed. A group of eighty students learnt such lists for a period of three weeks. It appeared that those who learnt more than the average number of words in a given time were also above the average in retaining what had been learnt when tested after a month's interval ; the rapid learners were also the better retainers. Further, in learning verse or prose where the psychological factor is still more prominent there has been found a positive correlation between rapidity of learning and retention of what has been learnt.

Indirect evidence of the distinction we are insisting upon has also been furnished by experiments on the direction of associations.[4] It was found that for physiological memory the associations are quite irreversible, i.e., they go forward only, as is seen for instance in the difficulty of repeating the alphabet or a sort of nonsense-syllables backwards. It is as though there were a forward conducting system so that the earlier the link in the chain the higher its potential with reference to later links. For psychological memory the direction of the associations is completely reversible. The former is a directional function, the latter signless.

In the previous chapter we saw that the attempt to explain the uniformity of habit by a series of fixed inter-central pathways in the nervous system presented almost insuperable difficulties. The assumption that psychological memory is wholly explicable by brain physiology is subject to further criticism still. In any case all that is known by direct observation about memory proper can be adequately described without reference to a physiological substratum as the rest of the chapter abundantly shews. Memory implies mental functioning and " if a given functional activity entirely ceases, it does not ' leave behind it ' a structural plasticity that survives independently. On the contrary when the function has completely lapsed the molecular structure has no longer any ' power ' to facilitate its recurrence. . . . The functional activity must surely be the formative principle. For to assign this priority to structure—meaning thereby molecular configuration—is to accept the materialists' *generatio æquivoca* of life and mind from inert ' stuff.'

" Again the attempt to get behind the psychical by talking about a physical arrangement of molecules *predisposing*, is to allow oneself to be misled by a metaphor, as if inert matter could ape the living mind. There is no predisposition in nitric chloride to explode if slightly disturbed . . . analogous to an irascible man's outburst when slightly provoked. Along with the explosion of the chloride there is no plasticity such as will facilitate its recurrence as there always is in the after-effects of exercise by living things." [5]

Yet the unwary are constantly trapped by such metaphors. No doubt the brain is necessary for memory, just as a brush is required for painting a picture, but neither the structure of the brush nor the state of the artist's muscles need be taken into account in a description of the painting. There is an easy way of avoiding all the difficulties in explaining the phenomena of memory beloved by those who are fond of pictures. When a mnemic phenomenon is studied by observation or introspection a diagram is drawn and the various lines are called brain-tracts. At a future time it is ridiculously simple to suppose that the brain-tracts are the result of observation and that memory is explained by them. And those who come afterwards and have forgotten how the diagram was made naturally imagine that observation of the brain-tracts came first. It is only necessary to fall back on brain-paths to account for the phenomena of memory when a psychological explanation in terms of mnemic causality is shewn to be inadequate.

It has been demonstrated repeatedly, and indeed is a fact of common knowledge that meaning is immensely more effective than association in enabling a person to reproduce what has been learnt. The meaning of a passage ensures a great economy of energy in learning by binding the different smaller units into larger significant wholes. In learning and reproduction these larger wholes serve as units. Mr D. O. Lyon [6] tested two persons with stanzas of poetry learnt at a single sitting with the following results.

Average no. of words .	.	60	150	300	750	1500
Average no. of repetitions .		6	15·5	17·5	19	26·5

These figures should be compared with those obtained by such practised learners as Ebbinghaus and Meumann who required 55 and 33 repetitions respectively to learn series of 36 nonsense-syllables. The enormous difference in the number of repetitions required in the case of nonsense and meaningful material is an indication of the disparity between the two factors previously described. The table also shews the great relative economy in learning longer passages, as though the meanings were synthesised into still larger wholes. Further, it has been shewn that after twenty-four hours the economy in relearning the same piece is greater with the longer than with the shorter passages.

REMINISCENCE

Important facts have been brought to light by the investigation of delayed recall as compared with the immediate recollection of what has been partially learnt. Dr Ballard carefully examined over 6000 subjects, mainly children, and his investigations are of great importance in this connection as they have served to bring to light a hitherto unsuspected recuperative power in memory. It is well known, both by observation and experiment, that there is a gradual fading or obliviscence of memory material; but reminiscence, or the process of improvement in the capacity to recall past experiences, escaped detection until experimental research made it clear. Dr Ballard [7] shewed that when a child has memorised a passage of poetry or prose, or even the shapes of a group of drawings he is, as a rule, able to remember more of it after a lapse of a few days than immediately after learning. The interest taken in the passage and its intelligibility determine the amount recovered, and under favourable conditions three-quarters of the children tested improved at the end of the second day. The degree of improvement varies with the age of the subject from 6 years and upwards, whilst adults over 20 years of age do not appear to improve in the aggregate. If, however, the number of subjects who improve is considered instead of the average amount of improvement, then it was found that nearly 90 per cent. of infants improve, 75 per cent. of older children and about 30 per cent. of training college students. Improvement was shewn not only in the quantity but also in the facility or speed of recall.

Now the total amount reproduced after an interval is the balance between what has been gained and lost ; consequently the degree of reminiscence is, as a rule, greater than the degree of improvement. Amongst the large number of classes of children in schools examined, although there was frequently a loss in the total amount remembered after an interval, in every instance some reminiscence was found.

The degree of reminiscence may be measured relatively by comparing the number of lines recovered after an interval with the number of lines originally remembered. Calculated in this way it diminishes amongst children with increasing age. If, however, the amount is measured absolutely by the total number of lines recovered without reference to those originally remembered, the power of reminiscence improves up to the age of 15 or 16 years and then declines.

The improvement in the amount remembered increases till about the third or fourth day after learning, with infants of six years of age ; it seems to attain its maximum after the

K

second day with children of twelve, and is not manifested with adults. Reminiscence, however, as distinct from mere improvement, persists, and is found in college students as well as in children. This power of reminiscence is more active amongst older memory material and a systematic attempt to recall has a stimulating effect on the amount remembered. With regard to recently acquired material, reminiscence measured *relatively* seems to vary inversely with the extent of the subject's general mental equipment ; being highest with mentally defectives. Amongst children of the same age there is, however, a distinct positive correlation between reminiscence measured *absolutely* and intelligence ; the reverse is true of adults. Immaturity rather than lack of intelligence is the basis of a high degree of reminiscence, and mental defectives behave in this respect like children of a lower age.

Dr Ballard maintains that this power of recovery in memory is due to an actual increase in strength of the memory impression after the learning has ceased. He has shewn experimentally, that neither fatigue nor retro-active inhibition, i.e. interference with what is previously learnt by what is learnt later, can satisfactorily explain the phenomenon.

Experiments have been devised to test the trustworthiness of memory in reporting what has been heard or seen, by reading a passage to the subject or shewing him a picture about either of which questions are subsequently asked. The evidence so far seems to shew that both in immediate and deferred recall tested in this way, women remember more detail than men and also remember a greater amount correctly, but men make less positive errors in reproduction.

THE EFFECT OF DISTRIBUTION

Experiments on learning nonsense-syllables have proved that the repetitions are more effective if they are distributed over several days than if they are continuous or made at one sitting. The most efficient method for any individual would be to distribute the repetitions at intervals corresponding to the times of his greatest reminiscent activity. In a long series of careful experiments on himself extending over a period of more than four years Mr Lyon investigated the *total time* taken for memorising passages of prose and verse of different lengths, and also nonsense-syllables and rows of digits. He compared the continuous method with the method of distributed repetitions (making one repetition only per day in the latter method), so as to discover the optimum distribution of time. A fundamental disparity was revealed between the results of learning material with meaning and that in which there is but little significance, namely the nonsense verses and digits ; thus establishing once more an opposition between habit and memory. The total time taken by the distributed method for poetry and prose was nearly always as long as that taken by the continuous method, whereas for digits and nonsense-syllables in which there is no logical connection, there was a considerable saving in time by the once-per-day method. A similar opposition between the power of brute retention by mere habitual association and the active function of memory has been found in French school children of 10 to 13 years.

For both verse and prose, up to the limit of about one-thousand words, the total time taken with either method varied very roughly as the length of the passage. An instructive reservation is to be made in interpreting this rule owing to the fact that we are dealing with units which have neither fixed length nor lines of demarcation between them, i.e. units of meaning. Such units are grasped as wholes in one span of consciousness. Within certain narrow limits, therefore, the length of the passage does not influence the time taken for learning it, provided that the meaning can be grasped as a whole. In consonance with this, it was found that by neither method did the addition of a couple of extra lines to a stanza of verse make any perceptible difference in the time taken for learning, allowance being made for the longer time required for reading.

The chief advantage of the distributed method for all kinds of material learnt lies in the better retention which occurs as a result of this procedure. A conclusion of great significance is that the most economical method of distributing single readings is to spread them over a rather lengthy period ; the intervals being in geometrical progression. For example, Lyon found that with a certain individual who memorised poems of twenty stanzas, the highest retentiveness was obtained by distributing the readings thus : 2 hours, 8 hours, 1 day, 2 days, 4 days, 8 days, 16 days, etc. Obliviscence is best prevented by reviving the memory when it is just beginning to fade away.

The following tables extracted from these researches illustrate some of the facts above stated.

Nonsense-syllables—

No. of syllables	8	12	16	24	32	48	72	104	200	300
Time taken in mts., learnt by *continuous* method	¼	6	9	16	28	43	138	...	...	...
Time taken (1 repetition per day)	⅛	1½	3¾	5	6	14	25	37	93	105

Digits—

No. of digits	8	12	16	24	32	48	72	104	200	400
Time taken in mts., continuous method	¼	¼	2	5	10	18	24	56	154	...
1 repetition per day	¼	½	1⅛	4	7	9	21	35	85	233

Poetry—

Average no. of words	25	105	125	245	300	450	625	875	1250	2500
Time taken in mts., continuous method	⅛	4	10	16	28	30	56	114	147	312
1 repetition per day	⅛	3½	5	18	23	46	58	98	146	385

Prose—

No. of words	25	50	80	100	175	300	600	800	1000	1200
Time taken in mts., continuous method	⅛	3	5	9	21	30	71	133	168	202
1 repetition per day	⅛	2¼	4½	9	22	36	84	136	165	186

A comparison has been made [8] of the rate of decay in psychological memory for material learnt by each of the above-named methods. The aim of the experiments was to discover whether the method of divided repetitions was more effective than that of accumulated repetitions for the purpose of retaining logically connected material. Passages of history and economics were chosen, each assignment being from two to four pages of a book. The assignments were carefully marked so as to get a record of the number of ideas contained in each and the scoring was done by counting the number of ideas correctly recalled. No attention was paid to the correct recall of words, but simply to the meaning, and the figures in the table below indicate the percentages of such units of meaning.

There were thirty tests in history and thirty in economics, the subject-matter being consecutive throughout each series of tests so as to maintain logical continuity. Each assignment was read through five times, either at one sitting on the same day or once a day for five days, and then dismissed from the mind. At varying intervals after the reading, the subject wrote all that could be recalled without any assistance, and the percentages of retention for each interval was determined. The figures in the table are, in each case, the average of ten tests, five in economics and five in history, taken under similar conditions.

The results were :

Read		Tested	Average amount recalled	
5 times in 1 day .	.	next day	66%	...
Daily for 5 days .	.	,,	...	64·4%
5 times in 1 day .	.	after 2 weeks	13·13%	...
Daily for 5 days .	.	,,	...	37·26%
5 times in 1 day .	.	after 1 month	11·49%	...
Daily for 5 days .	.	,,	...	30·59%

It should be stated that results similar to these had previously been obtained by experiments performed on other observers who were trained psychologists. In all cases accumulated repetitions are as effective as divided repetitions provided that the ability to recall is tested one or two days afterwards. With longer periods a different tale is told, for the effect of the accumulated method wears off much more rapidly. Forgetting occurs very rapidly at first, but more especially with the material learned by the massed method, and in both cases slows down considerably as time progresses. The method of divided repetitions is seen to be of far greater value for prolonged retention.

The reason for the superiority in retention obtained by the distributed method is to be sought in the facts of reminiscence. That the advantage is not due to the interference of fatigue brought on by the massed method has been shewn by experiments by Jost in which a number of repetitions of *other* material was made before each of the distributed repetitions so that the total work on each occasion was the same whether the divided or massed method was used. Nevertheless, the superiority still rested with the former method.

Some active change is going on during the periods intervening between the repetitions which leads to better assimilation and organisation of the material to be remembered. There is, however, a limit to this process so that if, for instance, a single repetition is made every week the effect would be lost, and repetitions every fourth day are less effective than those every third day, and so on up to the time of maximum reminiscence. In other words, if the repetitions are made before the strength of reminiscence has begun to wane, the effect of divided repetitions is beneficial and the memory is aided, otherwise the advantage of distribution is lost.

The author of these experiments thinks that the law for the decay of a habit formulated by Ebbinghaus applies equally to the obliviscence of memory. But although the general trend of the curves appears to be the same in both cases, calculation shews that the numbers given above do not confirm the logarithmic law, there being no more than the very roughest correspondence.

Different methods of memorising are employed by various individuals. Amongst them we may notice the ' entire ' or ' whole ' and the ' sectional ' methods which are both forms of the continuous procedure previously considered. In the entire method the lesson to be learnt is read through from beginning to end until it is known ; whilst in the other it is broken up into sections each of which is learnt separately. There are numerous idiosyncrasies in procedure in this piecemeal method. It will be easily seen that the sectional method introduces unnecessary and irrelevant associations between the beginning and end of each section. A ' mixed ' method is more frequently employed, especially by school children, in which each section is learnt separately and then the whole is welded together from the beginning.

The relative efficiency of the methods has been submitted on several occasions to experimental investigation. The most recent experiments [9] are those on London school boys and girls of the ages of $11\frac{1}{2}$ and $12\frac{1}{2}$ in different schools. By means of preliminary tests of memorising verse the various classes were divided into equivalent memory groups. One of the groups in each case then learnt selections of poetry by the ' whole ' method and the other by the sectional method of learning line by line. When both groups were tested it was found that the sectional method was better than the whole method; the amount that was retained being measured by the number of words correctly recalled. The conclusion arrived at was that there was a " conclusive victory " for the sectional procedure. However, in two of the schools it appears to have been the normal custom for the children to recite whole poems in chorus after the teacher; a procedure admirably calculated to destroy all interest and any desire ever to read poetry again. And in the case of one long poem which is stated to have had continuity of meaning and a coherent story the whole method proved to be the more advantageous. No doubt in this case the interest in the story was responsible for the result.

In fact where interest is aroused the method of learning is of far less importance than is usually supposed.

Before we discuss the relation of interest to memory it will be as well to consider briefly the question of forgetting. According to the school of psycho-analysts the process of forgetting is not a passive one but is a protective measure or repression by which we are screened from unpleasant recollections. Thus it is said by the founder of the school that : [10] " the forgetting of impressions and experiences shews the working of the tendency to ward off from memory that which is unpleasant." By this principle he accounts for the forgetting of words, intentions, resolutions, etc., and he extends it so as to cover all erroneously carried-out actions such as slips of the tongue and pen. At the back of every such error there is said to be an intentional concealment or repression. In an examination of Professor Freud's contribution to psychology in which he considered what was his chief claim to

originality, a very competent and sympathetic critic, the
late Dr Rivers [11] came to the conclusion that " there is much
to be said for a view which would regard as a distinctive
feature of Freud's system his theory of forgetting." He went
on to say that it is forgetting rather than remembering which
needs explanation and that " it is, perhaps, the greatest merit
of Freud's theory that it provides us with such an explanation."

Now it is notorious that we often acutely remember
what we consciously dislike and would much prefer to forget,
whilst, on the other hand, we frequently forget what we
would desire strongly to retain. It might be expected that
the distinctive contribution to psychological theory would
provide an explanation. All that is offered, however, for
normal persons is an examination of cases of forgetting *isolated*
impressions and never an investigation into the obliviscence of organised groups of ideas, which is what an explanation should attempt. In the case of such isolated things such
as proper names, it is maintained that a forgotten or distorted
name has some associative connection with an unconscious
stream of thought. Of course everything in mental life has
associations ; it needed no ideas from the vasty depths of un-
consciousness to tell us that. And it is undeniably true that
when ideas are associated the whole series fade away together.
When we demand a reason for remembering unpleasant
experiences in contradiction to the assumed principle we are
told that a conscious intention to forget is powerless against
an unconscious resistance. Dr Rivers endeavoured to rescue
the principle we are considering, by the clever distinction
between witting and unwitting repression, so that when we
forget pleasant experiences we do so unwittingly.

The whole principle is, however, a mere *petitio principii*,
for nothing more is meant by this school when they speak of
the unconscious than a dark repository for forgotten experiences. When submitted to the test of experiment the principle

that unpleasant feeling tone leads to forgetting, has been shewn
to be unfounded. The experiment was conducted in the
following fashion.[12] On the day after a half-term's holiday
nearly seven hundred girls in a school between the ages of
11 and 16 years were told to write down all the pleasant
experiences of the holiday and on the reverse side of the page
all the unpleasant ones. About a fortnight later, without any
intermediate warning they were asked to write similar reports
about the same holiday. Any experience found in the second
report which did not appear in the first was ignored. In this
way it was possible to discover the relative forgetting of
pleasant and unpleasant experiences. Of 6735 pleasant
experiences originally recorded 2700 or 40·1 per cent. were
forgotten ; and of 3491 unpleasant events 1406 or 39·8 per
cent. were omitted on the second occasion. The number of
children who forgot a larger percentage of pleasant experiences
was 345 and of unpleasant experiences 280, whilst 62 forgot
an equal number of both. The experimenter concluded
somewhat hastily, that there was no difference between the
two feeling tones, pleasure and unpleasure, in their effect on
memory. Similar investigations ought to be undertaken on
adults when the results could be checked by introspection.
However, feeling does affect memory, as the following account
of an experiment performed by the author of this book shews ;
but by no means in the simple way that the psycho-analytic
principle would suggest.

Twenty-four men took part in the experiment, their ages
ranging from 22 years to 38½ years, with an average of 26 years
3 months. They were all graduates, mostly in honours, being
members of a practical class in psychology and they displayed
great keenness on the experiment ; five of them were men of
considerable literary judgment. The material to be learnt
consisted of four sonnets from Hardy's *Collected Poems* named
" She to Him." The selection was determined partly by the

sonnet form, which is useful in such investigations owing to the rigidity of its construction which provides comparable tasks, and partly by the fact that these sonnets have exactly the same ' colour ' and deal with the same order of ideas.

Each subject was given two of the sonnets to learn in a prescribed manner. The first was learnt by a ' mixed ' method according to the following plan, which insured that each line was repeated exactly eight times :

Plan of repetitions			Total
First quatrain	4 .	.	8
Second quatrain	. 4	. 2	8
Sestette	. . . 6		8

The second sonnet was learnt by the ' entire ' method, being read through from beginning to end eight times ; so that each line in both sonnets was repeated the same number of times. In the former case, however, as the plan shews, there were several irrelevant associations formed during the course of learning between the beginning and end of each quatrain and sestette which, theoretically, should interfere with the process of recall.

After each sonnet had been repeated in the way described, a couple of minutes' rest was taken, and then the accuracy of learning was tested. Each subject heard his neighbour who had repeated a different sonnet. A score was kept by recording the number of times that the person had to be prompted in order to repeat the poem ; which serves as an index to the completeness of the learning. One minute only was allowed at any point of hesitation, at the end of which the person was prompted ; and every prompt was counted, even if it consisted only of a preposition or article. This rigid method explains the large numbers given later.

Everybody who has experimented on learning is well aware that there are certain places where different persons find exceptional difficulty in making associations. No explanation has been so far given of these ' refractory points,' but their existence calls in question the accuracy of any method of determining the completeness of what has been learnt, which relies on counting the number of repetitions which are required to learn a passage, or to learn a series of nonsense-syllables, by heart. All the extra repetitions necessary to break down the resistance at the refractory points are unnecessary as far as the rest of the passage is concerned, which is therefore overlearnt. Hence there is always considerable doubt in the comparative interpretation of results when the efficacy of a learning method is calculated by the number of repetitions necessary to insure perfect reproduction. The prompting method avoids this difficulty by fixing the number of repetitions in advance and by not insisting on complete recall. In this way, the refractory points do not affect the other associations, but all are treated alike.

The second part of the experiment was carried out exactly one week later. In the intervening period the subjects were told to avoid thinking of the poems as far as possible, and the instruction was successfully followed. At the end of seven days they were allowed to read each sonnet through once, from beginning to end, and one minute later the amount of retention was determined, exactly as before.

Immediately after the final record was made, each was asked to state which of the two sonnets he preferred. Nineteen subjects expressed a decided preference for one or the other ; one liked both equally well ; and four disliked both strongly, either because they did not appreciate them, or else because they thought them nonsense. If the different subjects are classified in groups according to the sonnets they prefer, the effect of subjective preference on memory can be investigated.

The results are more clearly seen when exhibited in

tabular form, where the average number of prompts for the group of five subjects who had no preference are given for the sake of comparison. The figures in heavy type in every case are those for the preferred sonnet :

	Immediate recall		Delayed recall	
	I	II	I	II
	'Mixed'	'Entire'	'Mixed'	'Entire'
Learned by—	method	method	method	method
8 subjects (preferring Sonnet I)				
Mean no. of prompts . .	**26**	40	**18**	33
11 subjects (preferring Sonnet II)				
Mean no. of prompts . .	43	**32**	40	**30**
5 subjects (no preference)				
Mean no. of prompts . .	47	57	44	51

It is easily seen that in all cases the preferred sonnet is not only better learnt but better retained. These figures seem to suggest that it is not the method of learning which affects immediate memory or retention, but rather the subjective preference for what is learnt. Statements have been made in conflict with this opinion, such as that of Myers,[13] who says that the mixed method, " although more economical as regards immediate memory, is surpassed by the entire method in respect of retention." Such a view appears to be the result of taking averages from disparate groups or for dissimilar material, where the preferences cancel each other in the aggregate.

It follows from our investigation, that any experimental evidence about memory which does not take the subjective factor into account must be rejected. For if the experiments are valid, it would appear that subjective preference is a *vera causa*. The objection will at once be raised that " there is no cause or effect in nature ; nature has but an individual existence ; nature simply *is* " ;[14] and cause and effect are convenient fictions serving the purpose of economy of thought.

The concept of cause, we are told, is now replaced by the concept of function, and with the abolition of the causal concept the idea of activity must also be abandoned.

However well founded this view may be in the realm of physical science, it is impossible to dispense with the notion of subjective activity in psychology. If the psychologist finds it necessary to take into account the fact of thinking at all, and none except the behaviourist fails to do so, he is equally bound to postulate the activity of thought. Neglect of this consideration is due, as we have seen, to a physiological bias in psychology, by which function is regarded as determined by structure instead of *vice versa*. Mental structure is, however, simply crystallised function. From the psychological standpoint function is always prior, as we saw earlier in dealing with habit and heredity regarded as mental phenomena.

Now subjective preference is but another name for *interest* and is a state of mind in which feeling-tone and conation are both prominent but in which the latter dominates the former. When we say that a person is interested in or has a preference for certain objects we imply that they arouse in him both feeling and desire. Whether the feeling is pleasurable or not is quite immaterial for the strength of the interest is dependent on the desire. Hence we are led to the conclusion that the desire or will to remember is the essential determining factor in memory. In this respect habit and memory are on a par, for in the preceding chapter evidence was brought to shew that the active attitude or the will to learn was necessary in order to acquire and retain a habit. Consequently whatever else is involved, effective memory training should ultimately be a training in sustained voluntary effort.

CAN MEMORY BE TRAINED ?

There is a dangerous complexity underlying this apparently simple question, which is really an instance of the logical fallacy of many questions. The man who is asked whether he has left off cheating would, if he were wise, refuse to reply in the negative or in the affirmative. Now when the question of training the memory is under consideration, several different things are mixed up together. First we have the two main factors in every concrete act of memory mentioned at the beginning of the chapter. If we confine ourselves to true memory alone we have to disentangle several other factors involved in it. Dr Carpenter [15] first pointed out that an act of memory depends not only on our ability to *retain*, but also on our ability to *record* ideas, i.e. to commit them to memory, and finally on our power of *recovering* what has been so committed. Each of these factors is relatively distinct and our simple question has consequently branched out into several directions.

As to retentiveness, the meagre evidence available for physiological retention has been presented in the chapter on habit-formation, but as regards the psychological retention of ideas there is, as far as I am aware, no evidence to shew whether this is improvable by education or not. Professor James, who believed that our native retentiveness was as much an unchangeable property of our nervous system as its chemical constitution, based his doctrine on the view that all association is due to the formation of ' traces ' in the brain, consisting of paths of low resistance between adjacent neurones, which implies that all associations are of the mechanical habit type. But, as Dr Carpenter says, the associations " which are most useful to us in the acquirement of knowledge, and over the formation of which we have the most power, may be distinguished as *rational ;* being based on the fundamental relations of the ideas themselves, the perception of which gives to the new idea a definite place in the fabric of our thought." Such connections as these between our ideas are the basis of all memorising that is truly educative and it is not necessary to invoke the central nervous system in order to account for them.

For educational theory it is fortunately hardly necessary to consider whether retentiveness is or is not improvable, since pure tenacity of retention is not *per se* a valuable power of mind. If it is allowed to take the place of organised thinking, sheer retentiveness may be a bar to progress. This is very aptly illustrated by Professor Lloyd Morgan [16] in the following example : " I ask a boy who can readily learn a lot of dates when Jonson's *Every Man in his Humour* was published. He answers glibly 1596. I say : ' Was Shakespeare still living ? ' He looks confused, and I continue, ' Was Cromwell dead ? ' to his still greater confusion. And yet he can give me pat, if directly asked, the dates of Shakespeare's death and Cromwell's protectorate. He does not think but trusts to parrot-like association." This unfortunate youth has had his physiological memory trained to the neglect of a systematic training in relationships with the result that what he knows has no educational value. " Another boy of whom the same question concerning Jonson's comedy is asked may reply : ' I do not remember the exact date, though I have seen it stated. But it was after the publication of the *Faerie Queene* and before *Bacon's Essays* appeared. I happen to remember those dates, so *Every Man in his Humour* must have been produced between 1599 and 1597.' His answer is less exact ; but it is more rational, and from the point of view of systematic knowledge of greater value."

There are, of course, a number of facts which must be learned by heart, such as the tables, but a rational procedure in explaining them is the best method for remembering them and for future advance, as the methods employed in the best kindergartens have amply shewn. Some other things to be remembered have neither rhyme nor reason, such as English spelling ; but whilst these must be learnt, they have in themselves no educational value except as a means to some further end. Rational associations within an organised system of knowledge are the only kind of retentiveness worth educational consideration. It ought to be added that the systematic organisation of knowledge enables the material to be retained more readily since each part of the system is retained by the combined suggestive power of all the rest. Moreover, as meaning is more readily assimilated than bare facts (as the work on retention of nonsense-syllables shews), and as the amount that can be retained in this way becomes incomparably greater, since a unit of meaning may contain many sub-units, the whole functioning as one without further effort ; it follows that for practical purposes more complete organisation is equivalent to an increase of retentiveness. Every new generalisation or law increases one's power of retention, provided that it is arrived at by considering the particulars ; for the mere statement of the law or rule implicitly revives all the particulars. The question of retentiveness has been much obscured by the false analogies used in discussing the subject, all of them drawn from the physical world, such as ' the store-house of the mind,' ' imprinting on the memory ' and so forth. All these which are comparatively innocuous when we are considering physiological memory are apt to lead to erroneous implications when true memory is discussed.

When we turn to the other factors, namely the recording and the recovering, further light is thrown on the subject of the training of the memory. There is no doubt whatever that the ability to record is improvable by practice ; this has been shewn experimentally and indeed is obvious from general

L

experience For it depends on factors which are largely subjective and under our control ; namely on properly adjusted attention, rhythm, control of imagery, etc. and also on our innate or acquired aptitudes. A problem of considerable educational importance emerges at this point, namely whether the improved ability brought about in this way is purely specific, or whether it is of a general nature so that it can operate in spheres outside that in which the improvement has been acquired. As this question is not confined to memory alone but concerns all the powers of the mind it is considered in the next chapter on mental discipline.

Finally we have the third factor, namely, the capacity to recall what has been learnt. The name recollect which is usually given to this power is significant, for it calls attention to the dependence of memory on the will to learn. Recollection is to be contrasted with the kind of reminiscence which takes place in reverie where we are relatively passive spectators of the flow of ideas. When, however, voluntary attention is concentrated on the details of an organised system of knowledge those associations are recalled which are relevant to the particular subject thought about. So that the condition of recollection, in so far as it is not subjective, brings us back again to the organisation of our knowledge, which is likewise the condition of its retention. " Most men," said Professor James,[17] " have a good memory for facts connected with their own pursuits. The college athlete who remains a dunce at his books will astonish you by his knowledge of men's ' records ' in various feats and games, and will be a walking dictionary of sporting statistics. The reason is that he is constantly going over these things in his mind, and comparing and making series of them. They form for him not so many odd facts, but a concept-system—so they stick. So the merchant remembers prices, the politician other politicians' speeches and votes, with a copiousness which amazes outsiders, but which the amount of thinking they bestow on these subjects easily explains." It is evident that the real reason for the retentive memory in all these cases is the organisation of the facts brought about by an intense interest in them. Putting it briefly we may say that in the will to learn lies the secret of training the memory. In other words there is no royal road to this goal and instead of looking to specific exercises for this purpose we see that the proper method is to stimulate a desire for what is to be acquired and to make our studies systematic.

CHAPTER VII

MENTAL DISCIPLINE

Historical Idea of Mental Training or Discipline—Experimental Evidence—Interpretation of the Experiments—More Evidence and Different Interpretations—Ideals

THE HISTORICAL IDEA OF MENTAL TRAINING OR DISCIPLINE

THE conception of mental discipline is at least as old as Plato, as may be seen from the seventh book of the *Republic*, in which Socrates is represented as persuading Glaucon in the following manner :

" And have you further observed that those who have a natural talent for calculation are generally sharp at every other kind of knowledge ; and even the dull, if they have had an arithmetical training, although they may derive no other advantage from it, always become much sharper than they would otherwise have been ? "

" Very true," he said.

Later on a similar conclusion is reached about geometry : "The inhabitants of your fair city," says Socrates, "should by all means learn geometry. Moreover the science has indirect effects which are not small."

" Of what kind ? " he said.

" There are the military advantages of which you spoke," I said ; " and we know, of course, that the man who has studied geometry will be wholly and entirely superior to the man who has not, with respect to the better apprehension of all subjects."

" Yes, indeed," he said, " there is an infinite difference between them." [1]

As soon as he appreciates the point Glaucon fully agrees with Socrates that not only does a training in mathematics make a man sharper at mathematics but more acute in all departments of knowledge.

This notion of the indirect effects of education persisted throughout the centuries, for Bacon, in his essay on " Studies," doubtless influenced by Plato, also approved the doctrine, thus : " Nay, there is no stond or impediment in the wit, but may be wrought out by fit studies ; like as diseases of the body may have appropriate exercises. . . . So if a man's wit be wandering, let him study the mathematics ; for in demonstrations, if his wit be called away never so little, he must begin again. If his wit be not apt to distinguish or find differences, let him study the schoolmen ; for they are splitters of hairs."

The training here, too, is assumed to be of a general nature rather than specific, in that the splitting of dialectical hairs is thought to be a good remedy for enabling a man to split hairs of other sorts.

Locke put the matter much more succinctly. " I have mentioned mathematics as a way to settle in the mind a habit of reasoning closely and in train ; not that I think it necessary that all men should be deep mathematicians, but that, having got the way of reasoning, which that study brings the mind to, they might be able to transfer it to other parts of knowledge as they shall have occasion."   There was a good deal of inconsistency in Locke's views as to the effects of training as he was largely guided by utilitarian considerations, maintaining in his *Thoughts Concerning Education* that mathematics should be studied for their great practical value.[2]   Nevertheless the above statement may be taken as implying that the effects of training are of a general nature and not confined to the subject in which the training is received.

This doctrine once known as that of ' formal education '

rests on the view that the assumption underlying the thought of all the above quotations has a solid foundation. In the great controversy in England in the middle of the nineteenth century concerning the claims of natural science and modern languages to be included in the school curriculum the warfare raged chiefly round this doctrine. It was claimed by the adherents of the classical tradition that classics alone could furnish a liberal education since they demanded a vigorous all-round exercise of the active, cognitive and æsthetic faculties. They rejected the view that knowledge which had practical utility or which might be considered as leading up to a profession could have any educative effect on the mind. The classics were " regarded primarily as a species of mental gymnastics, a method of developing the intellectual faculties, without reference to the permanent utility of the knowledge conveyed." [3] This seemed to carry with it the notion, from which the extreme supporters did not shrink, that it was a strong recommendation for these studies that they were dry and distasteful to the pupils.

Girls suffered equally with boys under the yoke of the tradition, as in several schools they did not, nor were they expected to, get beyond the Latin declensions and conjugations, but the régime was defended on the ground that rote learning was such good mental training. The following actual dialogue between Royal Commissioners and a head-mistress in the year 1866 illuminates the view :

" Do you find any difficulty in adequately teaching to a girl of ordinary intelligence three languages, such as French, German and Latin ? "

" No ; but then we confine ourselves to the elements of German and Latin, to the grammar of Latin, especially to the declensions and the verbs."

" With regard to Latin, does your experience lead you to attach importance to it as a means of preparing girls for the study of English or as a means of giving power to the mind ? "

" I think it is in every way an excellent mental training."

" You think Latin grammar a very useful instrument for that purpose ? "

" Yes."

" Do you find the girls learn it readily ? "

" As readily as they learn any grammar.   Grammar is a difficult subject." [4]

Other girls' schools, at that period, taught German in place of Latin, but, lest one should imagine that this was due to superior enlightenment, a distinguished head-mistress [5] said that the girls derived as much benefit as the boys, for " German, we think, answers the purpose of Latin, inasmuch as it has a complicated grammar."

A head-master propounded the theory much more bluntly, declaring that it did not matter a bit what you taught a boy provided that he thoroughly detested it.   The object of teaching the classics was, in short, to give the pupil a ' mental training ' rather than any positive knowledge of the languages, for it was believed that a boy who knew Latin had obtained a master-key which he could apply to many a difficult lock besides.   But the supporters of the claims of natural science put forward similar views to justify their studies, one of the protagonists stating [6] that " the student of natural science is likely to bring with him to the study of philosophy, or politics, or business, or his profession, whatever it may be, a more active and original mind, a sounder judgment and a clearer head, in consequence of his study."

We shall now examine the theory that the effects of training in one sphere of activity can be, as Locke said, transferred to other different spheres ; which as is now evident has at least the merit of respectable antiquity.   Is the wisdom of the ages justified ?

EXPERIMENTAL EVIDENCE

Cause and effect are especially difficult to distinguish in this connection and are frequently confused one with the other. As Plato observed those who are successful in certain branches of study or who have special aptitudes or abilities frequently have a better general capacity. Instead of the special skill, however, having produced a better general capacity it may simply be an expression of such original general power. Thus clever boys in English public schools were usually placed on the classical side and naturally did well there and afterwards, leading to the general belief amongst schoolmasters that there was some virtue in a classical training which fitted a boy to succeed in all departments of life.

With the advent of experimental psychology certain methods were devised to cope with the problem, and although they have not given an unambiguous answer, at all events they have helped us to realise more clearly the issues involved and the great complexity of the subject. The earliest experiment of this nature is due to Professor James.[7] He considered but one aspect, namely, whether training in learning one type of poetry would shorten the time taken to learn an entirely different kind of poetry. For eight successive days he learnt 158 lines of poetry by Victor Hugo, the total time required being 132 minutes. Let us call this the test material or series. He then learnt the whole of the first book of *Paradise Lost* in " 20 odd minutes daily for 38 days " shewing that he must have had astonishing powers of retentiveness. This constitutes the practice material or series. Finally he tested himself on Victor Hugo's poem again and found that for 158 additional lines " divided exactly as on the former occasion " he required 151 minutes for memorising. The loss in capacity was explained by the statement that he was

" perceptibly fagged with other work at the time of the second batch of V. Hugo." Quite apart from this explanation it is evident that the experiment is too crude and could not be regarded as evidence for transfer of the effects of practice even if the final conditions had been more favourable and the result positive. The method, however, is serviceable and indicates the direction along which experimental evidence has been sought.

Preliminary examination by the test material will hereafter be called taking the first cross-section, and the final test will be named the final cross-section. Any experiment on the transfer of the effects of training may be described as taking a first cross-section by means of suitable test series, then giving a certain amount of training by the practice series and finally a second cross-section is taken by means of material similar to the first test series.

In order to overcome the difficulty of varying physical states and moods which vitiates the experiment of James, a refinement in procedure was introduced by Mr Winch, namely, the method of equal ability groups. By dealing with numbers of individuals, if some are more fatigued others may be fresher and so on. School children were divided into groups of equal ability in memory, which was tested by their accuracy in reproducing a historical passage. One of the teams was practised for a couple of weeks in learning poetry by heart ; the other team had no practice of this sort. Finally the teams were combined and a second cross-section was taken again by means of a historical passage. The practised group acquitted themselves better than the untrained.

Dr Sleight [8] introduced further refinements into the experiments more especially in the statistical treatment of the results. The improvement of one equal ability group as compared with another, owing to practice is usually expressed as a percentage of the initial ability. Such percentages are,

however, misleading, for the greater the skill already attained
the more difficult does it become to make further improvement.
To meet this difficulty the amount of improvement is usually
calculated in units of standard deviation as was done in a
similar case in the chapter on *observation*. Another fact to
be taken into account is that the first test itself gives a definite
amount of training which as our study of *habit-formation*
shewed is likely to be greater than any equivalent amount of
subsequent training. In order to compensate for this, only
the differential improvement of the trained group over the
untrained should be considered in drawing inferences.

An experiment was made on 84 girls of average age
12 years 8 months, in three different schools. Each class was
divided into four equal teams by different test series, arranged
so as to be representative of the many different kinds of
mental processes involved in memory such as logical associations, reproduction of meaning, verbal and spatial associations,
etc., and immediate and delayed recall were taken into account.
The division into four groups of the same average mark
constituted the first cross-section. One group had no special
training, but the other groups were practised as follows :
group 2 learnt poetry by heart ; group 3 learnt ' tables ' of
various sorts ; group 4 were trained intensively to reproduce
the meaning of prose passages. Unfortunately neither in
the preliminary tests nor in the practice was any distinction
drawn between the habit factor and the memory factor, and
as we have previously seen it is unreasonable to expect a
training in learning ' tables ' to influence the ability to reproduce meanings. At the end of six weeks a second cross-section
was taken, each trained group having been treated similarly
in all respects as regards the technique of training. The conclusion of the whole matter was that there was nothing in the
final cross-section to warrant the assumption of a general
memory training as the result of specific practice. The effects

of ' direct ' practice, as might have been expected, were found to be incomparably greater than the effects of 'indirect' practice and the latter did not last much beyond the period of practice. Six weeks, however, is not a very great time to influence general memory capacity. and the failure to discriminate between memory and habit makes the conclusions of doubtful value. The appended table shews a few of the results, and in interpreting the numbers it must be remembered that no figure is significant unless it is at least three times as great as the probable error.

TABLE SHEWING IMPROVEMENT AND RETROGRESSION OF THE FINAL CROSS-SECTION COMPARED WITH THE FIRST CROSS-SECTION

(in units of standard deviation)

		Increased marks	Superiority of trained groups	Probable error
In learning poetry Group	1	42	—	13
	2	11	−31	14
	3	32	−10	14
	4	42	0	14
In learning prose Group	1	37	—	7
(literal production)	2	24	−13	8
	3	32	−5	8
	4	59	21	8

Experiments have been performed to try the effect of practising to discriminate shades of one colour on the subsequent ability to discriminate between shades of another colour ; and a clear transfer effect was shewn.

Practice in memorising the order of intensities of tuning-fork notes was shewn by one observer to produce transfer effects in memorising the order of shades of grey, other series of tones, poetry, etc. ; the effect being more marked in those cases where the test and practice series were similar in form.

Professors Thorndike and Woodworth made a variety of

experiments to find out whether there was any transfer effect
of training in estimating areas, lengths and weights of various
shapes and size, upon the ability to estimate areas, lengths
and weights, similar in shape but different in size ; different
in shape but similar in size ; and different in shape and size.
Also, they tried to discover the influence of training in various
forms of observation or perception upon slightly different
forms.   They found that practice in estimating the areas of
rectangles from 10 to 100 square cms. resulted in a marked
improvement.   The improvement for areas of the same size
but different shapes was 44 per cent. as great ; for areas of
the same shape but larger, the improvement was only 30 per
cent. as much.   For areas of different shape and different
size the improvement was 52 per cent. as great.   Training in
estimating weights from 40 to 120 grams produced only 39 per
cent. as much improvement in estimating weights from 120
to 1800 grams ; whilst training in estimating lines from ·5 to
1·5 inches long (resulting in a reduction of error of 25 per cent.
of the original amount) produced no improvement in the
estimation of lines 6 to 12 inches long.   Training in perceiving
words containing e and s yielded an improvement in the speed
of perception of other letters of 39 per cent. as much as in the
ability specially trained, but an improvement in accuracy of
only 25 per cent. as much.   Training in perceiving English
verbs yielded a reduction in time of nearly 21 per cent., and
in omissions of 70 per cent. ; whereas the transferred effect in
perceiving other parts of speech shewed a reduction in time of
3 per cent., but an increase in omissions of over 100 per cent.

The general inference drawn by these observers may be
given in their own words since it dominated educational
thought on the subject and is still widely accepted.   " Improvement in any single mental function need not improve
the ability in functions commonly called by the same name.
It may injure it.   Improvement in any single mental function

rarely brings about equal improvement in any other function, no matter how similar, for the working of every mental function-group is conditioned by the nature of the data in each particular case." They concluded further, that as there was some loss of function even with a very slight change in the material, and as this loss became greater the more unlike the material became, it is " fair to infer that there is always a point where the loss is complete."

Such a conclusion is very risky, unless it is assumed that a mental act is always a mathematical function of its object ; and even then the inference is not certain, as two values may approach each other asymptotically.

Results similar to those just considered have been found by other investigators.[9] Elementary school children were practised in multiplying numbers in their heads, whilst the first and second cross-sections were taken by means of standardised arithmetic tests, cancellation tests, learning vocabularies, etc. The second cross-section of the practised group, compared with equivalent control groups, shewed that the transferred effect was greatest in functions most closely related in content, and in functions where certain points of procedure were emphasised which were the same in the training series as in the test series. The gain from practice did not spread much to functions having little in common with the training either in content or procedure.

Another set of school children were trained to read paragraphs rapidly, and immediately afterwards to answer questions on what has been read, whereas the test material consisted of certain standardised reading tests and tests on the rapidity of perception of words, figures, etc. As before, the amount of transferred effect was small and depended on the similarity of the material and the method of scoring. Some of the transferred effect was due to better technique on the part of the pupils in dealing with tests, such as starting promptly, suppressing excitement, learning to reply under test conditions, etc. Hence it has been suggested that in future experiments the untrained control group should have practice in dealing with neutral tests, in order to make the comparison fair. It ought to be added that in the last two investigations just cited the practice periods were not more than two or three weeks ; a most inadequate period on which to base conclusions.

The present writer measured the individual variability of each of 17 adult subjects in the estimation of the length of a horizontal line, and of a vertical line, each of 12 cms. length. As a result of daily practice for a week in estimating the length of the horizontal line the average variability decreased by 36 per cent. No practice was given with the vertical line, nevertheless the average variability decreased by 34 per cent. of which it was calculated that about 14 per cent. was due to direct practice in the first test. This appears to shew a certain degree of transferred effect, although a week is not a very long period in which to display it adequately.

The improvement of adult students in drawing various objects and pictures has been roughly calculated, and the experimenter asserts that much practice did not make the subjects better observers in general or give them better habits of observing accurately.

Other observers [10] used as their practice material a code of simple geometrical forms. The principle of the code was explained to a group of students who, having learnt it, proceeded to transcribe prose passages into code symbols using their mental image as the key. For eleven days the group were practised for five minutes twice a day. The test series consisted of five different substitution tests, such as transcribing digits into code symbols, or substituting digits for letters, etc. One of the tests was the reverse of the practice material, consisting in transcribing code sentences into ordinary script.

These tests and similar ones were given before and after the eleven days' practice both to this group and to a control group of students. By a lucky chance the preliminary tests shewed that the experimenters were dealing with equivalent groups, though no precautions had been taken in the matter.

The average number of letters transcribed in the first five minutes by the practised group was 43 and the average of the highest records made during the practice was 239—a gain of 537 per cent. The common average of both groups in the preliminary test series were calculated ; and the gains in the final test series of the practised over the control groups were found, using the initial common average as the starting-point. For two of the tests there was either no gain or a negative result, whilst the other three tests shewed a gain of 5, 9 and 15 per cent. These percentages yield no evidence in support of a transfer of the effect of training. It is interesting to note that the figures shewed a negative correlation between the absolute gains in code practice, and the gains in the reverse process referred to above, indicating some interference between them.

An attempt has been made to discover whether the method of learning used during the practice period makes any difference to the transferred effects.[11] For this purpose a simple code was constructed in which all the letters were represented by the figures 1 and 2, and was built up on a definite, simple plan. One group of students had the letters in irregular order, and code figures before them whilst writing, but did not know the plan, nor indeed that there was any plan. The other group had the plan explained to them and memorised it, transcribing from the memory of the structure. Both groups were practised for 20 minutes daily for 12 days in transcription. It is evident that one group had a mechanical task, requiring little intellectual effort ; and the other a more rational task to perform, demanding concentrated attention.

Each group had a preliminary test, the mechanical group

in transcribing letters into digits and the rational in transcribing letters into a code. Similar tests were given at the end of the practice period. The mechanical group shewed a gain of 32 per cent. in the number of letters transcribed after practice, the other group gained 52 per cent. Control experiments, by two different sets of students, shewed that the gain due to practice by the tests themselves could be estimated at roughly 25 per cent. and 35 per cent. respectively for the two groups ; leaving a net gain of 7 per cent. (32—25) and 17 per cent. (52—35) unaccounted for. These results were interpreted to mean that a rational method of learning, which involves the higher mental processes to a greater degree, and demands greater concentration, yields a more definite transfer effect of training. It is unjustifiable, however, to subtract percentages in this way, and apparently there was no attempt to secure equivalent ability groups either in the experiment itself or in the control experiment. Strictly speaking, all four groups should have been of equal initial ability.

There is one obvious objection that may be taken to the experiments described up to this point. All pronounced mental change is subject to a law of inertia in that the results are not immediately apparent, but take time to manifest themselves. By this is meant not only the obvious fact that time is required for practice but also, and more important still, that time is wanted in the intervals of practice and subsequently in order that the effects of training may be displayed. During such intervals some change is going on in the unconscious mind whereby a better organisation of our experiences is assured and they are more firmly knit into the fabric of our mental life. This is true of bodily equally with mental activities so that, as it has been well said, we learn to skate in the summer and to swim in the winter. The results of effective training cannot be forced.

Again, objection has been urged against the artificiality of the experiments on the ground that the persons, however well inclined, take only a passing interest in the matter, and so the effects of the special training are sure to be negligible. It has been rightly insisted that in order to demonstrate the results of education we should try to evaluate the effects which are produced by the actual studies carried on in the schoolroom in a normal fashion instead of substituting artificial tasks under laboratory conditions. There is much force in these criticisms and an attempt to meet them has been made by Professor Thorndike, who is again to the front in these researches, by an elaborate statistical investigation.[12] He examined over eight thousand pupils in high schools in different towns, apparently between the ages of fifteen to eighteen. The first cross-section was taken by the teachers and consisted of a series of composite tests of intelligence of various kinds chiefly aimed at measuring the abilities employed in language and mathematics, but not confined to these. The final cross-section was taken by similar tests exactly one year later, so as to discover the difference made by a year's ordinary schooling in the abilities examined by the tests. In order to eliminate the differences of practice value of the tests themselves, certain schools employed the tests in their final cross-section which were used in taking the first cross-section in other schools and *vice versa*. A record was made of the school subjects studied by the pupils and the gains made in the test were put into relation with the subjects studied. Thus the pupils who studied English, history, geometry and Latin (say) were compared with those who normally studied English, history, geometry and shop-work. " If other factors . . . are properly equalised or allowed for, the difference in gain represents the difference between Latin and shop-work, as taught in these schools, in general training or disciplinary value."

The list of subjects studied by the pupils would appal any but an American teacher as they ranged over modern

M

drama, community civics, algebra, Greek, horticulture and radio (whatever this last may mean)! We learn also, to our dismay, that amongst a thousand pupils in one town there were over seven hundred different programmes of work. However, when we have recovered from all this we find that the average gain in marks in the tests for the year was 23 (these marks being standardised so as to be of equal value at all points of the scale) of which it was estimated that about 12 were due to special practice in the tests, leaving 11 as the gain due to maturity and the disciplinary effect of the year's schooling. Seeing that there was a greater gain by the bare practice of taking the tests once than was due both to maturity and training combined these figures gave little positive support to the doctrine of transferred effects. The final result shewed that there was a positive relation between the presence of French or Chemistry in a pupil's programme and gain in the tests, and a negative relation between the presence of cooking and sewing in a pupil's programme and gain in the tests. Some subjects such as Spanish and English shewed neither gain nor loss. To the positive side also belong trigonometry, physics, Latin, mathematics and history, in the order given ; and to the negative side, drawing, business, civics, biology, stenography and economics in decreasing order to merit. It is gratifying to learn that it is bad to learn stenography and business in school ; and economics and civics are also not above suspicion, if these statistical results are of any value. Though why English should have no effect at all is difficult to fathom unless the secret lies in the way in which it was taught in these schools.

INTERPRETATION OF THE EXPERIMENTS

It is now time to make some attempt to evaluate the evidence, which at first sight appears to be very conflicting. The currently accepted doctrine concerning the indirect effects of training is based on the following analysis. Both the test series and the practice series are believed to contain common elements of form or material or both and these common elements may be called objective identities. There can also be identity of procedure or attitude in coping with the various problems, by which is meant an identity in the methods or technique employed in learning, in dispositions, modes of directing the attention or utilising rhythm, control of mental imagery and so forth. In contrast with the former identities these may be distinguished as subjective identities, being more or less under the subject's control.

Now it has been asserted repeatedly that, in all experimental cases where transference of the effects of training has been found to take place, an essential condition is the occurrence of identical elements of one or both categories, which the subject makes use of consciously or unwittingly. In the experiments on memorising, estimating lengths, using codes and the like the identical objective factors are said to be obvious. The curious cases of transference of effects in discriminating colours as a result of training in distinguishing musical tones, etc. are said to be explicable by the presence of identical subjective factors, such as better modes of directing the attention or avoiding distractions. But whilst common factors are a necessary condition they are not by themselves sufficient ; for it is argued that the common elements must be separable from the complexes in which they occur if transfer of effects is to take place. As this process of disintegration can never be complete there must always be some loss in the transferred effect, as was indeed noticed in many of the experimental results previously considered. Some observers have pointed out that certain common factors tend to facilitate the acquisition of a new activity whilst others interfere with it, and any transference is due to a balance between them.

A modified form of the identity theory is a refinement of the view of facilitation and interference.[13] Improvement in any mode of activity is considered to be due to the selection and weeding out of elemental abilities. When a new form of activity is undertaken the so-called elemental abilities are regrouped. In so far as the individual recognises the similarity or partial identity between the two activities the elimination of the unnecessary elementary abilities and the regrouping of the others is more likely to occur. The analogy of a football side is used to explain this where improved play may be due to greater unity of action. If a new team is constituted with a proportion of players from the old team, there will only be transfer of the improvement provided that the new side shakes down into good team work.

On the whole the accepted view amongst experimenters is that identical subjective factors play the more important part, and these being given, differences in the material are of relatively little significance in hindering the transferred effect, which may take place in spite of great objective differences. The importance of the subjective factors has been well illustrated in an investigation on school children conducted by Professor Judd. Two groups of boys were dealt with, and one was given a theoretical explanation of the refraction of light whilst the other was left ignorant of the principle. The groups were practised in aiming with a dart at a target, seen at an angle, under twelve inches of water ; and both groups did equally well. Theoretical knowledge of the law of refraction did not seem to be a substitute for the necessary practical skill. Then the conditions were changed and the depth of the water was reduced from twelve to four inches. A marked difference was now manifested, for the boys who were ignorant of the principle of refraction were not aided much in coping with the new situation by their previously acquired practical skill. On the other hand, the boys who knew the principle fitted themselves to the new conditions very rapidly. The subjective control of their movements, made possible by their theoretical knowledge, helped to secure effective transfer of the effects of training. It will be remembered that similar results were obtained in the previously quoted experiments on the different methods of learning. For where a rational procedure was employed there was more evidence of transference. This provides experimental evidence, if that were necessary, that rule of thumb methods are devoid of general educative value.

There is one function which is common to all mental processes, however different. In considering such activities as remembering, imagining, perceiving, reasoning and the like it is popularly supposed that the mental activities are diverse whilst the objects referred to in the various acts are the same. But there is no ground for believing in diverse kinds of mental activity ; on the contrary when the supposed faculties are thought to be different it will always be found that there are differences in the nature of the objects apprehended.[14] The subjective activity involved is in all cases the same, namely, the act of attention. So that here we have, for what it is worth, a function which is common to all mental processes ; and it is impossible that any real training can take place without mental activity. No doubt facility of attention depends on the content attended to, and to that extent attention is specific. Experiments such as we have considered conducted for a period of days, weeks or even a year can hardly be expected to shew the influence of better adapted attention in yielding a better all round calibre of mind. At this point we seem to approach the limits of the experimental method in dealing with the problem of the permanent effects of education on general capacity, and we are compelled to fall back on the evidence of experience. It seems incredible that years of training with suitable intellectual material adapted at each stage to the interest and capacity of the pupil should fail to produce better all round capacity. Whether the results are measurable is another story, and the question is only confused by experiments if the attempt is made to estimate intellectual calibre without regard to subjective preference or interests.

But, if the experimental method has tended to narrow the issue unduly, the interpretation of the experimental results has made matters worse. All reference to common elements, factors and everything of that sort is psychological atavism of a particularly distressful kind. It is an attempt to breathe the breath of life into the dry bones of mental atomism. But these bones cannot live, for in place of a collection of disconnected elements somehow reduced to order by subsequent processes, a psychology which knows its own business ought to assert that continuity and form are present from the very beginning of conscious life. The whole argument of this book up to the present chapter has been a prolonged protest against the attempt to deal with ideas, images, sensations, etc. as though they consisted of isolated bits of mental furniture. Our conception of the continuity of the mental stream is equally valid for movements and it is erroneous to suppose that a bodily habit, for instance, can be formed by the union of previously disconnected movements. No amount of " shaking down into team work" can account for the unity of action observable in a habit if we suppose that the movements were originally disconnected.

NEW EVIDENCE AND DIFFERENT INTERPRETATIONS

The whole question of the effects of training has been given a new turn by the researches of the *Gestalt* psychologists. It is rightly assumed by this school that a psychological or experienced whole is something more than a mere sum of its parts ; in fact it may even stand in opposition to some of its parts. Thus an ape soon learns to secure a banana out of his reach, beyond the bars of his cage, by dragging it to himself with a stick. If, now, the food is placed in view of the ape in a drawer, with one of its sides missing, so placed that the open side is farthest from the bars of the cage, the animal tries to drag the food towards itself, but is prevented by the back of the drawer. Professor Köhler, who has observed the phenomenon very carefully, noticed that the more intelligent apes, after groping vainly for some time, *suddenly* changed their tactics, and pushed the food away from themselves out of the drawer and then round it towards themselves, in a smooth continuous curve.[15] The less intelligent animals required the drawer to be turned, so that the open end pointed more or less to the side, before they could grasp the situation. That ' part ' of the solution of the problem, which consists in pushing the food away, is not only in conflict with the instincts and previous training of the animal, but, regarded *by itself*, is in opposition to the problem of securing the food. We must abandon the notion of separate elements or parts, and in order to understand behaviour in which ends are attained indirectly, by making detours which in themselves are in conflict with the ends sought, we must assume that the whole situation has a certain configuration or shape. The solution of the problem only occurs when insight into the configuration is possible. It is usual to talk of a flash of insight and rightly so, for it has been shewn repeatedly that a true solution is always a sudden phenomenon sharply contrasted with the blind groping due to trial and error. The more one contemplates it the more one realises that the situation of the ape with the stick and the desired prize resembles that of a man with a pencil and a problem to be solved.

When the open side of the drawer in the above experiments is farthest away from the bars of the cage its position with respect to the body of the animal may be described as 180°, but some of the apes do not achieve insight into the configuration unless the open side is turned more towards the body, i.e.

into the position 135° or even 90°. Now it was found that, if the animal succeeds in solving the problem in one of the easier positions, it will subsequently transfer the solution to the more difficult position. One of the less intelligent apes proved quite unable to secure the food either in the position 180° or 135° but was successful at 90°. Immediately afterwards, when the position 135° was again tried, it achieved a prompt solution, and after that a solution at 180°. A month later an unhesitating solution was accomplished at 180° at the very first trial. The interest in securing food, especially bananas, is no doubt a very powerful motive for these animals, sharpening their insight into the problem. But, unless we assume that schoolboys have less wit than apes, it would be a sad confession of impotence to believe that there can be no course of study sufficiently tempting to enable them to attain insight into situations other than those in which they are trained. Possibly the absence of general capacity which used to be so much deplored may be due to a lack of interest in school studies, so that the effects of school training depend to a great extent on stimulating interest in what is learnt. Bacon was not so far out when he asserted that 'impediments in the wit may be wrought out by fit studies,' but only on the condition that we interpret 'fit' to mean those that are fitted to appeal to the interest or aspiration of the pupils.

Just as a melody is something more than a mere series of notes, or a sentence something different from a mere collection of words, so a problem is a different thing from the parts or elements into which it may be analysed ; it is a unitary whole. When a person or an animal learns to respond to a given situation, what determines his behaviour cannot be regarded as the elements of the situation but must be viewed as insight into the meaning of the configuration as an integral whole. Professor Köhler has indeed changed the whole problem by demonstrating the fact that insight into the relations within a configuration is the only means of securing effective general training.

The experiments which he has devised are extremely simple in their application. An animal is confronted with two stimuli and is trained to seek food with respect to one of them. Let us call the stimulus which the animal seeks the ' positive ' and the one which he is trained to ignore the ' negative.' The animal is taught, let us say, to select the brighter of two greys, which may be easily done by placing equal quantities of food on two adjacent papers of these colours ; and if he chooses the positive colour he is allowed to eat, if not he is chased away. The procedure is carried out, as long as necessary, with the colours in different positions until the animal unhesitatingly chooses the positive colour. This constitutes our old practice series. When the training has been brought to a successful issue a test series is given. This time the ' positive ' colour is retained, but the ' negative ' is replaced by a grey which is brighter than the positive of the test series, and which may be called ' neutral ' since it has not appeared in the training series at all.

On the view that considers that transfer of the effects of training takes place in response to identical elements or factors in the new situation we should expect the animal to choose the positive colour, as nothing can be more identical with itself than the same colour.

But four stupid hens observed by Professor Köhler refused to lend support to the theory as they chose the neutral tint in fifty-nine tests out of eighty-five. Our intelligent friends the apes chose a neutral-coloured box containing food practically every time ; and a child who had been trained to select a certain positive box containing sweets without making any false selection, a couple of days later invariably and unhesitatingly chose the neutral box. Educational psychologists unlike the child and the clever animals have chosen the identical elements in the training and test series in order to account for the cases of transference of the effects of training : whereas, these experiments demonstrate that the choice is determined by the configuration or pattern of the situation, the animals responding to the relations between the colours in any particular situation.   Obviously, they have acquired insight into the relations of a perceived situation and this enables them to cope with a new situation, in which they definitely *avoid* the identical element and respond to the configuration.   It is as though they recognise that the melody is the same though some of the notes are different.   Hence we may infer that unless a task is carried out with insight into the configuration as a whole, the effects of training cannot be transferred. Otherwise the theory of mental discipline is sound enough, for the relations are universal and insight into them places the individual at a standpoint from which he can view a new situation much more readily.   We see also that training which consists of mere practice, however prolonged, is not discipline, for the latter implies understanding.   Very valuable indirect confirmation in support of the view here taken has been provided by experiments on the establishment of conditioned reflexes.   Professor Pavlov [16] trained animals to respond with fully formed reactions to previously inadequate stimuli. His experiments led him to the conclusion that " any stimulus, after it had become a conditioned stimulus, *was generalised—* that is to say, the conditioned reaction was provoked not only by the specially chosen stimulus, *but by any other of the same type* " (italics mine).   If dogs and mice can respond to a generalised situation it is preposterous to assert that this is impossible in the case of human beings.

IDEALS

An important consideration has yet to be dealt with. In all mental states the material employed in exercising the activity can be considered from the point of view of its worth or value to the person. Experiments have been tried to discover whether the habit of producing neat work in one school subject, say arithmetic, will result in an improvement in the neatness by the scholars in other school subjects, e.g. language or spelling papers. Although a great improvement was shewn in the arithmetic papers " the results were almost startling in their failure to shew the slightest improvement in language and spelling papers." Another observer, however, by carefully cultivating a special regard for neatness on the part of the children and enlisting their regard for its value, found that improvement was shewn in directions other than the one especially trained.

A review of the evidence which has now been presented leads us to realise that the whole problem of the effects of training must be viewed from a different angle. We must turn from the sphere of psychology to the realm of ends. For, if immediate results are aimed at, without considering the ultimate aim of education, it is possible to acquire a high degree of particular skill without affecting general capacity. Where, on the other hand, an ideal is consciously pursued a motive is at work which is capable of changing the whole mental outlook, since it is of the nature of an ideal to engender a ' divine discontent ' with whatever falls short of it. To revert to our original example, a training in mathematics may produce exactness of thought in other departments of intellectual work, and a love of truth, provided that the training is of such a kind as to inculcate an ideal which the pupil values and strives to attain. Failing this, Glaucon's observation that he had " hardly ever known a mathematician who was capable of reasoning " is likely to be repeated.[17] In order to justify the universal tradition which decrees that everybody should be taught mathematics, modern mathematicians are taking the line that the Greek view of the object of such study is the correct one, namely, " to make more easy the vision of the idea of good." As an eminent authority has well said, " Every great study is not only an end in itself, but also a means of creating and sustaining a lofty habit of mind : and this purpose should be kept always in view throughout the teaching and learning of mathematics." [18]

The following remarks made by a man who left the University and shortly afterwards was engaged as a missionary in the remote parts of Southern India, illuminate this point of view.[19] " I entirely agree that Cambridge ought to provide us with learning, practical ability and character. Now Cambridge entirely failed to give me anything directly useful for my work. I learnt, for example, nothing whatever about South Indian devil-worship and demoniac possession ; and of the many things which I did learn, hardly one is of any direct service. . . . And yet I have not a shadow of ill-feeling towards the University. . . . It is true that the learning supplied by Cambridge is here almost useless. The knowledge of Greek may have no commercial value to a missionary ; and yet the learning of Greek must have had a share in producing a frame of mind which finds pleasure and satisfaction in mastering the intricacies of a language whose vocabulary is as large as that of Greek, and whose construction is as idiomatic as that of French. It is true that practical ability is not greatly fostered by the Secretaryship of many Cambridge societies. But after all, the ultimate problems of organisation are concerned much more with men than with figures and diagrams." These pertinent observations help us to realise that there are other ways than experiment and statistics of evaluating the effects of education.

All roads thus converge to the same point and it is evident that the ultimate aim of effective training is a moral one consisting in loyalty to ideals. A training which is confined solely to loyalty to an institution will not necessarily lead to moral conduct. The love of a school because it is ours or because it has a fine tradition and a long history is no doubt a stage in moral growth ; but only the first stage. If it stops at this point the training is of limited value. The idea of honour which is based on the approval or disapproval of a particular group of persons is not necessarily a sound basis for moral conduct. Co-operation in games and playing for one's side may indeed produce ideals of altruism and self-sacrifice in later years, but solely on the condition that the general tone of the school is sufficiently sound to make the pupils prize these as of exceeding worth. The motive must be religious, or, at all events, rest on the conception of honour for honour's sake if it is to affect a person's whole outlook. By this means alone does 'playing the game' constitute a sound preparation for playing the game of living. If the ethos of the school is not in harmony with these ideals very good team work is not incompatible with a subsequent narrow selfish outlook on life.

CHAPTER VIII

SUGGESTION

The Nature of Suggestion—Influence of Preperception—The Personal
Factor—Mental Content in Suggestion—Method and Suggestion

THE NATURE OF SUGGESTION

THE term suggestion is used with very different connotations
in different contexts. Perhaps the most frequent use in
ordinary discourse as opposed to psychological or medical
discussion is in the sense of stimulating ideas. Any book
which stimulates reflection along the lines laid down by the
author or kindred lines is said to be suggestive ; and in a
similar manner a suggestive teacher is one who arouses reflection on definite lines by making certain particular directions of
thought appear interesting or likely to lead to that which is
interesting. In such cases the author or teacher conveys the
impression that he has touched only the fringe of the subject
or has given a bare hint of possibilities. The essential feature
of this use of the term appears to be that the process of association goes on smoothly and unwittingly along novel paths
without appreciable effort on the part of the person suggested.
New lines of association are, as it were, opened up or new
points of view indicated which would not have occurred to the
person if left to himself, but which occur unwittingly and seem
luminously clear when the initial impulse is given by another
person. In this case the ideas aroused in the subject's mind
are, of course, his own, and he is exerting his own mental

activity though he would not have done so but for the suggestions given by the teacher.

When, however, the ideas themselves are introduced by
another person and their energy is not dependent on the subject's own activity we are approaching the region of abnormal,
or, at all events, of hypnotic suggestion. In this latter sense
suggestion has been defined as " the intrusion into the mind of
an idea ; met with more or less opposition by the person ;
accepted uncritically at last ; and realised unreflectively,
almost mechanically." [1] The point of contact between these
two different meanings of the term lies in the fact that the
impulse to activity or belief is insinuated by another person.
It is important to observe that the first of the two meanings
indicated above, i.e. the popular use of the term expresses
the more fundamental idea of the phenomenon of suggestion,
and the latter or medical use is an artificial one which tends to
obscure the nature of the process. Perhaps the common
meaning is best brought out by Dr Rivers' definition of the
word suggestion as " a comprehensive term for the whole
process whereby one mind acts on another unwittingly."
The latter meaning is then a specialised and artificial variety
of the general process of suggestion, the artificiality lying in
the witting use of a process which normally occurs unwittingly. [2]
For educational discussion the former meaning is the all
important one, but the latter is not to be neglected since there
are regions of conduct or belief in the moral world where
suggestion of the latter kind is educationally not only justifiable, but the most effective procedure to adopt. This is
happily illustrated by the saying attributed to Pascal that men
do not go to church because they are religious, but that they
are religious because they go to church. Nevertheless honour,
duty, loyalty, etc. may be cultivated by suggestions received
from those around us who are honourable and loyal and whose
example is infinitely more potent than any direct teaching can be.

Much of our knowledge of suggestion is derived from a study of abnormal suggestibility as illustrated by cases of hypnotic suggestion. Hypnosis is a drowsy or semi-drowsy state brought about by bodily relaxation and stillness accompanied by the fixation of attention on some monotonous sight or sound such as the ticking of a clock or a light. Now it is believed that in addition to the normal waking self every person, normal or abnormal, has a sub-waking or secondary self sensitive to external impressions. In normal waking life the two selves are so completely co-ordinated as almost to blend into one, and the relation between them has been well compared with that of a broad stream in which there flows a current, with no fixed line of separation.

The hypnotic state is distinguished by the fact of dissociation, by which is meant that the secondary self is cut off more or less completely from the waking or primary self. When the person wakes from the state of hypnosis there is complete amnesia for the suggestions made to him in that condition, until the time comes to carry them out, when he acts in accordance with them without realising their origin ; and is under the impression that he is acting without constraint. If then he is challenged to give a reason for his action he will usually invent one which makes his act more plausible to himself ; in other words he tries to rationalise his conduct. Conversely in the hypnotic state there is amnesia for the events in the waking state, but a memory of the ideas or suggestions previously experienced during hypnosis. There are, as it were, two disaggregated streams of mental life each carrying its own memory. Now, when a person is hypnotised, i.e. when the control of his critical waking self is removed by causing dissociation, any suggestion made to him may be carried out in the subsequent waking condition provided that it is given emphatically, and repeated. The more direct the suggestion is made the better, and as the suggestions are received uncritically and carried out literally any indirectness in the command will militate against the proper effect of the suggestion. These observations have been summarised in a so-called law of suggestibility, namely, that abnormal or hypnotic suggestibility varies as direct suggestion and inversely as indirect suggestion. In contrast with this an attempt has been made by Dr Sidis to prove that in the waking state the effectiveness of a suggestion depends on its indirectness; so that normal suggestibility varies as indirect suggestion and inversely as direct suggestion. The method adopted to arrive at this law was to exhibit to the persons certain series of letters or figures one at a time arranged in various ways, or to shew series of coloured cards of various shapes or positions. Immediately after the exposure of a complete series the person was required to write down whatever letter, figure or colour, according to the material used, occurred to his mind. By the arrangement, position or frequency of the letters or figures and the more or less abnormal position of the coloured cards or the surroundings it was hoped to influence the subject's choice in definite directions. Sometimes a colour or a letter was verbally suggested whilst the subject was being shewn the objects. It was found that the more the person realised that his choice was being determined, and this was especially the case with verbal suggestions, the more opposition was aroused so that the choice was contra-determined by the suggestion; hence the above rule.

The experiments, however, are not very convincing and common experience, apparently, shews that for the great majority of normal people direct and repeated suggestion is effective. How otherwise could the spread of advertising be accounted for? The purpose of an advertisement is to influence choice or belief uncritically. This is sometimes veiled by more or less ingenious attempts to present the advertiser's reasons in a plausible form. Yet the suggestion

N

to buy is followed by large numbers of people who are perfectly well aware that the advertisement is designed to produce
belief without critical thought. Thus, although normal
persons appear to be suggestible in any sphere of conduct or
belief in the inverse ratio of their knowledge, the rule is by no
means absolute. The utility of a transport company, for
example, ought to be estimated by the comfort and convenience of the travellers, but they usually attract travellers
successfully by publishing statistics of the large numbers who
travel daily, though the larger the numbers the less the
comfort of those who make use of the facilities. The common
" cold in the head " is the result of inflammation produced by
foul air leading to congestion of the mucous membrane and
may be alleviated by a current of fresh air ; yet the vast
majority of people avoid a draught because they are repeatedly
told that this will bring a ' cold,' though the only method by
which a current of cool air in a warm room can produce a
' cold ' is by suggestion. Professor L. Hill the most competent
authority on the subject has given the opinion that " A very
great influence for ill acting on the health and stamina of
children is the belief, current among all classes, traditionally
handed down by grannies and mothers, and still taught in
the advice given by many, if not most, medical practitioners,
that exposure to cold is the great cause of illness. This
belief leads to over-clothing and confinement indoors, over-
coddling and debility of body, and weakening of nervous
strength and stability."

THE INFLUENCE OF PREPERCEPTION

In the chapter on *observation* the influence of preperception
in determining our present thinking was described in detail
and the section should be read again at this point. It is shewn
there that our present perceptions and ideas are determined to

a considerable extent by expectation founded on our past experience. Binet [3] has made a special study of the influence of expectation by experiments on school children, and has thereby added to our knowledge of the process of normal suggestibility. His procedure consisted of arousing a preconception in the mind of the individual scholar, with as little personal influence as possible, so that the idea was apparently auto-suggested. In other words, the scholars developed an idea as a result of their experiences which was then applied to later perceptions where it did not fit. Such preconceived ideas which function more or less automatically in later perceptions are called by Binet directing ideas. He found that some scholars, and later observers have noted the same phenomenon in adults, behave like automata ; they act in accordance with the directing idea constantly without variation, whilst others who are also suggestible are not automatic, sometimes carrying out the idea and sometimes refraining.

It is, of course, obvious that all critical thought involves directing ideas by means of which the reflection is guided. The difference between critical thought and belief and suggested ideas or actions lies, not in the presence of directing ideas but in their origin, and also in the fact that in the latter case the directing ideas are dissociated from the main stream of consciousness, forming part of the sub-waking self.

Suppose a series of lines of the following length namely, 12, 24, 36, 48, 60 mms. are drawn vertically, side by side, at about one centimetre apart. Anybody looking at the series will immediately get the impression that the tops of the lines are growing in length at a uniform rate. It makes no difference to the impression of uniform growth whether the lines are exhibited simultaneously or one after the other at short intervals of time. Now Binet shewed such a series of lines successively followed by about twenty or thirty others all of the length of the last line, i.e. 60 mms. The children experi-

mented upon were asked to indicate by means of dots on a
sheet of squared paper, drawn at appropriate heights above a
base line, the length of each immediately after it was shewn.
Nothing was said about the lengths of the lines except that
they were to observe carefully and shew the lengths that
were exhibited as exactly as possible, and they were warned
that some people went wrong and mistook the lengths shewn.
Despite this warning, the great majority of the subjects
continued to make the lines increase after the fifth, when in
actual fact all the rest were of the same length. The idea
given by the first five that there is a regular increase of length
through the whole series becomes a directing idea against
which most of the subjects struggle in vain. Subsequent
investigation has proved that suggestibility as shewn by
this method decreases in a regular manner between the
ages of seven and twelve. Some children, indeed, especially
young children and mentally defectives, continue to make
the lines increase through the whole series. With the majority,
however, there is a continual struggle between the directing
suggested idea of increase and critical judgment as shewn by
the effort to draw what is actually seen. Examination of the
individual performances demonstrates that children belong to
different types and it is interesting to observe that the author
of this book experimenting in the same fashion found these
same types amongst University graduates.

Very few subjects resist the suggestion altogether, i.e.
one or more lines after the fifth continue to shew an increase.
Some progress in length for several lines after the fifth, and
then brusquely recover and throw off all suggestion in all the
subsequent lines. Others correct themselves after acting on the
suggestion for some time but the corrections are not as great
in value as the subsequent increases, i.e. the suggestion continues to act and correction is constantly made, but critical
thought is too weak to counterbalance the suggestive effects,

so that on the whole there is an increase in length till the end. A third type carry out the suggestion till the end of the series without correction, but the increments get smaller after a certain point. It is as though the suggestion had a certain momentum which it steadily loses, but there is no sudden recovery as in the case of the first type. The fourth or automatic type carry out the suggestion all through the series without correction, the increments being the same all through so that there is a steady and regular increase of length from the first to the last line exactly in accordance with the original model of the first five lines. But the most interesting group and the most frequent is that which may be called the rhythmical type. Just as with the first type these subjects brusquely correct themselves after carrying out the suggestion for a short time, but they immediately act on the suggestion again and then correct themselves and so on until the end. Here there is a constant alternation between automatic action and critical thought but unlike the second type there is no increase of length, but a sort of hovering round an average length. As was said above this is the most frequently occurring type of normal suggestibility and most subjects shew a tendency towards such a mode of reaction even when they can be definitely assigned to one of the other groups. In short, suggestion follows the law of all living processes in being rhythmical. The periodicity of the rhythm varies from individual to individual but the results shew a continual alternation between automatic and critical response.

An experiment similar to the one described above on progressive lines has also been devised with progressive weights. A series of weights looking exactly alike is placed on a table and the pupils are instructed to lift each weight in turn to a certain height and to say whether it is heavier or lighter than or equal to the preceding weight. The series is as follows, namely 20, 40, 60, 80, 100 grams followed by a further eleven weights all of 100 grams each : and it will be observed that the first five regularly increase so that a directing idea of progression throughout the series is suggested. In some experiments the method was varied slightly and the weight of the first box was stated to be 20 grams and the pupils had to guess the weight of all the succeeding boxes.

The sixth box in the series was frequently said to be lighter than its predecessor owing to the fact that the pupils expected a heavier box and made too much effort in lifting it. Such a contrast between expectation and realisation is not uncommon in psychological work. But the notable feature to observe is that not only was the weight of the sixth box mistaken but the tenth and fifteenth were also frequently said to be lighter than their respective preceding boxes. This affords another instructive example of the rhythmical nature of mental activity for an expectation once made tends to recur at periods, though the reality offers no justification for it.

If we compare the two different methods with the weights it will be seen that the latter is more difficult ; for the subjects have to estimate the weights instead of merely deciding whether one is heavier than another. It was found that the pupils were more suggestible when dealing with the more difficult task. For the theory of education this is a point of fundamental importance, since if a suggestion is to be given to normal persons the more difficult the task on which they are engaged the better. In fact a casual suggestion made when the pupils are exerting their mental activity to the utmost in some other direction is much more likely to be effective than one made impressively when they are attending to it alone. The reason for this lies in the fact that by the former method dissociation is brought about, so that the suggested idea appears as though it were auto-suggested. Hence it is often useful to introduce suggestions casually whilst the pupils are intently engaged in their ordinary school work.

An important characteristic of action or belief due to suggestion is seen in carrying out experiments of the nature described above and is equally evident both with children and adults. In the case of the progressive series of lines it will be remembered that the subjects are not only told to draw what they see, but they are also warned that many go wrong. Nevertheless, it is found that nearly all subjects invent absurd reasons for their errors when these are pointed out to them. If they are pressed they will give two or three different explanations of their conduct, none of which has any relation to the real reason which prompted them. The obvious reason for continuing to make the progression is either that they cannot help themselves or that they were paying insufficient attention, but neither of these is ever adduced. This feature of the suggestible state is much more marked in hypnotic suggestion but is a constant character of normal suggestibility. Again, it must be remembered that some persons take a suggestion for emotional reasons and others from intellectual causes, but in neither case is the real ground for action known to the subject.

THE PERSONAL FACTOR

Experiments of the kind we have been discussing are apt to obscure what is perhaps the most important feature of suggestion namely the personal element, this being the real ultimate ground of all the phenomena. In many cases some object such as a diagram, a picture or written instructions convey suggestions which the subject carries out, and it is customary to contrast these as impersonal suggestions with the more personal examples in which the suggestion is given verbally or proceeds by imitation. Sometimes, too, the suggestion appears to come directly from the subject's sub-waking self. But in all these instances, i.e. both so-called impersonal and auto-suggestion the personal factor is opera-

tive though, it may be, indirectly ; and the only proper line
of division is between direct and indirect suggestion. Binet's
progressive lines and weights give rise to an apparently auto-
suggested directing idea solely because Binet himself has
arranged the conditions and he is ultimately responsible for
the suggestion. When any subject accepts the suggestion
given by the lines what is really influencing him is not the
objective figure but the fact that he consciously or unconsciously supposes that the experimenter has drawn the lines
with some purpose.

Where the personal factor is at a minimum or operates
through a set of pre-arranged conditions we may call the
suggestion indirect, whilst suggestions which are effective
primarily owing to the authority or prestige of the person may
be distinguished as direct. In the former case the personality
of the experimenter is more or less in the background, whilst
it is in the foreground in the latter. The chief difficulty
ordinarily encountered in making a direct suggestion lies in
the fact that it is apt to arouse opposition and result in contra-
suggestibility. This is the reason that often makes direct
moral training so ineffective with normal schoolboys. They
resent any direct interference with their established code of
conduct or their customary ideals, and consequently direct
instruction about loyalty, honour, courage and so forth is
either ignored or derided with some contemptuous term. Let
them, however, encounter examples of these as they occur in
their normal school life, or in their reading of literature or
history, or in some admired hero and the state of affairs is
immediately changed ; they are now ready to approve of
them with enthusiasm and adopt them as their own.

The conception of schoolboy honour referred to in the
preceding paragraph is largely the result of tradition, and has
been responsible for a good deal of harm. Custom prescribes
that a boy must never give information of anything occurring in

the school which affects another boy, even though the happening is something evil.   There are indications that some schoolmasters are dissatisfied with the results of this tradition and are determined to challenge it on moral grounds.   To do so requires much courage and it will only be possible where there is a strong mutual affection between the master and his boys so that he is really in *loco parentis* and the boys are perfectly frank with him.   The practical method of dealing with the situation by direct instruction has been so admirably expressed in a recent book[4] that a somewhat lengthy quotation is permissible.   It must be premised that the author is speaking as a preparatory school master, but there is no reason to suppose that a similar procedure is not equally applicable by any house-master.

After dealing with the paramount importance in all education of religious instruction he proceeds : " As soon as a boy has been in the school long enough for the Headmaster to feel certain he has gained his confidence and that he will talk to him freely and truthfully, he has his first serious talk with him.   The period varies, of course, but usually it would be during a boy's second term.   At this first talk—the first of many—the Headmaster lays the foundation of all his future training.   He must explain exactly what is meant by Truth, Honour and Unselfishness, and what their value is in life.   He must shew *why* one should be truthful, *why* unselfish, etc. ;   it is not enough merely to lay down the law.   For instance, it is easy to explain that our tendencies either get better or worse as we grow older.   If a boy is inclined to tell lies and he continues to do so, he will grow up a man whom people cannot trust and therefore will lose his chance of doing his real share in the world.   If, on the other hand he learns how to be truthful, he will grow up a person in whom people have confidence and he will therefore have great opportunities for doing real good in whatever path of life he adopts.   This sort of idea, if developed with further examples, will very soon shew a child that telling lies for the sake of a passing or apparent benefit is a very poor idea compared to all that hangs on the habit of truth. He must be shewn too, how closely allied are truth and beauty, and that beauty of spirit could not go side by side with falseness. It is so easy in such a talk to develop theme after theme which appeals to the child's natural love of beauty and idealism. Honour, being a comprehensive term, includes such things as purity of speech and action, decency and so on."

Now follows the break with tradition. The boy having been shewn that the tone and reputation of the school depends on the character of the pupils, he goes on : " Each boy must understand how his actions react for good or bad on someone else. Having made all this clear in much greater detail and at much greater length than it is possible to put on paper, the Master comes to the most difficult part of all. He explains to the boy that in most ways it is by his own example that he can help most, that if he and others succeed in bringing their characters up to the scratch, they are doing their job up to that point, simply by the force of example, than which there is nothing more infectious ; his friends will quite unconsciously do what he does in a great many ways ; it is the herd instinct. *But* he will point out, there is another way in which they can help more actively by direct co-operation with him. If ever there were an offence against Honour, for instance, if ever the boy heard another speaking or acting in a low or vulgar way or doing a mean or dishonourable action, he is expected to come and tell the Headmaster. The boy naturally hesitates, thinking that this would be sneaking. The Headmaster thereupon assures him that the last thing in the world he desires is sneaking and points out, for example, what ' sneaking ' is, namely, when one boy reports another and gets him into trouble. If this should happen the former would be sent about his business, and deservedly so. What he is suggesting, however, is a very different thing ; it applies to questions of Honour as explained—not to such matters as ordinary school rules, etc., and, *mark it well*, for this is the kernel of the whole thing—*there is no punishment*. In other words, if a bad thing, however elementary, happens in the school, it is an understood thing among all the boys that the Headmaster shall know—for one reason only, *in order that it may be put right."*

The author of this quotation is firmly convinced on the basis of his experience, that the healthy schoolboy responds to such direct training, and he hopes by converting others to his view eventually "to root out the bad old conception of school-boy Honour and to substitute something higher, nobler, more inspiring," which will react on the whole of life.

All, however, depends on the personality of the master and his ability to impress the boys by his sincerity so that they trust him absolutely. In order that instruction in such matters may be received with the minimum of opposition the person giving it must be endowed with sufficient prestige to keep contra-suggestibility within bounds. Prestige may depend partly on position, authority, athletic ability and so on ; but above all to be effective in moral training it requires transparent sincerity and conviction. Again, despite a popular belief to the contrary, schoolboys by no means despise learning if it is carried easily and accompanied by ability to control them, and a scholar possessed of this power carries much prestige, especially with older boys. Always the person as a whole is involved and anybody lacking in personality and powers of discipline, however well endowed with other qualities, is incapable of any suggestive or direct influence on his pupils.

To return to our experimental observations which may appear as an anti-climax after the above digression. A variant of the progressive-line experiment was included by Binet in his

' mental tests.'   Six pairs of lines each pair being drawn in the same straight line are shewn consecutively ; and, whilst in the first three pairs the right-hand line is always longer, in the last three it is of the same length as the left-hand line.   The child tested is asked which of the two lines is longer in each pair. As a mental test of intelligence this particular example is now regarded as practically worthless and in some versions of the mental tests is accordingly dropped out.   Dr Burt who applied this test to a large number of children, in schools of different status, noted the curious fact that such a test of suggestibility and indeed other tests of critical shrewdness were relatively easier for children of inferior social circum-stances.   He explains the difference thus : [5]   " The shrewd slum child unblushingly recognises that the examiner is setting a trap for him.   The child of nicer manners hardly entertains such a suspicion, and conscientiously searches for minute differences."   We must be on our guard against attributing to bare suggestion what is due to mere complaisance.   This was amusingly illustrated by a French child of seven to whom a series of colours were shewn by a foreign lady working under Binet's directions.   As each colour was displayed the child was asked to name it and afterwards to write the name ; the suggestion that it was some other colour was made verbally whilst the child was writing, and he apparently accepted the suggestion.   Later he said to his teacher, " That lady is not French, in her country the colours are not the same as ours."

MENTAL CONTENT IN SUGGESTION

So far we have considered the effects of suggestion in influencing action or belief.   But a more difficult problem arises when an attempt is made to investigate the suggestive consciousness itself.   This may be illustrated by a tale told by Rayleigh in his observations on lighthouses.   Tests were to be made on a new type of lighthouse lamp which was to be substituted for the old at a prearranged moment. Several observers were on board a yacht taking notes and each wrote down independently his impressions. Some thought the new lamp was an improvement, others thought it was the reverse. But when they got back to shore it was found that owing to some misunderstanding the change had never been made at all.[6] Now, did these Trinity House brethren on the yacht experience a change in sensation, or did their mental imagery intervene so that they ignored the sensation and reacted to the image, or finally was the effect purely motor, so that they responded automatically at the prearranged moment by writing in entire independence of their mental content ? The last of the three possibilities named would imply that suggestion is merely an automatic response in which the verbal suggestion can do the work of an adequate sensory stimulus.

It is obvious that it is only by the careful introspection of appropriately trained persons that we can hope to get some light on this question, and all discussion about suggestion in the absence of knowledge concerning the suggestible person's mental content is apt to be hazy. In some experiments to elucidate the point the subjects were University students or lecturers highly trained in introspective psychology and the work extended over a period of two years.[7] The observers were informed that a stimulus would be given and then followed by a second, and they were to report when they felt the latter ; or that a continually changing stimulus would be employed and they were to respond when they observed the change. In every case where a stimulus or a change of stimulus was employed its intensity was supraliminal, but the suggestions always ran counter to the actual stimuli employed. The kind of stimulus or change will best be appreciated by a couple of examples. A series of ten balls were dropped successively from a height and the observer had to state whether he heard the noise of the fall in each case.   Eight of the balls were of lead giving a definitely supraliminal sound and two of them, used in varying places in the series, were of cotton.   Sometimes a white light of a given intensity was employed and its intensity was diminished so as to produce a noticeable change, but the observer was told that he was to report when he noticed an increase of brightness.   Or again, the experimenter started with a red colour on a colour mixer and gradually introduced yellow, but stated that he was introducing blue and the observer had to state when he noticed the colour change. Control experiments were employed in which the changes were what they were stated to be; but strangely enough this made no difference to the observer for the replies given were the same in both the experiments and the controls.

There were ten subjects, five men and five women ; seven were suspicious of the experiments and all shewed from time to time that they thought that the investigation was other than it purported to be, namely an examination of their sensory acuity.   Consequently they were ideal subjects to determine the point at issue.

The results of the experiments and introspections shewed that the observers were of three types ; though as usual in psychological classification mixed types occur.   The first kind of suggestive consciousness may be called the motor-type in which the verbal suggestion is, as it were, carried across to the motor response immediately, as though the sensory data were irrelevant.   Many so-called sensory suggestions are of this nature.   The muscular organs are in a state of tension ready to " go off of themselves " when the verbal suggestion is given by the experimenter.   With subjects of the second type there is stated to be considerable relevant mental imagery corresponding to the suggestions made, i.e. preperceived imagery which gives a new context to the stimulus.   The stimulus here is not the bare objective sensation, and the response made to it accordingly is the expression of an imaginally modified situation. Consequently, the subject is reacting not to the stimulus but to his own aroused images. Finally we have the sensory type where imagery is lacking, or is fleeting and irrelevant, and there is no motor preadaptation. An instructive case in point illustrating this last type was furnished by one subject who responded to a suggested unpleasant smell in the absence of any odoriferous stimulus by a watering of the eyes and the assertion that the odour was decidedly disagreeable. The conclusion of the whole series of experiments is summed up thus : " In certain departments of sense, a verbal suggestion may arouse conscious processes which are, phenomenologically, identical with those ordinarily aroused by an adequate stimulus or change of stimulus." Only this type of suggestive consciousness furnishes evidence of a truly *sensory* suggestion.

The importance of the above described observations lies in the fact that a similar state of affairs is probably met with on the ideational level, though there is no experimental evidence at present to confirm it. Investigation in this direction is the next obvious step to be taken in the understanding of the mental processes involved in suggestibility. When a person carries out a suggested idea we have no reason, at present, to assume that he has realised the idea or that he is not acting in accordance with some other idea ; since he may be of the motor type responding automatically or of the imaginal type acting in response to a self-aroused idea. Only when we are certain that he belongs to the last of the three types can we be assured that the suggested idea is really operative in influencing his action or belief.

There is a popular belief that women are more suggestible than men, which is founded partly on the rapid spread of changes in fashion and dress, etc. But there is no convincing evidence in support of the belief. In the experiments we have dealt with in this and preceding sections no difference has been discerned between boys and girls or men and women. Moreover, if women are more liable than men to copy fashions in dress we have no reason to suppose that they copy other things more readily. The assumption that a person who is more suggestible in one sphere of conduct or belief is therefore more suggestible in other spheres has no warrant in experimental observations, and it is in conflict with the trend of general psychology. We have long since abandoned the view that there is a general faculty of memory, imagination, reasoning and the like, but the notion of a general faculty of suggestibility dies hard. Common observation shews that a man may be abnormally suggestible in response to patent medicine advertisements purchasing every new specific which comes on the market, yet in his business affairs he may be overcautious to his own detriment. The study of physical science makes its devotees most critical in evaluating and accepting evidence for scientific phenomena, but some eminent physicists are notoriously hypersuggestible when dealing with such matters as telepathy. Where their emotional beliefs are brought into play

> " They'll take suggestion as a cat laps milk ;
> They'll tell the clock to any business that
> We say befits the hour."

It is, in fact, only when the suggestions closely resemble one another that a person who is highly suggestible for one idea is apt to be suggestible for another. But there are limitations to this rule so that even when the form of the test is exactly similar but the matter varies we must not assume that their suggestive effect is equal. Experiments on a large number of men and women, in which each individual was tested with progressive lines and weights in which the form is strictly comparable, shewed that " in spite of the close resemblance of the two tests, the coefficients of correlation (men ·16, women

·17), do not indicate that they are particularly apt to affect the same persons in a similar manner." [8]

METHOD AND SUGGESTION

From what has been said it will be apparent that some of the more important of the characteristics of hypnotic suggestion are to be found in the ordinary waking state. The chief of these is the uncritical acceptance of beliefs, moral standards, fashions, etc., which prevail in the various groups with which our life is bound up. Post-hypnotic suggestions are, as we have seen, realised unreflectively and almost unconsciously, for they appear at the time of acting to be the obvious course to adopt and need no other justification than their own luminous self-evidence. And many of our ordinary beliefs are so much part and parcel of the very texture of our nature that the challenge to produce a reason is apt to lead to a natural irritation. We feel, rightly, that there are good enough reasons though we are unable to state them ; and in consequence if we are forced to justify ourselves we, like the hypnotised subject, give any reasons which will make them appear more or less rational to other people.

This has been wittily expressed in the following paragraphs.[9] " If we examine the mental furniture of the average man, we shall find it made up of a vast number of judgments of a very precise kind upon the subjects of very great variety, complexity and difficulty. He will have fairly settled views upon the origin and nature of the universe, and upon what he will probably call its meaning ; he will have conclusions as to what is to happen to him at death and after, as to what is and what should be the basis of conduct. He will know how the country should be governed, and why it is going to the dogs ; why this piece of legislation is good, and that bad. He will have strong views upon military and naval strategy,

O

the principles of taxation, the use of alcohol and vaccination, the treatment of influenza, the teaching of Greek, upon what is permissible in art, satisfactory in literature, and hopeful in science.

" The bulk of such opinions must necessarily be without rational basis, since many of them are concerned with problems admitted by the expert to be still unsolved, whilst as to the rest it is clear that the training and experience of no average man can qualify him to have any opinion upon them at all."

Mr Trotter, who is the author of this quotation, states that the only rational attitude towards these beliefs is that of suspended judgment. But surely such a position would be intolerable. If I have good reason to suppose that experts have demonstrated that boric acid (say) is a bad preservative for food, why should I not believe this and act on it until I can follow their arguments ? No doubt it is wiser for me to be ready to abandon a view when experts say that it is no longer tenable, but that is no reason for refusing to have a belief until I can prove it to demonstration. Experts on relativity prove that the velocity of light is the maximum velocity that any body can possibly have. It is easy enough to picture in imagination a velocity greater than this, but the fact that such a concept leads to conclusions which the experts can shew to be absurd, though I cannot follow their arguments, is a good enough reason for adopting their beliefs. In most of the practical affairs of life it would be ridiculous to suspend judgment until sound reasons can be brought to light. Many of our beliefs rest on reasons which we have long since ceased to envisage and which in consequence would be difficult to produce, as they have lapsed into our subconscious life. There may nevertheless be valid reasons and we are justified in acting on them. If a person has a sovereign remedy for influenza the best thing for him is to use it with complete assurance in its efficacy, as in that way he may, at all events, get the benefit of a cure by suggestion. All this gives point to the advice tendered to a man of practical good sense, who, being appointed governor of a colony, had to preside in its court of justice without previous judicial practice or legal education. The advice was to give his decision boldly, for it would probably be right ; but never to venture on assigning reasons, for they would almost certainly be wrong.[10] Every man is justified in acting on the assumption that he knows what should be the basis of moral conduct even though the experts in ethics have never yet reached agreement, nor seem likely to do so. His real reasons are his conviction that the course of his education and the approval of those whose opinion he values are safer guides than any philosophical argument in all the ordinary affairs of life.

The question has sometimes been asked as to whether a teacher is justified in making suggestions about belief and conduct. The considerations dealt with previously have shewn that he cannot help himself ; whilst, if he is fit to teach, he is thereby fitted to make suggestions and the professional spirit of the teacher can be trusted not to abuse this authority. No pupil can be kept isolated from suggestions from those around him whether in the sphere of religion, literature, history and so forth. The attempt to teach the humanities impartially in the school would lead to a dull, uninspiring and worthless treatment. But the effort to make direct suggestions during the teaching of these subjects is more likely than not to arouse a spirit of contrariance and so defeat its own end. This is the real safeguard of the pupil and the public against all biased instruction and is much more effective than any regulation of the teacher's authority ; for the scholars have an acquired immunity against direct suggestion more powerful than any artificial restraint on the profession.

A topic of considerable interest to teachers is the suggestive force of a question or the extent to which the nature or form of the question produces a non-critical answer. Here, as in most of the topics concerned with suggestibility in normal persons Binet did pioneer work. His method was to exhibit a card, with certain objects attached to it, for a definite period and then to ask a variety of questions about them. He had three forms of questionnaire which were written out and presented to the children who took part in the experiments, and they wrote their replies. Now one of the objects was an intact round button with four holes which was stuck on the card with gum. With regard to the button the following questions were asked in the three questionnaires. (1) How is it fixed to the card? Is it broken or whole? Draw it. (2) Isn't the button fixed to the card with cotton? Isn't it broken? Draw it. (3) There are four holes. What is the colour of the cotton which passes through the holes fixing the button to the card? Mark on a drawing the place where it is broken. It will be seen that these three forms are of varying suggestiveness and when the proportion of errors to the number of resistances was taken into account they were found to be progressively suggestive in the order here given.

The present author has tried experiments on this sort of suggestibility in a somewhat different manner. A series of six drawings was made in each of which some object or part was missing. The subjects tested were sixty-three University graduates; and a couple of questions, one of them suggestive, was asked about each drawing. In every case the first question either demanded a certain amount of critical thought or else called attention to some actual feature in the picture. Thus one picture represented an artist standing in front of an easel, with a brush but no palette, and the subjects were asked, in the first place, to determine the nationality of the artist, and when this was done to state the shape of the palette. All the questions were given orally so that the personality of the experimenter was in the foreground, and at the end of

the series they were invited to revise any answers which they
thought were wrong. Only seven of the subjects proved to
be completely non-suggestible right through the series. In
several cases they grew suspicious at some point in the series
as they were being repeatedly asked to describe something
that was not there. Nevertheless it frequently happened
that a subject, who suspected at some point in the series that
suggestions were being made by the questions, was trapped at
one or more later points. The following figures shew the
number of subjects who accepted the suggestion for each of
the six pictures in the order in which they were shewn :

19   40   10   32   10   18

There is a rough kind of periodicity exhibited by this table
indicating that periods of suggestibility alternate with intervals of resistance ; thus yielding further evidence of the
rhythmical nature of the suggestive state of consciousness.

The suggestiveness of a question depends to some extent
on its form. An important difference of form is seen by a
comparison of the questions, " Did you see (hear, perceive,
etc.) . . . ? " " Was there . . . ? " The former have been
called subjective-direction questions since they direct the
attention of the subject to his relation to the object ; whilst
the latter are objective-direction questions since they direct
the person's attention to the object observed instead of to
his observation. All questions belong to one or other of
these forms and it has been shewn that, on the whole, the
suggestiveness of the former type of question is much greater
than that of the latter. The introduction of the definite or
indefinite article, or of a negative, into a question form also
affects its suggestiveness in a somewhat complicated way.[11]
Thus the change from the indefinite article to the definite
decreases suggestiveness, whilst the introduction of a negative
increases it.

We may pass next from the technique of questioning to the wider problem of method in education. Now there is no one method of teaching any topic since method is relative not only to the subject-matter but to circumstances of age, capacity and so forth.

" There are nine and sixty ways of constructing tribal lays
      And every single one of them is right."

Nevertheless, there are certain principles underlying all teaching which Dr Keatinge was the first to point out and these may be considered as the foundations of general method.[12] There is first of all the principle of grading and demonstration whereby the teacher arranges his material systematically in such a manner as to make it suitable to the capacities of his pupils at any stage, the order and arrangement being fixed in advance. The order in which knowledge has grown in the history of the race offers much guidance here, for in the mental just as in the physiological realm phylogenesis offers the best clue to ontogenesis. A rigorous adherence to the order of the growth of knowledge is, however, to be deprecated since the individual may be a mutation from the stock. Moreover it has happened more than once that racial development of knowledge has taken a wrong or unfruitful direction. Thus the additive principle of arithmetic preceded the more fruitful development of the arabic notation with values determined by position ; and it would be absurd to teach the former method because it was the first in order of time.

The second general principle of method is that known as heurism, i.e. the method of placing the pupil, as far as may be, in the position of the discoverer. This method had a great vogue a generation ago and was responsible for a complete change in the method of elementary science teaching, substituting the more fruitful plan of dealing with problems for the more formal plan of dealing with the subjects in a strictly concatenated series of topics. Thus the pupil would be set the problem of discovering why, for instance, iron rusts, instead of waiting to deal with the matter until he studied the oxides of iron systematically. The difficulty of such a plan is that the pupil can never really be placed in the attitude of the original discoverer since he lacks the background of knowledge which the originator brings to his task. The fundamental error of the heuristic method consisted in the assumption that scientific method could be learnt by discovering the facts of science, whereas the facts of science can only be obtained by an application of scientific method. For scientific method like all methods does not work *in vacuo*, but is appreciated by studying the actual processes whereby science has grown. Consequently it is often valuable to allow pupils to work through some original investigation, not in ignorance of where it is leading or in order to acquire a knowledge of facts, but in order that he may discern the methods by which great discoveries have been made.

The third principle is that which is dealt with in this chapter, namely that of suggestion. " Method, then, as a whole comprises these three factors: demonstration, heurism, and suggestion. Their proportions may vary, sometimes one, sometimes another, taking the lead ; but in all teaching which is to be effective, and especially for the guidance of conduct, suggestion must be given its due place. . . . When we are dealing with a train of reasoning heurism is our surest method. In the elementary theory of arithmetic, for example, the pupil with a minimum of guidance can be made to do his own reasoning, and this holds good of experimental science, though to a smaller extent. In literary subjects, while heurism is by no means ruled out, demonstration and suggestion play a large part, and in all ethical teaching suggestion must be supreme. The whole art of the teacher consists in finding the exact blend of the three ingredients that will just suit his subject, his pupils and himself." [13] It must be borne in mind that whilst moral training may be an incidental product of good teaching in the humanities, yet the most suggestive moral instruction in school is that absorbed constantly and unconsciously from the general atmosphere and the personalities of the staff.   The ethos of the school founded on its aspirations, traditions and history is essential in all moral education and the most potent means of suggestion. It acts in a personal way, for it is through living persons that the characteristic spirit of the school community is brought to bear on its pupils.   Everything which helps to keep the past alive such as memorials, records, old boys' clubs, etc. gives a sense of continuity which is important in quickening the spirit.   Sooner or later the feeling that he is a member of a community with a record of service and achievement and a bearer of the tradition makes itself felt as a powerful motive in all his conduct.   For this reason schools with a long history and a roll of great personalities have a much greater chance of suggestion in determining action and belief than any other human institution, owing to the fact that they begin to exercise their influence at the most impressionable age.

CHAPTER IX

PSYCHO-ANALYSIS

Word Association—Complexes—The Unconscious—Psycho-analysis
—The Sexual Theory

WORD ASSOCIATION

THE easiest approach to the doctrines of psycho-analysis is by
way of experiments on word association. In the course of
the preceding chapters we have seen the havoc wrought by
mechanical association in the application of psychology to
education. The interest in association, which would undoubtedly have died down, was revived by the introduction
of the experimental method into the field by Galton in 1879.
He selected a random word as a stimulus and by means of a
stop-watch measured the time taken for two other words to
be revived by it ; and in this way found the average rate of
recall of associations to be 1·2 seconds per word. He distinguished between associations aroused by the meaning of
the stimulus word and those aroused simply by its sound
(clang-associations). With over-elaborated measuring
apparatus Professor Wundt's pupils measured association
times under various conditions, such as free and constrained
associations. By the latter is meant associations limited by
certain conditions, e.g. the stimulus word being (say) *money*,
the subject had to respond with a particular instance of it,
such as *shilling ;* or being given a word like *sorrow*, he had to

find a contrasting word such as *joy*, and so on. The study of word associations on Galton's plan took a new lease of life when Professor Jung [1] shewed that it could be used as a method of diagnosis in abnormal mental states.

Before describing the technique of word association it is necessary to sound a warning note. When a person responds to a stimulus word, such as *tree*, with the first word that occurs to him, e.g. *river*, it is correctly assumed that these words are associated with each other in his mind; but nothing is revealed as to the actual formation or process of association which is simply inferred with more or less acumen by the experimenter. Such inferences are very dangerous unless they are assisted by careful introspection by the subject, and even then cannot be accepted without reserve since the ability to introspect is a difficult art. But the original association as we have seen over and over again is the result of subjective selection by the person and not of natural selection amongst the words themselves. Word associations are objective phenomena due to subjective causes. The associationists were consequently wide of the mark in believing that education had unlimited power to determine a person's associations. Nor is frequent occurrence of impressions or words sufficient to establish an association between them. No doubt repetition does aid the process, but as we insisted in the chapter on habit-formation the rôle of repetition is to provide frequent opportunities for the subject to exercise his mental activity. The study of divergent lines of association shews the importance of subjective preference or interest in determining the particular direction of association. Consider the following lines from the "Ancient Mariner":

> The fair breeze blew, the white foam flew,
> The furrow followed free;
> > OR
> The furrow streamed off free.

If I know both versions the direction of association at the end of the first line will depend on a large number of considerations, the chief of which is the particular ' set ' of mind at the time of recall which depends on my prevailing interest or mood of the moment. Any attempt, therefore, to draw conclusions is very risky unless this ' set ' is definitely ascertained by precise introspective analysis.

Professor Jung studied both normal and abnormal people by the word-association method. The technique is fairly simple consisting in the preparation of a list of words which are repeated singly to the subject who responds with the first associated word that occurs to his mind, and the time between the stimulus and the response is recorded by means of a stop-watch. The predominance given to verbal reactions and speech facility explains the paradoxical results obtained by the method, namely that educated persons exhibit a more superficial type of reaction than the uneducated as they have a more ready command of words which come trippingly to their tongues. The subject is instructed to react to the stimulus words as quickly as possible with the first word that occurs to him. The reaction words are subsequently classified and irregularities in response are carefully recorded. It sometimes happens that the subject fails completely to react with a word and this is called a ' fault.' Again the word is sometimes misunderstood and the subject responds to a word which was not given, but to one similar in sound or meaning. When a list of one hundred words has been given, the stimulus words are repeated and the subject is asked to reproduce his former reaction words, which are recorded as ' reproductions,' or if he gives a different word as a ' failure ' in reproduction.

The association is sometimes due to the stimulus word producing a reaction by virtue of its sound only as in rhymes, word-completions (sing-song) and so forth. When there is some affinity in meaning between the stimulus and reaction words, i.e. when they are in some way similar the association is called *inner*. An association due to practice or repetition, i.e. mainly to contiguity is described as *outer*. Finally, there is a *residual* group composed of mediated or indirect associations (e.g. red-fragrance, mediated by the word ' flower '), meaningless responses, faults, repetitions of the stimulus words, etc. Other reactions are determined by associations previously or recently made and are known as *perseverations*, as when the same word is given as a response to several different stimulus words.

Clang and outer associations are the signs of lowered or disturbed attention ; consequently they are frequent in states of drowsiness, fatigue or distraction. By comparing a number of half-educated with educated people Professors Jung and Ricklin obtained the following percentages of reactions for the various categories :

			Educated	*Uneducated*
Inner associations	.	.	35·8	43·4
Outer associations	.	.	55·3	52·4
Clang reactions	.	.	3·4	·5
Residual group	.	.	4·0	2·2

These differences, which apparently shew that the educated belong to a shallower type point to differences of attention ; such persons regard the word merely as a word and react to it with the minimum of attention. The half-educated apprehend words as part of significant sentences and fix their attention more on the meaning, hence the inner associations predominate.

It has been found that, on the whole, normal persons tend to give one or other of a small group of common reaction responses to the same list of test words whereas the feeble-minded give more individual and varying responses. This shews the effect of the environment in producing common modes of activity. The same point is brought out by the observation that, as compared with adults, children give a

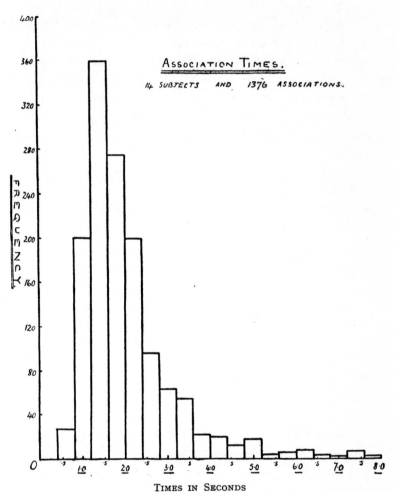

TIMES IN SECONDS
The subjects were University graduates and Jung's list of
association words was used

larger number of individual reactions with a corresponding reduction of the common reactions. Thus age and culture tend to produce more uniformity of response, for education and a common mental environment tend to force us all into a common mould.

The median time of reaction for men is, according to Professor Jung, 1·6 seconds, for women 2·0 seconds ; but it varies individually with the state of culture of the persons. The author of this book found that the median time for University men graduates was 1·7 seconds, with a quartile deviation of ·6 seconds. It may be thought that the speed of association would increase gradually with age. Experiments on school children with concrete nouns as stimulus words yielded a median reaction time of 2·6 seconds for children of eight years. A recent investigation of children between the ages of 7½ to 14½ years failed to shew any relation between the speed of association and age within this age range. The children between ten and twelve reacted to concrete nouns in times ranging from 2 to 5·6 seconds, whereas to abstract nouns the times of reaction varied from 3·4 to 6·2 seconds, without relation to age differences. Word completions and clang reactions occurred but seldom with these children. With constrained associations, the time for causal dependence (e.g. heat—melt) was greatest, and for the whole-part relation (e.g. table—leg) least.[2]

COMPLEXES

The theory of ' complexes ' was evolved independently of the use of word-association experiments, but such experiments have been employed as an instrument of psycho-analysis in order to detect complexes in the technical sense of the word. Much discussion has centred round the idea of a complex, and its connotation remains obscure in several points, though the man in the street employs the word with assurance. The term is used in both a narrower technical sense and with a wider general meaning, but the two shade off into each other imperceptibly. In the wider use of the word there is nothing essentially morbid about a complex which may be regarded as a constellation of psychical elements having their centre in a common emotion and functioning as a single whole with a definite conative trend. According to this usage any persistent idea or group of ideas coloured with a strong emotional tinge would be called a complex. This meaning of the term closely resembles the technical meaning of the word sentiment which is described by Mr Shand as an organised system of emotional impulses centred round some object, such as loyalty to one's school or college.[3]

Now a sentiment is a perfectly healthy and normal mental product reducing to order and disciplining the emotional life, which without this organisation would be a chaos. A complex, on the other hand, has a certain irrationality both as regards the emotion which is its nucleus and as regards its impulse. The action to which it leads is inexplicable to an outside observer, and often to the subject himself, owing to the fact that the complex is not completely integrated with the man's personality. If we regarded lack of integration amongst a person's ideas as morbid we should be forced to conclude that everybody is more or less pathological in his mental make-up, seeing that there is no sharp dividing line in this respect between the normal and the abnormal. As far as his specific complexes are concerned, a certain degree of irrationality is a universal characteristic of human nature. Everybody can easily detect complexes in others, but it is a property of a complex to prevent him from seeing those in his own constitution. The features of a complex, by which we recognise it in others, are that it disables the intellect from functioning normally in relation to any matters which touch the complex. The person refuses to entertain ideas in conflict with the central thought of the complex ; for instance, those who have a materialistic-complex refuse to see any evidence of spiritual forces in the universe. Evidence which runs counter to the complex is rejected or neglected or trifling excuses are made for avoiding it.   On the other hand for conclusions in conformity with the complex, any evidence is sufficient; thus sufferers from a telepathy-complex will accept as proof of their pet theme the wildest statements of notorious deceivers. This last phenomenon is due to the fact that although his opinions on matters touching the complex are entirely moulded by it the person himself remains in ignorance of the fact that he is labouring under a complex.[4]

The characteristic just named leads us to the narrower meaning of the term in which a complex is considered as a pathological phenomenon.   In this sense it is *completely* disintegrated from the rest of the personality and functions in isolation of the remaining mental content.   Thus Professor Freud[5] defines a complex as " a circle of thoughts and interests of strong affective value of whose influence at the time nothing is known " to the subject ; that is to say it is an unconscious product.   Such complete dissociation from the rest of the mind, which is said to be the result of suppression, gives to the complex considerable functional autonomy and the subject's behaviour is unpredictable to an abnormal degree.   As a result of his studies in word association Professor Jung came to the conclusion that the following irregularities in word response could be regarded as indicating the existence of complexes either in the wider or narrower sense.   (1) Prolonged reaction times well above the median ; (2) Faults ; (3) Failures in reproduction ; (4) Stimulus words taken in a rare or peculiar sense or misunderstood ; (5) Perseverations.

All such abnormalities of reaction are thought to be due to the influence of some strong emotion preventing the free flow of associations.

The term ' complex ' is peculiarly unfortunate since the distinguishing feature of a complex compared with any other

state of mind is its extreme simplicity, and it ought in strictness to be called a ' simplex.' There is one complex, however,
occupying a sort of intermediate position between the normal
and pathological to which the name is applicable owing to
its wide ramifications, namely the inferiority-complex.[6] It is
probably universally found in some form or other amongst
children and persists in many adults. Dr Adler who has
described it very fully maintains that it is the kernel of every
neurosis or psychosis ; and there is good reason to believe
from the study of children in ordinary schools that it is the
nucleus of many childhood fears.[7] Children who suffer from
some form of maldevelopment or arrested development, such
as squint, errors of refraction, stuttering, deafness, adenoids,
eneuresis nocturna, defective endocrine glands, or any other
childish organ inferiority may, if not properly attended to,
shew a tendency to neurotic or psychopathic states. If, as
sometimes happens, their companions or relatives call attention to such somatic inferiority and they feel their defect
keenly they are prone to contrast themselves with their more
fortunate fellows and, feeling themselves insecure, they lose
self-esteem and a sense of inferiority ensues. They are then
apt to turn from reality and take refuge in protective devices
and day-dreams as a sort of compensation. As they grow up
they dwell more and more on their weakness, their malforma-
tions, they blame their education, their parents, their heredity
and so forth. Neurotic symptoms arise as a security against
the too vivid realisation of their inferiority—anything in
order to make life bearable rather than face reality squarely.
The normal person also has his protective devices and his
flights from reality into phantasy, but in his case they are
harmless fictions, whereas the neurotic fosters them and
lives constantly in an imaginary world. As a compensation
for his inferiority-complex he strives for mastery by devious
routes and is unable without medical help to cope with life's

P

situations. By perpetually relying on others he attains what to him appears a dominance over them by securing their constant attention.

Dr Adler has painted the picture of the neurotic constitution with a few bold strokes. " The consciousness of the weak point dominates the neurotic to such a degree that often without knowing it he begins to construct with all his might the protecting superstructure. Along with this his sensitiveness becomes more acute, he learns to pay attention to relationships which escape others, he exaggerates his cautiousness, begins to anticipate all sorts of disagreeable consequences in starting out to do something or in experiencing an injury, he endeavours to hear further and see further, belittles himself, becomes insatiable, economical, constantly strives to extend the boundaries of his influence and power and at the same time loses that peace of mind and freedom from prejudice which above all guarantees mental health. His mistrust of himself and others, his envy and maliciousness, become gradually more pronounced, aggressive and cruel tendencies which are to secure for him supremacy over his environment, gain the upper hand, or he endeavours to captivate and conquer others by means of greater obedience." [8]

THE UNCONSCIOUS

It is now time to consider what ought to be the meaning assigned in psychology to the much-abused term the unconscious. Many writers on psycho-analysis have the most fantastic notions about mental processes. Their view of the mind is the compartment theory described in our first chapter in accordance with which ideas, images, feelings and so on are stored up in receptacles ; the receptacle being most often regarded as constituted by the nervous system. But an unconscious image, if its existence had any meaning, has no more power of activity than a dead horse has of winning a race. It is possible, however, to give a meaning to the term without having recourse to pre-scientific psychology. The best definition of the word is that given by Dr Rivers who said that in so far as the term is applied to experience it ought to be " limited to such as is not capable of being brought into the field of consciousness by any of the ordinary processes of memory or association, but can only be recalled under certain special conditions such as sleep, hypnotism, the method of free association, and certain pathological states." [9] According to this usage of the term the difference between conscious and unconscious is one of degree of difficulty in bringing an idea or image into the mind. When faced with a given situation in which an object is not present a person may react in a manner similar to his action on a previous occasion when the object was present. Thus if I make a friendly response to a man whom I meet because I like him I may experience a similar friendly emotion when I think of him later in his absence. In the latter case it is usual to speak of reacting to the image of the man. If, however, I forget him completely so that his name arouses no image in my mind I may still greet him in a friendly manner in a dream, and on awaking I may recall his name and remember him. Images which only function under such special conditions may be called unconscious, just as I might loosely call objects in a mist invisible because I have to peer hard in order to distinguish them. The case is exactly analogous with the attempt to solve a mathematical or any other problem. I may be totally unable to arrive at the ' solution ' at one time, but at a later period when certain difficulties have been cleared away by a persistent effort the solution suddenly emerges into consciousness. It would be preposterous to suppose that the ' solution ' existed in my mind all the time in exactly the same manner in which I subsequently apprehend it. But this absurdity is the sole psychological furniture of some psycho-analysts. What really happens is that owing to the removal of certain obstacles to thinking, or, it may be, to more effective attention to the given conditions, my mind functions effectively and smoothly. The ' solution ' is nothing but the smooth functioning regarded from an objective standpoint. Similarly when I get up and walk my legs function smoothly unless they are cramped or diseased, but this surely does not mean that I keep stored up in my muscles a set of motor images which were suppressed whilst I was sitting. Walking is not bringing into use unconscious motor images ; it is simply the name for the functioning of my leg muscles. It is possible to think of myself as walking when I am sitting down, which is not to think of unconscious motor images but simply to consider an organ as functioning when it is actually at rest.

In order to make clear what is implied in the difficulty of functioning under abnormal conditions I may quote the case of a pupil of mine, a student of the German language, who suffered from intermittent amnesia. On one occasion he met the following sentence in a German book : " Stunden der Not vergiss, doch was sie dich lehrten, vergiss nicht." The idea appealed to him strongly, as it expressed concisely a thought of which he approved but had never quite formulated to himself. He repeated the lines a few times in order to learn them but found shortly afterwards that not only had he completely forgotten them, but he had forgotten the idea enshrined in them. After an interval he again made the attempt to learn them with the same result. A prolonged examination extending over a few weeks revealed the fact that during the war the whole of his platoon except himself was killed in a night attack, and just before he himself was hit in the head a particularly distressing incident involving his dearest friend had occurred. The combined shock of the wound and the mental distress brought about amnesia for the incident referred to lasting for two and a half years. It was evident that he had connected the words " Stunden der Not " with the terrible incident of the night attack, to which, in fact, they were peculiarly appropriate. The association thus established made it difficult for his memory to function smoothly with reference to the lines owing, no doubt, to the agitation which made it difficult to concentrate until, in the dreamy state preceding sleep, the agitation subsiding, he remembered the forgotten incident, when normal functioning was re-established.

Now how does an experience become unconscious in the sense here defined, i.e. why is a process difficult or impossible at one time which was previously carried out easily ? It is as reasonable to expect a single answer to this question as to the analogous one ; why is walking difficult or impossible ? Possibly because the man has rheumatism, or because he is tired, or his leg is broken, or he is paralysed, or there may be a hundred other different reasons. There is similarly no reason to suppose that there is only one method by which memories are suppressed. Nevertheless the psycho-analytic doctrine of the unconscious rests on the belief that an experience which is forgotten " either belongs definitely to the affective aspect of the mind or, when intellectual in character, has been suppressed on account of its association with affective elements." [10] Now in so far as it is impossible to separate the affective from the cognitive attitude of any mental process this theory is a truism. But as we saw in the chapter on Memory, what is really meant is that we forget only that which is unpleasant. Yet who has not blushed for shame at the thought of some *faux pas* which he would gladly consign to oblivion if deliberate repression were within his power ? The attempt to get over such difficulties by using a distinction made by Dr Rivers between repression and unwitting suppression over-simplifies a very complex problem. Suppose I have learnt a piece of poetry by heart and some time later

attempt to repeat it, I find frequently that I am blocked for
several lines because I am unable to remember a particular
word. The cue which gives me the forgotten word enables
me to recover the lost lines by virtue of the law of association,
whereby if one member of an associated group is presented
the others tend to come into consciousness. There is no
reason whatever to suppose in such cases that a particular
affect is attached to one part of the poem which is absent from
the rest. The supposition, that there is such an affect for one
section alone, is merely an attempt to save the theory at any
cost. Moreover it is in flat contradiction with everyday
experience to assert that unpleasantness has anything to do
with forgetting, for the unpleasant emotion may be the last
thing to survive when the intellectual components are difficult
to recover. It is a common occurrence for instance to feel
an intense dislike for a book or a play long after one has forgotten the reasons for the emotion or at all events when it
would be a matter of considerable difficulty to state the
intellectual grounds. And, on the other hand, the reasons may
survive in recollection whilst the emotional tone tends to
disappear, as when we cease to dislike a person though we
remember the original grounds of our aversion. Pleasant
and unpleasant experiences are forgotten (or remembered)
with equal facility, but since in the course of a normal life
the pleasant experiences must outweigh the unpleasant the
odds are greatly in favour of forgetting a greater number of
pleasant experiences. A passion for experimental work which
obsesses modern psychology has supplied unnecessary confirmation of this last observation. Nine subjects of approved
introspective ability kept a careful record of their normal
affective life for a month. In every case a predominance of
pleasure over unpleasure was observed, the degree varying,
of course, from one person to another.[11]

PSYCHO-ANALYSIS

With the above preliminaries we are in a position to discuss the doctrines of psycho-analysis which we are assured, by its professors, are of immense importance to education. It was at one time supposed that every nervous person must have something wrong with his bodily organs, although physicians could not discover what it was. Such persons often complain of diverse specific pains, curious feelings, morbid fears and obsessions and it was assumed that bodily causes were necessary to account for them. When it was repeatedly found that they had neither heart nor lung nor digestive nor other visceral weaknesses it seemed natural to suppose that their nerves were weak ; and Dr Beard an American physician accordingly described all such cases by a term denoting nerve weakness, namely neurasthenia.

It was discovered by Professor Charcot that when hysterical persons were hypnotised they could develop the symptoms of ' neurasthenia ' by suggestion, and it was reasonably supposed that therefore they could be removed in the same way, i.e. by mental as opposed to physical means such as drugs. Professor Freud studied under Charcot and his interest was thus directed to mental therapy. Apparently, however, it was a patient of Dr Breuer's who hit upon the talking method of treating hysteria. This patient had been treated by various doctors by various approved methods such as hot and cold baths, electricity, drugs, etc. without success. It seems that she insisted on coming to Dr Breuer regularly to talk to him about all her symptoms, her domestic and other intimate troubles, her dreams and so on ; in fact to talk at large without any suppressions whatever. After the patient physician had submitted to this course of talking without shewing undue signs of distress he was surprised to find that the talker was beginning to lose all her hysterical symptoms. As he himself did not acquire them despite the provocation, and the patient lost them, he naturally inferred that they had disappeared. When Professor Freud was called in he conceived the happy idea of tapping the subconscious strata of the mind by the talking method under the influence of hypnotism, for he thought that in this way he could arrive more rapidly at the origin of the symptoms. Accordingly Professors Breuer and Freud, working together, came to the conclusion that many symptoms were entirely due to emotional causes without accompanying physical nervous traumata. Subsequently the suggestion part of the treatment by hypnosis was abandoned, but it is highly probable that in all cases, though they stoutly deny it and whether they are aware of it or not, psycho-analysts do make use of suggestion.

The idea underlying Professors Breuer and Freud's treatment was that hysterical symptoms were due to forgotten emotional experiences of a highly painful nature ; and it was believed that the recall of such memories would release the painful emotions associated with the experience and thus the symptoms would be lost. They believed that if the patient could discover the origin of the symptom, the mere dragging it into the light of day would be sufficient to cause it to evaporate. Just as Aristotle thought that the representation of a tragedy, despite its horror, produced a healthy catharsis of the emotions so it is said that this method of treatment leads to a healthy unburdening of the mind. The method has consequently been called the cathartic instead of the more descriptive but less implicative talking method, and the process whereby the talk is more or less distorted is known as psycho-analysis. It is, of course, assumed that only functional and not organic diseases of the mind can be treated in this way. I have no doubt too, that a serious talk with an adult who is trusted, as a parent, teacher or doctor is infinitely preferable to brooding over disturbing experiences such as may occur during the early stages of adolescence. Such unburdening of the mind if associated with a strong moral or religious appeal and the necessary explanation of the facts of sex is the healthiest method of dealing with sex difficulties. But nobody who believes in the views of the Freudian school should be allowed to undertake this task lest he corrupt the youthful mind wittingly or unwittingly by suggesting his own theories. The reason for refusing to trust the psycho-analysts is that they apparently believe in what they call the Pleasure principle. Professor Freud says : [12] " We may put the question whether a main purpose is discernible in the operation of the mental apparatus ; and our first approach to an answer is that this purpose is directed to the attainment of pleasure. It seems that our entire psychical activity is bent upon *procuring pleasure* and *avoiding pain*, that it is automatically regulated by the *PLEASURE PRINCIPLE*." Both the italics and the capitals are Professor Freud's, and his followers repeat this doctrine *ad nauseam*, apparently under the impression that it is a great discovery instead of a theory long since exploded. It seems rather late in the day to protest against psychological hedonism seeing that the whole modern doctrine of instinct is in direct opposition to it. But the following few sentences, written over thirty years ago [13] at which time the view was beginning definitely to be abandoned by competent persons, are sufficient refutation. " Important as is the influence of pleasures and pains upon our movements, they are far from being our only stimuli. With the manifestations of instinct and emotional expression, for example, they have absolutely nothing to do. Who smiles for the pleasure of smiling, or frowns for the pleasure of a frown ? Or who in anger, grief, or fear is actuated to the movements he makes by the pleasure which they yield ? . . . Or what shall be said of a shy and unsociable man who receives point-blank an invitation to a small party ? The thing is to him an abomination ; but your presence exerts a compulsion on him, he can think of no excuse, and so says ' yes,' cursing himself the while for what he does." Disraeli defined a practical man as one who practised the mistakes of his forefathers and it looks as though the new psychology is a repetition of the errors of a bygone psychology.

THE SEXUAL THEORY

So much for the reversion to obsolete psychological doctrines. We shall next turn to one which is completely new, the sexual theory, for it is on this ground that psychoanalysis is said to be necessary for education. Professor Freud points out correctly that the sexual impulse is an appetite analogous to hunger and uses the term libido (craving) to express this resemblance.[14]

Now there are certain people called inverts who have sexual impulses towards members of their own sex and in many cases the direction of their libido has been determined by something that occurred in their childhood, or at all events that is what they say during a psycho-analytical investigation. It is assumed that these and other sexual perversions, being so widely spread, are congenital ; and that normal sexual life is a mean between the extremes of perversion and repression. On the assumption of their congenital nature it is urged that we must search for the roots of perversion in the child or in neurotics who " conserve the infantile state of their sexuality or return to it." Freud's views about infantile sexuality are either speculative or else based on the study of neurotic persons with perverted sexuality. In other words it is a theory of psycho-neuroses based on neurotic persons' recollections of their own childhood and not founded on the observation of children. From this point of view he challenges the popular belief that the sexual impulse is absent

in childhood and appears only in puberty and maintains that
this impulse is normal in childhood. He strives to shew that
only in this way can we account for the widespread perversions and the homosexuality which was a feature of highly
civilised Greek life. If this view were correct we should
expect to find that the main cause of juvenile delinquency
was sexual. Yet Mr Clarke-Hall[15] a Metropolitan magistrate,
in giving evidence on the subject, said that out of 49,915
youthful delinquents under 16 years of age proceeded against
in children's courts in 1918 only 101 were for sex offences,
i.e. roughly 2 in a thousand. Normal persons know nothing
about their infantile sexuality owing, it is said, to the
amnesia of most childish experiences in later years brought
about by suppression. Such amnesia " is responsible for
the fact that one does not usually attribute any value
to the infantile period in the developments of the sexual
life." But psychopathic people distort their childish
recollections and, as Adler has shewn, sometimes do this
with a purpose.

There is, according to Freud, a double wave of sexuality,
the first crest appearing at three to five years of age and the
second beginning to appear at puberty. Between these periods
there is a time of latency brought about by a combined
conspiracy of all normal parents to do everything to repress
the infantile sexuality. During the period of latency certain
opposing forces are brought to play such as shame and moral
and æsthetic demands and " the erection of these dams in
the civilised world is the work of Education." It is further
assumed, without any attempt at proof, that all the energy
of a human being is derived from the sexual impulse, i.e.
diverted sexual energy ; and this diversion into other channels
begins to take place during the period of latency. " Such
deviations of sexual motive powers from sexual aims to new
aims, a process which merits the name of *sublimation*, has

furnished powerful components for all cultural accomplishments." That is to say that the energy which goes to the development of an individual from his babyhood onwards, is derived from sexual sources.

The process of sublimation, the diversion of energy into social and moral directions instead of dissipating it or using it for lower ends is one of the aims of education, and the purpose underlying such organisations as the boy scouts, girls guides, church lads' brigades, and so on. These admirable outlets for activity undoubtedly appeal to an urgent demand of youthful human nature as is indicated by the fact that they have spread over the whole globe. The assumption that all the energy is diverted sexuality is a mistaken inference of the Freudian school, due to the too-ready acceptance of their patients' statements and the belief that such people are fair representatives of normal human nature. Fortunately we have the statement of a psycho-analyst of other views who, with the same kind of patient takes a much more reasonable attitude, and is consequently able to evaluate the evidence. Dr Adler says : " It is easy for the neurotic to convince himself that he is the subject of a high sexual tension by means of a more or less purposeful arrangement, and especially by means of a concentration of attention in this direction the moment he begins to seek proof of how much injury sexuality works to his feeling of security and how much his personality is threatened from this source. . . . The later psychic perverse tendencies derive their material and impulse from the harmless bodily sensations and misjudgments of childhood which when occasion arises are given an extraordinarily high value, or some chance pleasurable sensations are perceived as analogues of sexual sensations. The psychologist must not assume the same point of view, must not maintain such a mode of apperception as valid, not substitute real sexual components for a fiction as the patient does. His task, on

the contrary, consists in revealing to the patient the super-
ficiality of his attempts at orientation, to tear it apart as a
mere product of the imagination." [16]   Our task also as teachers
is to reveal to our pupils higher goals towards which they should
strive and, whilst respecting individuality and their point of
view, to refuse to be led aside by any doctrine which teaches
that perverse or immature human nature should set the
standard for healthy living.

Freudians are convinced that babies are sexually active at
three or four years of age.   But as there are no facts to support
this strange belief we are presented with a few terms and
theories to fill the gap.   Any portion of the skin or mucous
membrane which yields a feeling of pleasure when stimulated
is described as an erogenous zone, which is at once a question-
begging epithet of a particularly daring nature, and a theory
that all pleasure is sexual.   Certain definite parts of the body
are obviously erogenous, but this is not enough to demonstrate
infantile sexuality, so we are stimulated to accept the theory
by applying the question-begging epithet to other parts, for
we are told [17] that " any other region of skin or mucous membrane may assume the functions of an erogenous zone."   All
parts of the surface inner or outer may thus be erogenous zones.
Little wonder, then, that the typical instance of infantile
sexuality which Freud examines at length is the innocent
but annoying pastime of thumb-sucking !   This, which we
have hitherto regarded as neutral from the point of view of
propagation of the species turns out to be very type of a sexual
act.   Not only is thumb-sucking of this nature, but as the
skin is pleasurably stimulated by the jolting of railway
carriages, travelling too must be sexual.   Lest anyone should
think that this is a manufactured illustration I quote Professor
Freud's own words.   " The shaking sensation experienced
in wagons and railroad trains exerts such a fascinating influence
on older children, that all boys, at least once in their lives,

want to become conductors and drivers. . . . The desire to connect railroad travelling with sexuality apparently originates from the pleasurable character of the sensation of motion." Comment on this seems entirely superfluous, but the complete lack of humour displayed is due to the fact that Freud apparently knows nothing of children beyond what he infers from analysing sexually perverted adults ; for, he admits [18] that his views on "infantile sexuality were justified in the main through the result of psycho-analytic investigation in adults." He maintains, however, that the results are confirmed by the study of nervous diseases in children. His evidence for this has recently been examined by Dr Wohlgemuth [19] who has shewn conclusively that the case on which Professor Freud relied was due to the outrageous suggestion of morbid sexual ideas by a psycho-analytic parent to his innocent small boy.

The followers of Professor Freud have not attempted to add observation on healthy children to his doctrines but have contented themselves with repeating their master's *dicta*. The most prominent English exponent,[20] for example, maintains without a shadow of an attempt to justify the view that ignorance of the facts of sex " is never primary, but is based on repression and forgetting of earlier knowledge and speculation in childhood." Speculation on sexual matters before the age of five ! In order that there may be no doubt in our minds as to the activities of these speculative philosophers the same authority tells us that psycho-analysis shews (he means, of course, that Professor Freud has stated it) that, " It is almost a regular occurrence for children of the age of four or five to turn from their parents, to withdraw into themselves, and to pursue private speculations about the topics concerning which they have been denied information, whether by direct refusal or by evasion."

To a complete absence of a sense of humour many psycho-analysts add a complete ignorance of what is meant by sex, and an abysmal inability to understand children's ideas. It will sorely perplex this school to learn that there is as little that is sexual even in a young child's masturbation as in his playing with his toes or his toys. And when a child asks " Where do I come from ? " it is perfectly stupid to imagine that this is a sexual question ; for he is equally interested to know where birds come from and who made trees ; and this boundless inquisitiveness all has its origin in the same root of natural instinctive curiosity. The only way to discover what a child's questions mean is to observe children closely, and not to infer their meaning by what neurotic adults tell us from distorted recollections of their own childhood. Fortunately we have a record of a close study of his own children by a very competent Danish observer who brought up his girls at home and made careful notes of their development for the first few years, thereby making a valuable contribution to child psychology.[21] At the age of four years one month one of the girls asked her mother, " How are ladies made ? " The rest must be given in the father's own words. " Her mother, startled at the question, inquired : ' Why do you ask ? ' But R. had her good reasons, and said : ' Because there's meat on ladies.' To make sure of her meaning, her mother demanded : ' Which ladies ? ' and received the answer : ' You and other ladies.' It being thus placed beyond all doubt that what R. desired was general information relating to the origin of ladies, she received the unsatisfactory answer : ' I don't know.' R. being thus thrown back on her own resources remarked : ' I think it's a meat-man, don't you ? ' It is rather obscure what she meant, but I assume that she possessed a vague notion that ladies—in whom ' meat ' struck her as a salient characteristic—were manufactured by a person analogous to what she called a meat-man."

Luckily the father was not a psycho-analyst and so the

child's responses were not distorted, consequently we are able dimly to see what the child is speculating on, and it is perfectly clear that it has nothing whatever to do with sex. The same child at the same time wanted to know "Who made the birds?" and it was obvious that she regarded creation and birth as a kind of *fashioning*. What is there sexual about this? At the age of four years and ten months she made the inquiry : "Where's the child now which the lady is going to have in the summer?" "Her mother replied: 'In the stomach of the lady.' This evidently appeared to R. somewhat peculiar, for, after a pause for reflection, she asked: 'Has she eaten it then?' Her mother answered: 'No'; but R. persisted: 'Does it come out of the mouth?' Her mother, realising that there was no escape, at last answered: 'No, it comes out of the tail' (this was the children's expression to indicate the part in question). This truthful explanation contented R." If anyone will compare this conversation of healthy-minded parents with Freud's account of the analysis of a five-year-old boy [22] to whom an unhealthy minded father made the most repulsive suggestions he will be wary of expecting guidance in education from psycho-analytic sources. The Danish father rightly remarks that he cannot see why a child should feel shocked at being told the truth and his children were obviously satisfied and pleased. He observed too, " that the birth of children is connected with the *marriage* of the parents is not understood at all by the child of the age under discussion." In other words there is nothing sexual about the child's idea of marriage ; and the less that is said about infantile sexuality the nearer we shall approach to the child's point of view.

If the view taken of the child's mental life is completely distorted the same can be said of the psycho-analytic view of the adult's moral life. There seems good reason to believe that the various forms of psycho-neurosis such as anxiety neurosis, hysteria, etc., are due to a conflict between instinctive impulses and the forces by which they are controlled. Mental health depends on the presence of a state of equilibrium between these conflicting tendencies.[23] Such a state is normally brought about by the social environment and the education by means of which the individual is fitted for the society in which he lives. The educative process, in its widest sense, is in fact one long means by which a balance is maintained between instinct and ideals, between raw human nature and the human nature which fits a man to live in harmony with his fellows. Now the conflict between instinct and social morality in which every human being takes part at some time of his life may be fought out in a variety of ways. Those who believe in the pleasure principle are apparently under the impression that all suppression of instinctive tendencies by education is harmful. It never occurs to them that the repression of moral standards may be still more harmful. It is true that such repression may not produce the symptoms of psycho-neurosis, but it may produce other effects of a much more serious nature.[24] It is the supreme function of education to implant ideals of moral conduct and moral responsibility; so that when the time of conflict between sexual desire and moral conduct arrives the individual may choose the right. If the desires are satisfied and the moral standards repressed, by the operation of the law of habit subsequent relapses are made easier and moral fibre is sapped. The view that harm necessarily comes from suppressing the instinctive appetites is one which education must reject as inconsistent with morality. It would be a sad confession for teachers to make that in such conflicts the forces of morality have no power over the individual. The process of education is an unending course during which the individual instinctive tendencies and appetites should be opposed by ideals and social traditions.

The evidence on this matter from those who are in direct

Q

contact with boys and girls is always in opposition to the psycho-analytic doctrine. Thus Dr F. A. Sibly [25] who for over thirty years systematically gave sex guidance to boys from 9 to 19 years in school and to several hundreds outside, summed up his experience thus: " The neuro-pathologist looks at pathological cases not from an ethical but from a physiological standpoint, and, if he is a disciple of Freud, his chief aim is to put an end to the conflict between conscience and the libido. The simplest way to do this is to persuade the patient that erotic satisfaction in some form or other is natural and blameless. We must beware how we attempt to oppose scientific theory merely because it menaces cherished ideals. Men of large experience assert positively that most psycho-neuroses arise from sexual repression, and there are certainly cases in which the expert cannot hope for a *cure* of abnormal erotism, and it is quite clear that palliative measures are alone possible. We have, however, a right to demand that measures appropriate to extreme cases shall not be recommended in milder cases.

" A far more serious menace to our cause comes from the vogue of Freudian views among general practitioners and the lay public. Whether the subliminal self is, as F. W. Myers believes, a region of our being in which unfolded powers of the soul are hidden, in which we are in touch telepathically with other beings, and into which we draw inspiration from the Infinite and the Etern ; or whether as Freud represents, it is a moral cesspool in which the spiritual excreta of the soul collect from infancy, and from which they send their noxious vapours through our waking life and our dreams, research may presently shew. Meanwhile, Freud's theory of a libido which *will* manifest itself in an open or disguised form, and his theory that evil repressed is not conquered but merely driven as a noxious influence into inaccessible parts of the mind is certainly giving, both in medical and lay circles, a pseudo-scientific authority to the idea that *ex*pression of the passions is less dangerous than *re*pression : that strict chastity is not merely impossible but undesirable.   The harm such an idea can do is incalculable, because the sinner eagerly appropriates a theory which not merely excuses his sin, but presents it almost in the light of a duty.   In justice to Freud one must admit that this deduction from his theory is not warranted. He admits that evil influences may be transmuted into beneficent ones by the process which he calls sublimation. Every intelligent spiritual worker knows that inhibition alone is valueless, that earnest direction of energy into the right channels is death to sin and life to virtue."

The overwhelming body of opinion amongst teachers, both men and women, is that youth should be given a knowledge of the facts of sex, but there is no such consensus as to the proper person to give the instruction.   The duty naturally rests with the parents but many, even if they did not shirk the task owing to its delicacy and difficulty, are by no means competent to impart the knowledge.   Everybody is agreed that the knowledge should be given when curiosity in regard to these matters appears or when there is an indication of bad habits.   But it is a great blunder to allow the information to come as a shock at the age of puberty without previous preparation ; the knowledge should gradually be woven into the fabric of childish and adolescent experience.   Since the mind unfolds gradually the instruction must be suitable to the age, and it should be remembered that premature sexual experience mental or physical must not be forced. " Premature sex knowledge, into which the *emotional factor* enters, is premature sexual experience.   Moral prohibitions of undesirable practices *given with emotion* on the part of the parent or teacher form a case in point." [26]   The desirable thing is to build up the knowledge of organic life including the facts of sex without emotional bias, and whilst not omitting, yet not unduly stressing the processes of reproduction. The content of the instruction is so varied and complex that for the majority of pupils it must be left to the school. Courses of biology spreading over three or four years including plant and animal life and ending with the human body and its functions are now attempted with excellent results in some schools. They should be accompanied with instruction in personal hygiene including especially the care of the body and modesty and reticence with regard to bodily functions. Responsibility for the complete care and feeding of pets is an integral part of the training. The outlines of such a course are beyond the purview of this chapter, but good suggestions may be found in such a book as *Youth and the Race,* and above all the instruction should only be given by fully competent teachers with an objective habit of mind.

In the long run the spread of such knowledge will create a healthier public sentiment by removing the aura of mystery which surrounds childbirth. But those who think that knowledge of the facts of sex is in itself a guarantee of normal sexuality know little of human nature. Medical students as a class are not more or less moral than the rest of the population and village children and all the children of warmer climates have the relations of sex obviously presented. Does anybody really imagine that this knowledge is sufficient to secure a sounder morality ? What is of essential importance is a moral environment due to the combined influence of the home, the school, and religious institutions, and mere knowledge of the facts of sex is not sufficient. Respect for morality is the guarantee of a moral life and there are no substitutes though there may be aids. The following extracts from an actual dialogue in which the replies are given by the head master of a public school may serve to emphasise this fundamental side of enlightenment.[27]

"Is it your opinion that knowledge is not a safeguard any more than ignorance ?—I believe in instruction in these matters; but I do not attach so much value to knowledge as some people do.

Do you advocate knowledge as of importance under proper circumstances ?—As useful ; of that I am quite certain.

You consider that everything depends immensely on the kind of way knowledge is given ?—It depends immensely on the right kind of knowledge being given at just the time when it can be assimilated.

Do you think that the atmosphere is much more important than the amount of knowledge imparted ?—You may give the definite instruction in a school where the atmosphere is wrong, and that instruction, however good, would be more likely to have ill effects than good. You have got to get the atmosphere ready before you do anything else. . . .

Who creates the atmosphere ?—I do not think I can answer that. But I think that the head master has to think more of creating atmosphere than of imparting knowledge.

But you think that the home ought to make the beginning ? —There is no substitute for the home, either in religion or in any part of education."

CHAPTER X

ÆSTHETIC APPRECIATION

Æsthetic in Education—Perceptive Types—(a) The Objective Type—
(b) The Subjective Type—(c) The Associative Type—(d) The
Character Type—Psychical Distance—Appreciation of Music and
Literature—Rhythm

ÆSTHETIC IN EDUCATION

NOTHING is more characteristic of modern reform in education
than the change which has come over the teaching of languages.
A play of Shakespeare is no longer regarded as a cloak to cover
exercises in formal grammar and philology, nor a sonnet simply
as an excuse for a lesson on prosody. The best exponents of
the teaching of English take the view that theirs is not a
scientific study but an art, a means of arousing æsthetic
appreciation and creative expression. Teachers of modern
languages using the direct method aim ultimately at making
their pursuit a training in language as a fine art and a cultivation of imaginative sympathy with foreign peoples. With
these objects in view the writing of verse and the acting of
plays form an integral part of the work in schools where the
ideal of a liberal education is kept in view.

It is trite and unnecessary to emphasise the æsthetic appeal
of drawing, painting and music in the school, unless it be to
point out that the cultivation of technical skill is subsidiary
to this purpose. Ultimately no doubt all appreciation rests
on executive ability, but it is only a secondary aim of general
education to develop such skill. It is also becoming recognised

that the masterpieces of music, painting and sculpture should take their place side by side with the best literature and drama in the appeal to the æsthetic feeling of the pupils.

The means for the cultivation of æsthetic appreciation are not lacking if the value of such training is approved. Some indeed in the revolt against a utilitarian outlook in education would search for æsthetic values in the most unexpected directions. " Mathematics, rightly viewed," says an eminent authority, " possesses not only truth, but supreme beauty— a beauty cold and austere, like that of sculpture, without appeal to any part of our weaker nature, without the gorgeous trappings of painting or music, yet sublimely pure, and capable of a stern perfection such as only the greatest art can shew." [1] Only a select few are capable of such appreciation, yet Mr Russell maintains that this aim is the sole justification for the universal tradition that decrees that every educated person should be acquainted with the elements of mathematics. Astronomy indeed bears in its train the whole gorgeous choir of heaven, and tradition for centuries demanded its study as one of the Seven Liberal Arts. [2] Some of the present over-loaded curriculum of schools might well be sacrificed to make room for a pursuit so admirably calculated to stimulate appreciation of the universe as a whole, and entirely barren of any taint of practical appeal.

The nature of the material or subject-matter is, then, but a subsidiary consideration in dealing with our present topic, and we shall be concerned in this chapter mainly with the mental processes involved in æsthetic appreciation. For artistic training is not confined to particular subjects, but depends on the attitude of mind adopted in dealing with its material. All educational values, in fact, are relative to the mode of presentation, but it is in the field of æsthetic that the full force of this doctrine is felt.

The objective nature and constitution of artistic products

are special and distinct branches of æsthetic study outside the
scope of psychological treatment which is limited to the subjective point of view.   According to Croce the subjective
essence of art is vision or intuition.   The artist discovers a
new point of view and æsthetic appreciation consists in looking " through the chink which he has opened."   A beautiful
example of this is given by the consideration of Whistler's
set of etchings of the Thames.   Prior to 1860 nobody had
realised that the mud flats and dun-coloured brick buildings
of the riverside wharves had any artistic significance.   Whistler
fairly gloated over the silhouettes of the warehouses, the lines
of the barges, the riggings of the vessels, and by delineating
the light and shade effects he created a new set of values which
everybody now realises.

Appreciation rests on the intuition or recognition of such
values, and is distinct from the contemplation of the world
of scientific realities which involves reflective judgment.
This distinction is well stated by Thomas Hardy who in the
preface to *Tess* says that his novel is intended to be neither
didactic nor aggressive, but that in the scenic parts it was
meant to be representative merely and for the rest charged
with impressions rather than convictions.   We may apply
to art generally his dictum that " a novel is an impression,
not an argument."   But a bare impression, the mere contemplation of a crowd of images is not the essence of artistic
intuition which needs the touch of affective consciousness to
give it organic unity.   The imagery must be coloured with
some feeling, producing an emotional resonance or sympathy
in the observer, to give the impression æsthetic significance.
For perfect æsthetic enjoyment of a musical composition
for instance, there must be no conflict between the emotions
of the listener and those inherent in the character of the music.
" An aspiration enclosed in the circle of a representation—
that is art." [3]

PERCEPTIVE TYPES

The prerequisite of all appreciation is, then, an intuition or perception of the admired object leading to the æsthetic attitude as opposed to the critical outlook of scientific thought. But it would be a mistake to regard such artistic perception as an ultimate unanalysable faculty. Psychologists have long since abandoned explanation by means of faculties and no longer refer, for example, to a faculty of imagination, but analyse this partly into the various kinds of imagery involved, such as pictorial, auditory, etc., and partly into affective and conative constituents. It is fatally easy to perpetuate the blunder and to talk of artistic appreciation as though it were some primordial power, unique and therefore indefinable. We can avoid the error by shewing what factors are involved in such appreciation.

In attempting to analyse artistic perception, much help may be obtained by a study of the psychological significance of speech forms. When we consider that language is the universal medium of communication it is reasonable to expect that the varieties of perception will be embodied in speech. Now, active participles of transitive verbs, in their adjectival use, have a peculiar psychological function which may be seen from the following examples : a *thrilling* book, an *irritating* pain, a *dazzling* light, an *inviting* prospect, an *affecting* spectacle, a *chastening* experience. Logically, no doubt, all these participial adjectives characterise their corresponding substantives. Primarily, however, all language has a psychological basis, and if we examine the function of such adjectives from this point of view it is evident that the purpose of the speaker is to call attention to some subjective or organic effect produced by the object on a person. Passive participles on the other hand appear to have a very different function. Contrast the examples given above with the following : a *swollen* river, a *broken* reed, a *diffused* light, a *chastened* man, a *prolonged* pain, a *thrilled* audience. In all these instances the speaker intends primarily to convey to his hearer some characteristic of the object named. If it is permissible to use the terms in a somewhat loose sense we may say that, psychologically considered, the function of the active participle of transitive verbs is subjective and of the passive objective.

Amongst the oldest devices of language are the use of metaphor and simile, bearing witness to a deeply seated trait of human nature. By the use of a simile two things are associated together and compared with respect to certain common features. Sometimes the common feature is perfectly obvious so that the perception of one thing immediately suggests the other as when Shelley describes the stars peeping through a rift in the clouds " like a swarm of golden bees." Often the things compared are remote when it is necessary to keep both steadily before the mind in order to discern the similarity, as in the simile used by Hardy in the "Dynasts" comparing the creeping of the Austrian army " with a movement as of molluscs on a leaf." Or again in Shelley's " Adonais " :

> " Life, like a dome of many-coloured glass,
>   Stains the white radiance of Eternity,
>   Until Death tramples it to fragments."

Here the delicacy of the comparison is gradually felt as one lingers over the image. But, whether the common character leaps to the eye or is only subtly suggested, the outstanding psychological character of a simile is the association of similars. Such association marks the man of responsive sympathy, who discerns in a flash of insight a remote yet inevitable connection between things widely sundered. Hence Professor James regarded the ready recognition of these similarities as distinguishing the man of genius from the prosaic creatures of habit and routine thinking.

Metaphors reveal the most penetrating of all modes of human perception, for they arise from the intuition of a similarity between objects or ideas or acts so fundamental that one is thereafter identified with the other. The great majority of the words in a language, except those naming physical objects, are metaphors or the débris of metaphors ; but the identification is usually so complete that all sense of the metaphor is lost.[4] What is crooked has become the symbol of all that is perverse (pravus) and motives to conduct which serve to hide one's real motives are borders to conceal the faults of the stuff (prætextum). So too the valuation of money lends its name to all kinds of estimation (æstimare). And astrology with its belief in a fluid which flowed from (influere) the stars and acted on men, provided the word for all imperceptible action. But these metaphors are dead, for who thinks of these words now as metaphors except the philologist ? The identity is so complete that the metaphorical sense is unconscious. In the last example (influence) the metaphor was still alive in the time of Milton who wrote in " L'Allegro " :

> " With scores of ladies, whose bright eyes
>   Rain influence."

The process still continues, for as soon as a new metaphor is introduced and its aptness discerned it becomes common property, passes into current discourse, and its metaphorical significance vanishes. Nor is it restricted to one language, for the most striking metaphors enter into different tongues, as may be seen by a comparison of the words *discover* and *entdecken, comprehend* and *begreifen.*

In some cases the process has not carried language to this point so that it is easier to discover the metaphorical sense of the expression. Instances of this occur when an epithet suitable to one domain of sense or feeling is transferred to another. We talk of a *deep tone*, a *loud colour, black care, bitter grief,* etc., and the aptness of the expressions is evident to all at first sight. Again we have cases in which the metaphor is less completely assimilated, so that its borrowed sense is still evident as in Milton's " motes that *people* the sunbeam," and Browning's " The air broke into a *mist* of bells," or when we speak of petty annoyances as *pin-pricks*. Whether a metaphor is living or dead in every case its distinguishing psychological function is the attribution of some quality or action peculiar to one object or idea, to some other so as to lend it a character which is thenceforth regarded as its own property.

The most illuminating instances of transference are those in which our own feeling, emotion or mood is read into inanimate things so as to give them human character. This tendency has received the technical name of empathy,[5] ' feeling into,' coined to correspond with the word sympathy ' feeling with.' Examples abound in poetic diction : thus the psalmist sings :

> " Let the sea roar, and the fulness thereof ;
> The world, and they that dwell therein ;
> Let the floods clap their hands ;
> Let the hills sing for joy together ; "

And Shakespeare :

> " The rude sea's enraged and foamy mouth."

And Milton :

> " The stars with deep amaze
> Stand fast in steadfast gaze."

The whole realm of nature is viewed in this way by the poets whose perceptions are strongly tinged with their own emotion. Wordsworth regarded this as the distinguishing mark of a poet who is " a man pleased with his own passions and volitions, and who rejoices more than other men in the spirit of life that is in him : delighting to contemplate similar volitions

and passions as manifested in the goings-on of the Universe." [6]
The following lines of Coleridge though suitable for descriptive
verse may, as he points out, by a slight alteration of rhythm
be regarded as prose :

> " Behold yon row of pines, that shorn and bow'd
>   Bend from the sea-blast, seen at twilight eve."

Yet the same image ' will rise into a semblance of poetry if
thus conveyed ' :

> " Yon row of bleak and visionary pines,
>   By twilight-glimpse discerned, mark! how they flee
>   From the fierce sea-blast, all their tresses wild
>   Streaming before them."

Though this metrical experiment is only a ' semblance of
poetry ' yet it serves to illustrate the magical transforming
effect of empathy.[7] It is important to realise that whilst
the origin of these feelings is in ourselves and they are read
into nature by a translation from our own consciousness it is
nevertheless erroneous to suppose that the process is a
deliberate one. Rather, such emotions and volitions, as
Wordsworth says, are directly discerned in the objects as soon
as they are perceived and they are seen at once as endowed
with a life of feeling similar to our own. How little conscious
purpose has to do with empathy may be inferred from the
fact that it is coeval with humanity, being the basis of universal
primitive animism. Neither can time wither it nor custom
stale its freshness, since the capacity to perceive in this manner
is the supreme form of æsthetic intuition.

Approaching the matter from an entirely different standpoint, Dr Jung has observed that in some cases of mental
disease there is an exaggerated intensity of feeling and in
others extreme apathy. In normal persons, too, we may trace
the existence of similar psychological types characterised by a
predominance of feeling and of abstract thought respectively.[8]
The libido or *élan vital* urges the individual to respond to the

world in one or other of these ways. " The one who feels his way transfers himself to some extent to the object ; whilst the other withdraws himself from the object to some extent, or pauses before it and reflects about it. The first is called the *extroverted* type, because in the main he goes outside himself to the object, the latter is called the *introverted* type, because in a major degree he turns away from the object, withdrawing into himself and thinking about it." In extreme cases the one limits himself to observation and reflection, the other to feeling. The latter finds æsthetic satisfaction in empathy whilst the former, as in the case of Mr Russell previously quoted, discovers beauty in the rigidity of abstract law. Empathy is the result of warmth of passion which is carried over into the object in order to assimilate it or pene-trate it with emotional values. Abstraction on the other hand despoils the object, even when it is organic, of living qualities and grasps it by purely intellectual thought crystallised and fixed into the rigid forms of universal law. In fine, the intro-vert abstracts from the object and deals with it by concepts concentrating upon the inner world of thought, whilst the extrovert goes forthwith to the object and feels himself into it.

This instructive and useful distinction of psychological types has been expanded by its author into a large volume with elaborated detail thereby robbing it of much of its value. For he has attempted to shew that practically every twofold distinction between human beings that has ever been made, and their name is legion, ultimately reduces to a difference between introversion and extroversion. For instance, Pro-fessor James drew a distinction between the temperaments of philosophers whom he described as tender-minded and tough-minded respectively, the former being rationalistic, intellec-tualistic, idealistic, religious, etc., in contrast with the latter who are empiricist, sensationalists, materialistic and irre-

ligious. The philosophers of tender-minded temperament are
only interested in inner life and spiritual things whilst the
tough ones lay most stress on material things and objective
reality. But it is absurd to call the tender introverts and the
tough-minded extroverts as Dr Jung does, seeing that in all
essential respects idealists and religious-minded persons are
more akin to the poets by virtue of their characteristic
empathy; and the poet, as we have seen, goes out to the
objective world to endow it with living reality.

The experimental study of æsthetic appreciation confirms
the existence of four different modes of perception to which
we have been led by the examination of various universal
forms of language. Before an object can be appreciated,
whatever its nature, its meaning must be grasped, and it is
clear that for experimental purposes a work of art, such as a
picture or a musical composition, is far too complex. Experimental work has accordingly been confined, in the first place,
to the simplest material, such as colours or tones, but the
results, as far as music is concerned, have been verified by
dealing with finished compositions.[9] By presenting single
colours or simple colour combinations to different persons,
and recording their comments, Mr Bullough has shewn that
different people range themselves under one or other of four
non-exclusive classes. These represent differences in the
attitude of the subjects towards the colours, in that they
apperceive them and other æsthetic objects from different
aspects. As with all other mental differences rigid divisions
between the types or classes do not exist since the majority
of individuals belong to mixed types, but shew a tendency to
a more consistent adherence to one of them. Such differences
of adaptation to an object form the foundation on which all
æsthetic experiences are constructed. Ultimately the difference of adaptation rests on the temperament and personality
of the individual and, to a lesser extent, on his momentary

mood. Thus the appreciation of æsthetic values touches the very core of human individuality. The types of perception distinguished by Mr Bullough, which should be compared with our language types, are here set forth roughly in the order of their æsthetic worth.

(a) *The Objective type*

Persons belonging to this group primarily emphasise the purity of a colour or a tone, its brightness, saturation, poorness, etc., and they have a tendency to compare it with some standard of purity. Their appreciation, in so far as it can be said to exist, for their attitude is almost extra-æsthetic, is intellectual rather than emotional. They are the most critical but the least appreciative, and adopt conformity with some standard as their reason for æsthetic valuation. The critical attitude seems to interfere with the free flow of imagination.

(b) *The Subjective or Physiological type*

Persons of this class refer to the stimulating, soothing, exciting or temperature aspects of the object. A colour or tone produces organic and affective changes in them, and so they call it warm, cold, depressing, exhilarating, and so forth. For the same reason they sometimes complain that the colour is glaring or trying to the eyes, or that a tone is piercing or makes them shudder, or appealing and makes them sad. It may be thought that these effects are due to suggestion or association, but this is negatived by the observation that whilst red, yellow and orange are described as warm colours, red is always the warmest, whereas if the effect were due to association with the sun we should expect yellow or orange to be the warmest. Moreover those who take the associative attitude are not necessarily sensitive to the temperature effects.

There are other emotional states and moods, such as repose, feelings of desolation, or even mystical feelings which are typical of the present attitude. And finally there are certain conative effects or active endeavours to interpret what is presented, the subject being dissatisfied until a meaning is found.

(c) *The Associative type*

This variety is common enough, being the type which in the sphere of language creates similes. Such persons, on being faced with an æsthetic object, promptly and unconsciously pass to associated things. A colour suggests a sunset, a landscape a storm at sea, and so on, whilst a tone may recall a symphony, a church service, the face of an absent friend, and a host of other associations immediate or remote. It may happen that the associations are symbolic, a musical note suggesting looking through a misty veil, or a narrow streak of light streaming in a particular fashion ; and this kind of association shades off into synæsthesia or coloured hearing, where every tone has its distinctive tint. Just as with some people every vowel is coloured. The poet Heine had a similar faculty in a peculiarly marked degree. He speaks of the " gift of seeing with every note which I hear its corresponding figure of sound : and so it came that Paganini, with every stroke of his bow, brought visible forms and facts before my eyes ; that he told me in a musical picture-writing all kinds of startling stories ; that he juggled before me at the same time a show of coloured Chinese shadows." [10]   Finally there is

(d) *The Character type*

Subjects belonging to this class tend to personify the colour or tone. They perceive in them characteristics which in the case of a human being would be called his mood, temperament or character. A colour or tone may be described by

R

them as insipid, stubborn, jovial, energetic, gentle, solemn, grotesque, fidgety, etc. Persons belonging to this class, on the whole, agree remarkably well in the characters they assign to the same colour or tone, thus shewing that the phenomenon is not due to association. They agree for instance in perceiving a temperamental contrast between red and blue and colours containing these tints. Red is described as sympathetic, affectionate, and its character is open and frank, whereas blue is reserved, distant and unsympathetic. The origin of this type is to be sought in empathy, a projection into the object of affective characteristics which are essentially human. But it must not be supposed that the projection is a conscious process, or that the subject recognises that the characters are transferred. No sooner is the object perceived than the character aspect is evident and *there*. The case is exactly analogous to the perception of distance by vision which since Berkeley's day is regarded as having its origin in muscular and tactile sensations ; nevertheless no sooner do we open our eyes than we *see* the distance of any object in our neighbourhood. On occasions it may happen that an object is perceived as solemn or melancholy at a time when the percipient himself is jovial and gay, when it would be palpably absurd to talk of consciously projecting his own mood. As previously observed the tendency to regard æsthetic objects from their character aspect is the same as that which produced animism amongst the primitives, and is the distinguishing mark of poetic insight. To ascribe such a faculty to a conscious translation of feelings is totally to miss its significance. Its essential feature is a mystical discernment of identity with oneself in the object, which gives rise to a peculiar emotional response leading to sympathetic understanding. Artists who belong to this class have no abstract preference for any particular ' subjects ' ; all may be beautiful in their eyes. Some indeed do not hesitate to assert that the character aspect alone is what art should seek to display. "*Character* is the essential truth of every natural spectacle whatever, beautiful or ugly," said Rodin,[11] "it is the soul, the feeling, the idea which is expressed in the traits of a face, the gestures and actions of a human being, the tints of a sky, the line of a horizon. Now for the great artist everything in nature exhibits some character : for the uncompromising sincerity of his observation penetrates into the hidden sense of everything."

Whilst the objective type is determined, as was said, by conformity to some standard in accepting or rejecting a work of art, the character type are guided in their judgments by sympathetic resonance with it and are therefore likely to be the least critical but the most appreciative. This must not be interpreted to mean that the study of the highest standards of art can be neglected in æsthetic education since the contemplation and reverence of these is the surest way of stimulating the finer perceptions. For the great artists in striving after ideals have revealed the character aspect to less discerning minds. Doubtless this is what Rodin intended in his testament to young sculptors when he admonished them to study diligently the great masterpieces. "Love the masters who preceded you with devotion. Bow before Phidias and Michael Angelo. Admire the serenity of the one and the fierce anguish of the other. Admiration is a generous wine for noble souls." [12] As sincere admiration can only come as the result of perfect understanding and familiarity those teachers are justified who strive to inculcate at an early age the great masterpieces of literature so that the pupils practically know them by heart and have them as a permanent part of their mental structure.

PSYCHICAL DISTANCE

It is said that the best descriptions of mountain scenery have been written by those who are not mountaineers. Certainly support is lent to this view when we consider that Ruskin, who has given some of the noblest descriptions of the Alps in literature, regarded mountaineering with haughty disdain, and Kipling in *Kim* has invested his descriptions of the Himalayas with a feeling for the infinite far to seek in those who have tried to climb Everest.   Doubtless the recollection of the physical effort and the dangers involved in climbing great heights is a bar to the detached view necessary for æsthetic contemplation, for an indispensable condition for all appreciation is such cutting loose or release from the practical standpoint.   Thus a thunderstorm on a summer night appears beautiful if we can ignore its possible destructiveness and contemplate simply the vivid effects on the landscape lit up by momentary violet flashes of sheet-lightning.   By eliminating the practical attitude and adopting a completely disinterested standpoint the experience is brought to the æsthetic focus and given what has been called ' psychical distance.' [13]   Such an attitude is closely akin to the attitude of play, and may develop out of it.

The remarkable success of the Play Way [14] method of teaching literature shews the importance of this attitude in developing appreciation.   It has been conclusively shewn that for boys under ten years of age the dramatising of traditional ballads and for those over ten the acting of Shakespeare's plays with all the joyous freedom of play is the most efficient means of securing æsthetic appreciation.   Schoolboys have a special power of projecting and imagining themselves as characters seen and heard,[15] and this faculty, rendered definite by acting, enables them to get that insight, vision or intuition into character which is the essence of dramatic art.   Moreover the elimination of the school atmosphere obtained by having the plays performed in a specially adapted room helps to secure the ' distance ' experience. As in other arts a true feeling for drama can only arise out of the trial practice of the art. If the objection is made that school is meant for work it may by pointed out that by the Play Way boys under fifteen years of age have been led to understand and appreciate Shakespearean tragedy in a manner incredible to pedagogues who do not realise that a play is meant to be acted. Although the attitude of detachment from practical considerations is essential it must not be supposed that æsthetic appreciation consists in taking an impersonal view. Rather, it is a peculiar kind of personal relationship with the object often highly emotionally coloured, but the personal character of the relation has been ' filtered ' or cleared of its practical concrete nature. Æsthetic intuition is diametrically opposed to any sort of practical appeal. In drama, for example, the characters " appeal to us like persons of normal experience, except that that side of their appeal, which would usually affect us in a directly personal manner, is held in abeyance." Such detachment, however, must not be too great or the artistic effect is apt to be lost. Both in appreciation and in artistic production what is required is " the utmost decrease of distance without its disappearance." This concept of ' distance ' serves to make clear the distinction between the agreeable and the beautiful in art. The agreeable is a pleasure which has not been cut loose or distanced from our practical interests ; its centre of gravity lies in the self, whereas the centre of gravity of an æsthetic experience lies in the object. For this reason the consideration of pleasure is as foreign to the æsthetic appreciation of a work of art as the question of its money value since ' distance ' raises the work of art out of the realm of practical systems and ends. In the attempt to drive home the importance of this conception of art to his generation, Whistler with his usual directness and emphasis insisted that art should stand alone and appeal solely to the eye or ear. It must not be confounded, said he,[16] " with emotions entirely foreign to it, as devotion, pity, love, patriotism and the like. All of these have no kind of concern with it ; and that is why I insist on calling my works ' arrangements ' and ' harmonies.' "

Allowance being made for the exaggeration of missionary zeal this standpoint of the autonomy of art may be conceded. But a serious difficulty arises when the question of the relation of art to morality is considered. It would be vicious to maintain that morals like emotions can be distanced, yet there have not been wanting those who believe that art is outside the realm of morality. Nothing could well be farther from the truth, yet the view is one which has frequently been found to appeal to immature minds ; and modern teachers of literature anxious above all things to stimulate the imagination and arouse appreciation sometimes fall into the same error.[17] But there can be no holidays from morality even in imagination. In literature the blunder arises from a failure to distinguish between two distinct things, namely the moral point of view which is an organic part of the artistic conception and a morality imposed upon it from without. " It is clearly a mistake," says Drinkwater, "to suppose that moral judgment did not come within Shakespeare's scheme. Every one of his plays from the dark and terrible pity of *Lear* to the light and gracious revelry of *Twelfth Night* is charged with moral judgment, but it is a judgment that is strictly complementary to the action of the characters within the play, and as organically a concern of the poet's creative function in the play as are the characters and actions themselves. In other words the moral judgment becomes inevitably a part of life itself, and is an altogether profounder thing than a merely abstract moral point of view." [18] Drinkwater rightly maintains that in respect of making morality an integral part of poetic creation instead of fitting the latter into a prearranged scheme the Shakespearean era was definitely superior to the Victorian ; and the reaction against the later conception has led some modern poets and teachers to the absurd misconception " that supposes it to be outside poetry's function to have any moral purpose whatever." He shews that it is the chief glory of Elizabethan poetry to be intensely concerned with moral consequences which flow inevitably from the poet's conception of life. And though Milton in constructive grandeur and poetic imagination is on the same level as Shakespeare yet in seeking to " justify the ways of God to men," he would have risked the integrity of his art but for the supreme intensity of his moral conviction. So far from dramatic art (and the same is true of all literature dealing with humanity) being outside the realm of moral judgment it only justifies itself when its moral character develops inevitably as it grows, being an essential feature of its creation.

APPRECIATION OF MUSIC AND LITERATURE

The existence of the various perceptive types was demonstrated originally for what may be called the alphabet of the arts. It is interesting to learn that Dr Myers found that in listening to music as one would in a concert hall the same types were displayed.[19] The subjects who took part both in the experiments on tones and in listening to the more complex material of musical compositions (played on a gramophone) judged the material from the same aspect in either case. With the more complex as with the simpler material hardly any person was of an absolutely pure type, and moreover different kinds of music evoked different aspects in the same person ; so that even for the same individual there are different ways in which music may be appreciated. The ordinary person, in listening to music, has associations which may aid his appreciation, provided that such associations blend with or melt into music, whilst this associative aspect is absent in the unmusical.

Those who are predominantly of the subjective type, surrendering themselves to the sensory, emotional and conative effects produced on them, may derive pleasure from the musical composition, but they fail to appreciate its beauty. If, however, the emotions can be ' distanced ' they may appear not merely agreeable but beautiful.

The impossibility of complete separation of the types is well shewn by the observation of technically trained musicians. These were found to adopt the objective attitude which, it will be remembered, is that taken by unmusical persons with regard to tones. But in the case of the musicians this aspect is artificial, and is evident only because the others have been suppressed, as is shewn by the observation that when taken off their guard the character aspect emerges, having been there all the time but inhibited by their critical attitude in the experiments.

In describing ' empathy ' we saw that the poets enjoyed, as it were, a mystic insight into nature's moods, and it is probably the case that all appreciation of beauty has in it some touch of mystical character. Despite this there is no doubt that appreciation can only be developed by suitable training. Many schools in England now include in their curriculum lessons on musical appreciation and by help of the gramophone and wireless installations all may do so in the absence of an executant. Short preliminary discourses on the distinctive work of some composer are given and subsequently illustrated by the music. A word or two prior to each composition on its structure, the use of different instruments, the way the effects are obtained, etc., has been found sufficient to lead boys to take an intelligent and cultivated interest in the best music. Such lessons given once or twice a week and spread out over three or four years are sufficient to introduce the pupils to all the best music and lead them to prefer and enjoy it. For in the realm of art the good tends to eliminate the bad. When the pupils are encouraged to perform the music themselves the results in the hands of an enthusiastic teacher are most striking, shewing that the ability to appreciate the finest music is very widely if not universally spread. Mr C. T. Smith, working in one of the worst districts of London in an elementary school with no previous tradition either in the home or the school, has demonstrated that children under fourteen years are capable of appreciating and even performing grand opera.[20] His course lasts six years, and the time devoted to music is not greater than that in other schools. It begins with folk dances and song, and proceeds according to the historical development of music ; the technique of oratorios and operas and the values of the various instruments being carefully studied in detail. " An incident in the experiment was the production by the children of a grand opera, viz. Gounod's 'Faust,' the recitatives practically without ' cuts ' and the choruses in four and occasionally five parts." The children also performed "The Magic Flute" and read Wagner at sight with great enjoyment. It should be added that the course involves an elaborate study of technique and a detailed explanation of the varieties of musical composition and the points to be looked for, since Mr Smith believes " that the appeal of the best music is intellectual rather than physical . . . it must be understood by the head as well as the heart ; and the knowledge necessary for such an appreciation must be taught." There is no doubt that his results justify his method and the genuineness of the appreciation is evidenced by the fact that several parents in the district replaced their music-hall gramophone-records by records of first-rate music, owing to the pressure of their children. Good art universally tends to drive out bad.

There is no reason why the composition of simple melodies should not form a part of the ordinary school programme in music ; and there is no doubt whatever that such composition is a first-rate means of stimulating the understanding and appreciation of the best music. If it be objected that the results of such attempts at composition are bound to be worthless the reply may be made that pupils are universally expected to compose in language and that this is regarded as essential to understanding and appreciation. Moreover, children in Welsh schools are taught to compose in music and the results justify the attempt. The outline of the procedure may be learnt by consulting a pamphlet by Sir Walford Davies on melody-making.[21]   The basis of the method is the explanation of the structure of melodies beginning with scales, chords, rhythms, etc., and proceeding by the analysis of adventure (the first thought) balance and cadence, all illustrated by examples from the great composers. Experience has shewn that children under fourteen are capable, after such a course, of composing simple and enjoyable melodies. As was said previously, the best introduction to the enjoyment of the fine arts is the trial practice of them.

In the realm of literary appreciation some excellent work has been performed both with primary and secondary school children. The work of Mr Lamborn in a primary school in Oxford, and that of Mr Caldwell Cook in the Perse School, Cambridge, are of first importance in this connection, and have given a new turn to the teaching of English. Their books should be consulted for the methods they employ in stimulating a taste for literature.[1] It needs to be stated, since it is apt to be overlooked, that both these teachers by no means neglect the more scholarly and formal parts of language study, but their astonishing results are due to the fact that the emphasis is not placed on them ; they are but a means to the aim of cultivating appreciation and creative expression. Mr Lamborn, indeed, believes that as far as poetry is concerned there is a mystic insight necessary to perceive the beauty which cannot be intellectually explained. And although he thinks that explanations are only permissible when they increase enjoyment he by no means neglects the thorough study of stanza forms, metre and rhyme. He has good exercises for developing the power of word description, the pupils being set to describe some scene and the result is judged by the ability of the class to recognise the exact place described. The use and abuse of simile and metaphor are also taught by employing them, and the children are encouraged to take similes and compress them into metaphors. Other figures of speech are learnt by studying the effects produced by them in good poetry and by original exercises founded on these. Similarly, rhyme arrangements and stanza forms together with the whole architecture of verse are carefully studied, and writing in verse forms make these a delight to the children. Exercises in verse properly conducted compel boys to discriminate nicer shades of meaning, to weigh values and in fact to get a ' feeling ' for correct language. Rhythm is emphasised and practised in its varieties and the boys are made to feel the distinction between rhyme and assonance. As the results of the original exercises in verse and prose have now been published, it is unnecessary to do more than refer to them here. But it is important to note that these teachers believe " that poetry, its rhythm, its music, its imagery, its figures of speech, are instinctive in children, that they have a natural appetite for them, and an intuitive gift of using them. . . . I suggest that children [under fourteen] can express themselves better in verse than in prose." [22] The conclusion of the whole matter is that the thorough study of form, in so far as it is undertaken for the purpose of assisting creative expression in verse, is the most effective means of securing appreciative enjoyment of poetry. And the method is the Play Way.

No doubt in the pre-adolescent stage of a pupil's career the imagery of poetry is an essential factor in securing appreciation. But for later stages its importance is greatly overrated.[23] It is only in a limited kind of poetry, where the meaning is largely embodied in the imagery, that the arousal of images in the mind is an aid in appreciation. Just as with music, however, such images must fuse completely with the poet's meanings, and this fusion must be unconscious if appreciation is to be aroused. If the images are isolated and refuse to blend they may be a positive hindrance to enjoyment. Any deliberate attempt to awaken imagery apart from that which develops spontaneously as the poetry is read or heard, as is sometimes done in class teaching by emphasising the images, is apt to defeat its own purposes and to interfere with appreciation. There is no reason to suppose that, for older pupils at all events, poetry whose meaning is mainly dependent on imagery is easier or more enjoyable. Anything, in short, which obstructs the easy flow of a literary work militates against the æsthetic attitude. Not only is the unified emotion destroyed, but more important still the sense of rhythm is baulked. So subtle is the effect of the rhythmical unity of emotional mood and thought that some of the best teachers of literature refuse to give any explanation of poetry at all ; but, having selected a piece within the comprehension of the class they trust to good reading in order to awaken appreciation. They maintain that any intervention of the teacher between the poem and the pupil for the purpose of explaining allusions, linguistic or historical, or arousing images, destroys the artistic unity and prevents the adoption of the æsthetic attitude.

The author of this book has made an attempt to investigate the various factors which influence the appreciation of poetry amongst adults. A number of selections from a classical poet were given one at a time to each of the thirty-seven University graduates,[24] who were asked to say simply whether they thought each piece, considered by itself, to be good, bad or indifferent. No indication was given as to the name of the author, nor was it suspected by any of the persons who were examined. Some time afterwards the selections were again presented to the students and they stated in detail what affected their likes or dislikes. Those who had graduated in literary subjects shewed a marked tendency to admire the extracts which appealed to their sense of rhythm. Nine men and six women were influenced in their appreciation partially or wholly by the imagery suggested by the verse ; and of the men, delight in the images themselves was the real ground of preference in only four cases. In one of these latter persons the imagery gave rise to feelings which were felt to be congruous with the feeling aroused by the poem so as to blend easily with it, and this feeling was the basis of his enjoyment. Four men and two women admired certain poems on account of the associations called up, and in every instance the sights or sounds evoked were similar to those described by the poet, so that complete fusion was possible. The appreciation of the remaining subjects was influenced by linguistic or emotional factors difficult to disentangle from each other. Amongst the linguistic elements determining appreciation were apt or striking metaphors or similes, appropriateness of the language, energy of phrasing, clearness and smoothness of expression, the music and beauty of the words. The emotional appreciation was variously described as a feeling of exaltation, a sense of grandeur, pleasing unity of sound and idea, emphasis on passion without loss of harmony, sincerity of the poet's love of nature, complete sympathy with his emotion—all these were recorded by women. The men were mostly affected by the crescendo or diminuendo of passion,

the working up to a climax and the gradual fall, sympathy
with the poet's emotion, sincerity and truth of expression;
and in one case by pure pleasure which increased at each
reading without any specific reason. On the whole the depth
and intensity of emotion appeared, in these students, to be
less amongst the women than the men.

RHYTHM

We have seen above that a literary training tends to influence appreciation by developing a sense of rhythm. Now,
the rhythm of poetry, music and the other arts is an essential
factor in the subjective adaptation to artistic values on which
all appreciation ultimately rests. Nor is this to be wondered
at when we consider that the external influences of nature
which affect life are rhythmical. Seasons and tides, spring-
time and harvest, night and day, occur in periodic alternation
producing a rhythm of responsive movements in the organic
world. And superadded to these externally imposed rhythms
there are innate rhythmic activities peculiar to each species
so that the very daisies of the field which close their petals at
nightfall continue to do so periodically when deprived of
external stimulus. Even the inhabitants of the depths of
the ocean, far removed from all external influences display a
physiological periodicity in their vital acts. Not only is
the organism as a whole rhythmical but the various parts
carry on their separate functions as breathing, heart-beat,
walking, each at its own characteristic periodic rate. And
the sucking of the new-born child involves the accurate co-
ordination of muscular movements of expansion and contraction in a definite rhythm, timed to correspond with the
acts of swallowing. The essentially rhythmical nature of

vital activity is discerned most clearly when we turn to the functions of the nervous system. Thus certain reflex actions occur in periodic series independently of the nature, the rate, or the intensity of the stimuli which evoke them; and should the stimulus be continuous the rhythmic character of the response is nevertheless unaffected. In short, nervous activity proceeds according to its own rhythmical laws whilst the external stimulus is not a determinant but simply a call to action.

Voluntary attention, too, is not a continuous function, but tends to be rhythmical. In the last resort then our *experience* of rhythm rests on our nervous and mental constitution. Life is rhythm. Sequences of acts of attention yield accentuation, thereby breaking up the most monotonous series of sounds, such as the beats of a metronome, into regular groupings.[25] Each person is possessed of a vital *tempo* based on the periodicity of his vital functions, and it would seem reasonable to suppose that the rhythm of art must in some way correspond to the vital time measure. The nature of the correspondence, however, is very obscure and stands greatly in need of further careful investigation. There is a close relation between vital *tempo* and temperament or at any rate between *tempo* and mood. Thus, Vernon Lee has compared listening to the " Ring " with finding oneself in a world where the time unit is bigger than our own, owing to the extreme slowness of Wagner's vital *tempo*, whereas in listening to such an opera as "Carmen" the mind is made to work quickly, due to the incomparable briskness of the rhythm and phrasing. In the former case one feels slothful and in the latter braced to imminent action. So there are persons who have temperamental preferences for artists who are endowed with a similar vital *tempo* to their own and to whom, therefore, they are prepared easily to respond. But this view of a temperamental correspondence has been challenged and it is maintained that the delight of artistic contemplation is due to subtle changes of rhythm involving departures from one's vital *tempo*.   Art selects and emphasises.   In a dramatic work such as " Macbeth " the rhythm of actual life is departed from, owing to the exigencies of the stage ; there is further the music of the verse varied by lyrical digressions which introduce changed rhythm, and so forth.   These digressions or departures from vital rhythm are, it is asserted, the chief sources of our emotional enjoyment, which comes from the novelty of adjusting ourselves to changes skilfully introduced by the artist.   Whatever view may ultimately be taken of the relation of the rhythm of art to vital *tempo* it is clear that the appeal of poetry is a call to the inmost depths of our nature.   The metre may be regular or irregular, accented or unaccented, but the one essential feature is the rhythmic experience and its artistic unity with the underlying thought.   Use may be made of the dependence of rhythm on muscular movement by teaching boys under fourteen to express the rhythm of poetry by waving short pointers held in the hand accompanied by swaying motions of the body.   By such a course of " stick wagging " it has been shewn that the most subtle rhythms can be delicately expressed and *felt*.[26]

To M. Jaques-Dalcroze belongs the credit of developing a new and beautiful system of rhythmical education.   As a teacher of music he was impressed with the fact that no amount of auditory training, however closely accompanied by finger exercises, gave the capacity for estimating exactly variations of time and rhythmic groupings which are essential to real musical feeling.   For " musical sensations of a rhythmic nature call for the muscular and nervous response of the *whole organism*."   Hence he developed a system of special training, happily called eurhythmics, designed to effect a co-ordination of muscle and nerve in all parts of the body ; to harmonise mind and body. He is convinced, and the above discussion shews that he is right, that it is only by means of movements of the whole body that we are able to perceive and appreciate rhythm.[27] The training in eurhythmics is a successful attempt to express all the nuances of time—*allegro, andante*, etc., and all the nuances of energy—*forte, crescendo,* etc., in movements of each and all parts of the body. It is a special system of musical gymnastics by means of which sound rhythms are transposed into plastic rhythms of movement. After a year's rhythmic training the pupil's subconscious mind responds unhesitatingly to any variety of rhythm ; he develops, as it were, a limb and trunk speech, resulting in a bodily *feeling* of rhythm. Such training is distinguished from other forms of gymnastics, not only by being a part of musical education but by its æsthetic value in developing a form of bodily expression which realises the Platonic ideal of physical combined with intellectual culture to produce harmony of the soul. In the words of M. Dalcroze, " Rhythmics aims at the bodily representation of musical values, by means of a special training, tending to muster in ourselves the elements necessary for this representation—which is no more than the spontaneous externalisation of mental attitudes dictated by the same emotions that animate music. If the expression of these emotions does not directly react on our sensorial faculties, and produce a correspondence between sound rhythms and our physical rhythms . . . our plastic externalisation will become mere imitation. It is this that distinguishes eurhythmics from the old system of callisthenics, musical drill and dancing."

S

CHAPTER XI

MENTAL TESTS

ORIGIN OF THE TESTS

MENTAL tests of the type discussed in this chapter have been widely used in recent years for a variety of purposes ; to distinguish the lower levels of intelligence, to discover the causes of juvenile delinquency, to select children for transference from one grade of school to another, in some cases in order to select candidates for Universities and the Civil Service, and to give vocational guidance. In order to estimate the value of such tests some knowledge of their origin is essential as otherwise their application may be misconceived. In the year 1904 the Minister of Public Instruction in France appointed a Commission to inquire into the training of mental defectives. Mons. A. Binet and Dr T. Simon, two French psychologists, set to work in order to establish a scientific diagnosis of grades of intelligence below the normal. Up to that time three grades of inferiority had been recognised, mental defectives, imbeciles and idiots. Further, idiocy had been distinguished from dementia arising at puberty, which was not necessarily permanent. The French have always been the pioneers in the investigation of mental disease. Two French physicians whose work we considered earlier, Dr Itard and his brilliant pupil Dr Séguin, laid the foundations of the educational treatment of mental deficiency. The latter published a treatise on idiocy in which he put forward the results of his observations : " Man being a unit is artificially analysed for the sake of study, into his three prominent vital expressions, activity, intelligence and will. . . . The predominance of any of these functions constitutes a disease ; their perversion leads to insanity ; their notable deficiency at birth constitutes idiocy, afterwards imbecility, later dementia." [1] There was, however, no accurate differential diagnosis of such states, although suggestions had been made for grading by means of the greater or less facility in the use of words, or by the degree of derangement of bodily movements. The classification by symptoms was so arbitrary and subjective that no agreement was possible. Dr Sollier had proposed a psychological classification on the basis of attention, according to which imbecility was to be judged by highly unstable attention and complete idiocy by the absence of attention. The chief objection to such a means of diagnosis, even if its principle were sound, would be the impossibility of measuring voluntary attention *per se*. Every mental operation necessarily involves attention which is the presupposition of all mental life. Consequently, any test of perception, memory, judgment, or any other faculty whatever is indirectly a test of attention, but no test can be devised which isolates attention.

The most fruitful plan for mental testing was suggested by Dr Blin who conceived the idea of examining persons of low levels of intelligence by a series of prearranged questions referring to such concepts as time, place, number, etc. The questions, however, were arbitrarily chosen as no control tests were made and the marks assigned to them were purely subjective, so that the value of the questions for diagnosis was not great nor could comparison be made with the results of other observers. The credit of developing the method scientifically, by standardising questions and orders and securing an objective system of evaluating them, belongs to Messrs Binet and Simon. The new conceptions introduced by them will be considered later. Here it is sufficient to emphasise the fact that the inception of the idea of mental testing was due to the practical need of classifying the lowest grades of intelligence.

It was thought at one time, that experiments on the acuity of sensation would yield a measure of intelligence. Theoretical writers also shared in this conviction. Thus Bain [2] wrote : " We can from the outset discriminate, more or less delicately, sights, sounds, touches, smells, tastes ; and in each sense, some persons much more than others. This is the deepest foundation of disparity of intellectual character, as well as of variety in likings and pursuits. If, from the beginning, one man can interpolate five shades of discrimination of colour where another can feel but one transition, the careers of the two men are foreshadowed and will be widely apart." It is worthy of note that psychologists who regard Bain as hopelessly out of date, nevertheless hold this very opinion with regard to differences of mental imagery ; and there is as little justification for the one view as for the other. Measurements of the ' spatial threshold,' i.e., the smallest distance to which the points of a compass must be stretched in order that the two points may be distinguished by touch, were made on this assumption. It was found, curiously enough, that primitive peoples were more sensitive to this kind of test than civilised and that the sensitivity varied inversely with the state of culture. Other attempts to correlate intelligence with simple processes such as visual or auditory acuity, reaction times to various stimuli, rapidity of muscular movements, discrimination of colours and tones, etc., have all yielded results either difficult to interpret or conflicting with one another.

A little reflection should be sufficient to convince anyone that acuity or integrity of sensibility can stand in no direct relation to intelligence. Persons like Helen Keller and other blind deaf-mutes, who lack what might be regarded as essential sensations, are nevertheless capable of developing very high degrees of intelligence. Again the attempt to estimate the level of intelligence by the accuracy of memory would be futile for there is no necessary correlation between intelligence and memory, as imbeciles may have good memories. Similarly, all single tests seem bound to fail. With these considerations in mind Messrs Binet and Simon attempted to solve the difficulty by selecting a number of heterogeneous tests in order to explore as large a part of mental life as possible. They produced, in fact, a battery of tests which could be aimed at different heights so as to determine the intellectual level of the individual. So much importance was attached by them to variety and number of the tests that Binet, comparing the relative importance of a number of tests with a single one, states that he would almost be prepared to say : " no matter what the tests are provided that they are numerous." Now, it is obvious that the degree of education of a person will make some difference to his ability to deal with certain tests. Thus a test involving the power to calculate will, other things being equal, be answered best by one who has been taught arithmetic. It would be desirable, therefore, as far as possible, to eliminate acquired knowledge if a measure of intelligence is desired and to devise tests to discover ' mother wit ' only ; unless indeed the capacity to acquire education is part of what is meant by intelligence. This ideal method, however, has proved impossible of attainment.

A large number of tests were selected by Binet and Simon in 1908 and revised by M. Binet in 1911. Their idea of what is meant by the intelligence which is tested by the tests is best stated in their own words, thus, " To judge well, to understand properly, to reason well, these are the essential springs of intelligence." They also include certain other powers, chiefly initiative and "practical sense" or adaptation to novel circumstances.

It was pointed out above that any test which is to have a diagnostic value must be standardised. We owe to Binet and Simon the ingenious device of standardising their tests by the ability of normal children to cope with them. This can best be illustrated by considering an actual test and the method of dealing with it. Suppose a number of ordinary children are asked whether they know what a butterfly is, and what a fly is ; and then are asked to state " In what way are they not the same ? " Experiment shews that at the age of 5 years normal children are not capable of making the comparison neces- sary to distinguish such a simple difference. Although they know the two things quite well, they are not able to under- stand in what way the two things differ. By the age of 7 years the transition has been made and about two-thirds to three-quarters of normal children are able to make the reasoned comparison. In order to make the test more complete and fair, three such differences are asked namely between a fly and a butterfly, wood and glass, paper and cardboard. It is found that the majority of normal children of 7 years are able to state two out of the three differences. In consequence this degree of correctness is accepted and the test is assigned to the age of 7 years. Normal children of this age have therefore tested the test, and if they are a fair unselected sample of children it is assumed that any other normal child of seven will be able to supply at least two out of the three differences. A separate collection of such tests has been standardised in the above-named manner for each age from 3 to 16 years. In this way the conception of mental age arises ; for if a hild answers all the tests up to and including those of the age of 7 (say) and not any beyond this point then he would be said to have the mental age of seven years. A curious fact has been observed which shews the superiority of this experimental method over any *a priori* procedure. Normal children of the age of 7 years can state a difference between two things, e.g., paper and cardboard, yet they find it much more difficult to say how they are similar to one another, so that the majority fail, and the statement of resemblances between common things cannot, therefore, be used as a test for this age.

For the various ages Binet and Simon used a collection of tests, involving various tasks, such as verbal memory, memory of digits, power to understand and carry out an instruction, comparison of length of lines, arranging small weights in order, tests of suggestibility and a number of tests involving the correct use of language. Having tried all these on normal children they then proceeded to use them to test mental defectives, imbeciles, etc. In this way it was possible to compare abnormal children with normal by tests which were objective and therefore impartial and to which a more or less definite value could be attached ; thus securing a reasonable diagnosis.

It is necessary to draw a distinction here, the neglect of which is likely to lead to serious error. The tests we have been describing do not measure mental ability in the same sense that a test of skill measures a particular kind of talent ; hence we must distinguish between ability and maturity. The tests are intended to shew that an individual displays intellectual activity of a more or less mature type.

It does not necessarily follow that a child who does well in the tests will certainly acquit himself with credit in school work, for the ability to do well in school tasks depends on a large number of factors of which intelligence is only one. Thus, scholastic ability demands docility, regular habits; continuity of effort over prolonged periods, and so forth.

Such factors hardly come into the tests at all, and the personality of the examiner is usually sufficient to secure maximum attention to the task in hand during the short time that the tests are being given.

A distinction must also be made between maturity and accuracy of intelligence. Intelligence may be mature without necessarily being correct with regard to particular processes, owing mainly to lack of interest in certain directions. Nevertheless we may agree that, on the whole, want of rectitude in a very simple process, provided that we are sure that interest is sustained, is an indication of immaturity.

MENTAL RATIO

In the final rearrangement of his tests Binet had standardised a set of five for most years up to the age of 15 and a final set of five for adults. To find the intellectual level of any individual he gave the tests in order, and found the extreme upper set in the whole series which the person could pass with but one failure; beyond this point a credit of one year was given for every five tests, chosen from any of the higher sets, which were answered correctly. By this method a mental age could be assigned to any child. A similar procedure, with variations, has been used by subsequent investigators; so that we may roughly define a mental age as the ability to cope with most of the tests which normal individuals of that age can deal with, provided that credit is given for successful attempts with tests that are usually answered by normal persons of a higher age.

If an individual's mental age is divided by his chronological age the quotient obtained indicates his level of maturity compared with that of normal individuals. This number has been called the ' intelligence quotient ' or the ' mental ratio.' [3]

Thus a child of eight years who has a mental age of 6 has a
mental ratio of $\frac{6}{8}$ or 75 per cent. of normal maturity. We
may, perhaps, say that the mental ratio is a measure of the
brightness of a child ; for one who is above the normal
maturity for his age would usually be called brighter than the
average and one below the normal, dull. It is believed on
the evidence of mental tests that maturity of intelligence is
practically complete at the age of 16 years ; consequently
in finding the mental ratio of adults 16 is taken as the denom-
inator of the fraction for all persons above 16 years of age.
As the rate of progress towards complete maturity is not
constant but slackens down, it must be remembered that a
normal individual of mental age 15 is much nearer to one of
16 than a child of mental age 5 is to one of 6.

REVISION OF THE TESTS

The Binet-Simon tests have been subjected to a thorough-
going examination, rearrangement and revision. Two of the
revised scales are sufficiently noteworthy to be considered in
some detail. Professor Terman of the Leland Stanford University produced a revised scale called the ' Stanford revision.' [4]
He compared all the tests that had been previously used in all
countries and included several others for the purpose of experimenting. By choosing schools of average social status, and
taking all the pupils of different ages in such schools who were
within two months of a birthday, he examined a thousand
children between 5 and 14 years selected simply on the ground
of age. Using the old and some new tests he arranged them
in sets for each year in such a way that the median mental
age of the children of each group coincided with the median
chronological age. If the median mental age at any point

of the provisional arrangement was too high or too low, the location of some of the tests or the standard of marking was changed to secure the above result. Some 400 adults were treated in the same way ; so that finally sets of standardised tests were obtained for each age from 3 years to 14 years and sets for adults and ' superior ' adults. The tests, as a whole, treated in the above manner are, therefore, arranged so that the average individual of those examined obtained a mental ratio of unity. Each single test within a set was further standardised by arranging the children of each age level in three groups, thus : inferior with a mental ratio below 90 per cent., superior with a ratio above 110 per cent., and an inter-mediate group. The percentage of successes for each test at or near the age level was found for all three groups, and if a test failed to shew a decidedly higher proportion of passes in the superior group than in the inferior it was not regarded as satisfactory.

Not only were the tests standardised but the procedure for giving each test was carefully elaborated and the method of marking was strictly defined. In brief it may be said that the attempt was made to standardise the examination and the examiners. This rigidity of procedure applied to the Binet-Simon tests was found to reduce the mental ages in the lower part of the scale and to raise them in the upper part, i.e., above 10 or 11 years.

When the mental ratio for the separate age groups from 5 to 14 years were plotted on a frequency diagram it was found that their distribution for each age was fairly sym-metrical. The similar nature of the distribution at each age suggests that an individual's mental ratio remains constant and re-tests of the same children at different ages seemed to confirm this, i.e., bright children do not deteriorate nor the dull improve. The coefficient of correlation between the estimates made by teachers and the results yielded by the tests was found to be ·48 as measured by the Pearson formula ; not a high figure for this kind of work. As far as the average mental ratios at each age were concerned very little difference was found between boys and girls from 5 to 14 years.

The frequency of the mental ratios was not only symmetrical above and below the median but decreased gradually on each side, so that there appeared to be no definite dividing line between the normal and the mentally defective. Consequently, the number of mental defectives in any population would appear to depend on what particular mental ratio is chosen as the standard of defectiveness. Professor Terman regards a mental ratio below 70 (i.e. $\frac{7}{10}$) as shewing definite feeble-mindedness ; and amongst his thousand cases, one per cent. were marked as low as this.

A most scholarly and thorough revision of the tests has been made by Dr Cyril Burt who has introduced certain refinements of procedure and analysis based on modern statistical theory. He found that in their application to English children the tests required much re-assortment both in the order of difficulty and in the age assignments. He insists more strongly than others that in giving the tests the examiner should adhere with meticulous exactitude to a standardised procedure, for the tests are not intended primarily to discover how the individual carries out certain operations *but how he responds to certain standardised formulæ.* The examiner should neither teach nor criticise nor give any clue as to whether the answer is correct or not ; and further all emotional excitement other than encouragement should be avoided as far as possible.

With these ideas in view careful standardised directions for giving each test were worked out, mainly based on M. Binet's procedure but supplemented by that of other competent investigators. Dr Burt believes that for English children, in the present state of our knowledge, the Binet-Simon scale should be used as far as possible as Binet left it and his revision

consequently is very conservative.   His procedure is set out in
detail in an excellent book called *Mental and Scholastic Tests*
which should be studied by all who wish to use the Binet-
Simon scale ; and the statistical methods employed are described simply and clearly in his *Distribution and Relation of
Educational Abilities*.[5]

He examined over three thousand five hundred children in
London schools, comprising above 2600 normal children in
ordinary elementary schools, over 700 in mentally deficient
schools, and more than 100 juvenile delinquents in industrial
schools, etc.   The tests were given to children of all ages from
$3\frac{1}{2}$ to $14\frac{1}{2}$ years and the average percentages of all the children
at all ages who passed each test were calculated.   The figures
so obtained made it possible to arrange the various tests in
order of increasing difficulty as estimated by the percentage
of passes.   Now an ideal scale of intelligence would be one in
which there was equal difference of difficulty between any two
tests at all points on the scale, i.e., in which all the units were
of the same size.   Such accurate graduation is not possible
with the Binet scale ; but Burt shewed that if the percentage
of passes is converted into terms of units of standard deviation
there is a rough equality of units between the tests assigned to
the intermediate ages from seven to twelve.   An approximate
scale of difficulty comprising sixty-five tests was accordingly
constructed by using these units.

There are serious discrepancies between Binet and other
investigators in the assignment of various tests to the different
ages ; for Burt in comparing his age assignments with those
of twenty other investigators found that only four out of his
sixty-five tests were allotted to the same age-group by all of
them, so that the concept of a mental age is not as precise as
it is usually supposed to be.

A very interesting fact was brought to light by this revision,
namely, that the order of difficulty of the tests is not the same

for normal as for defective children. The order varies greatly with the nature of the test. Thus the following were found to be relatively easier for normal children ; scholastic tests, especially those involving the use of language and other tests of a linguistic kind, scholastic tests which are learnt early by normal children such as counting backwards, etc., tests of immediate memory and tests of reasoning. Whereas those which proved to be easier for defectives were tests of suggestion and general information, such as naming coins and common objects, picture tests involving description and interpretation, mechanical counting, simple money tests such as giving change for twopence out of a shilling by the use of coins of different value and so on. Consequently, scholastic tests turn out to be among the best tests of intelligence ; and linguistic disabilities are, on the whole, the distinguishing feature of defectives. It will be remembered that some of the investigators who preceded Binet proposed to classify the lowest levels of intelligence by defects in the use of words, and apparently they were on the right lines although their methods were crude. Moreover, it would appear that inability to profit by ordinary school instruction, in so far as it is not due to emotional or moral defects, is a clear indication of lack of intelligence. The application of the scale to defectives yielded the result that they advanced only just over half a year in mental age for each chronological year, so that the absolute amount of mental retardation increases steadily.

The extent to which individuals may deviate from the average was investigated. Until the age of ten the standard deviation was found steadily to increase, approximately in arithmetic progression, and to bear a fixed ratio to the mean age, i.e., the range of variability shewed an absolute increase together with a relative constancy. Beyond this age up to the time of puberty mental variability continues to increase but with diminished rate. On the whole, the variability as measured by the standard deviation, was for all ages from three to fourteen about one-eighth of the chronological age. Hence the difference between individuals (and this is also true of defectives) is larger as the individuals grow older. In educational ability which was tested by examinations in the ordinary subjects of the curriculum, the standard deviation was discovered to be about one-tenth of the corresponding age. Accordingly children appear to be more variable in intelligence than in educational attainments.

This conclusion, however, of the greater variability with advancing age is by no means to be regarded as definitely proved. A coefficient of variability may be calculated by dividing the number denoting the average performance of a group of persons by the standard deviation ; and by means of such coefficients we can compare the variability at different ages. An examination of the results obtained by different observers using various sorts of mental tests on normal subjects of both sexes yielded the table set out below.[6] It will be seen that the period of greatest variability is during the early years of childhood and not at adolescence as is often supposed. There is on the whole a decrease of variability with advancing age. Of course the persons were selected, in that abnormal subjects were not examined, and this partly explains the results. Moreover it is probable that all normal subjects, especially at adolescence and later, shew results below the level they could attain if an adequate stimulus to do well were offered ; so that it is still possible that individual differences may increase at adolescence, but there is not sufficient evidence at present that they actually do so.

age (years)	7	8	9	10	11	12	13	14	15	16	17	18	adult
coefficients of variability	.42	.36	.31	.28	.28	.27	.26	.25	.26	.25	.27	.21	.20

It was stated above that the idea of a mental age was not an exact conception. This is further evident from the fact that any particular chronological age-group trenches very deeply in mental age on its successors ; even in the lowest age-groups this overlapping is considerable but it becomes greater still in the higher ages ; between the ages of thirteen and fourteen the amount of overlapping is as high as 77 per cent.

The frequency diagram for mentally defective school children constructed on the basis of the revised tests considerably overlaps the diagram for normal children. In general intelligence, as measured by these tests, more than half of the defective children could be easily matched by children in ordinary schools : there is thus no break between the two groups. Accordingly Burt defines a mentally defective child " as one who for intelligence ranks among the lowest one and a half per cent. of the school population of the same age." As tested by his scale this was shewn to be equivalent to a mental ratio of 70 ; in other words a deficient child is backward by three-tenths of his age. The fact was previously noted that this mental ratio was found by Professor Terman by a less rigorous method.

We noted that those who rely on mental tests to measure intelligence usually assign a mental age of sixteen as the limit of growth. A mental ratio of 70, therefore, would be equivalent to a mental age between eleven and twelve for mentally deficient adults. Dr Burt, however, thinks this is much too high, for an adult who is not capable of coping with the tests or with school work may yet be able to adjust himself to the demands of practical life so as to be self-supporting, especially in the lower grades of labour. Comparatively little weight should be given to mere mental age as far as adults are concerned since success in practical affairs makes greater calls on other factors such as temperament, emotional stability, physique, environment, etc. A mental ratio of 50, corre-

sponding to a mental age of eight may be regarded as the border-
line for adult mental deficiency.   This means, in practice,
that for the adult population of the country between three
and four per thousand are defective.

Using the evidence provided by the revised Binet scale
together with that obtained by the reasoning tests Dr Burt
concludes that a mental ratio above 115 or 120 indicates Central
school ability at least, and a ratio above 130 or 135 scholarship
standard for secondary schools.   These figures may be compared with those of Professor Terman who regards ratios of
110 or 120 as indicating ‘ superior intelligence ’ whilst ratios
between 120 and 140 indicate ‘ very superior intelligence.’
A mental ratio above 150 is very rare indeed and Burt has
never, in all his researches, found a ratio above 160 in a Public
Elementary school, though he discovered a boy of seven years
with a ratio of 190 in a private school.

The use of the tests has shed some light on the causes of
juvenile delinquency.   By examining over one hundred
individuals in industrial schools and other places of detention
Burt concluded that these potential criminals were technically
‘ backward ’ but not ‘ deficient.’   They were retarded by
nearly two years in general intelligence, but by four years in
educational attainments.   The low estimate for general mental
level discovered by several observers amongst criminals
generally is largely to be explained by the educational back-
wardness of such offenders.   For the chief factors in the causation of delinquency are, as a rule, mainly emotional rather
than intellectual, and the share contributed by real mental
defect has been greatly exaggerated.

Messrs Yerkes and Bridges [7] decided to adopt a new mode
of marking, more especially in the case of psychopathic individuals in whom they are chiefly interested.   They constructed three ‘ point scales for measuring ability ’ for infants,
pre-adolescents and adults, each consisting of twenty tests.

The pre-adolescent scale has been most widely used and the tests in this scale, with one exception, are closely modelled on, or exactly like, those of the Binet-Simon scale. All the tests of a similar nature, as for example those for the immediate memory of digits, which Binet placed in different years according to the number of digits remembered, are grouped into a single test and given together, in increasing order of difficulty. In the Binet-Simon method of marking the all-or-none principle is used on the whole, i.e. the subject either succeeds or fails; whilst in the point scale there are graduated subdivisions so that the twenty tests consist of over fifty questions and credit is given for partial successes. The results of the examination are expressed in total scores ranging from 0 to 100, and by the help of a table of norms, constructed from the results obtained from normal individuals, a test score may be converted into a mental age. Theoretically the entire point scale is given to each individual examined, but in practice this is not necessary with very young children who break down with the earlier subdivisions of any test so that the later are unnecessary. The idea of giving the same tests at all ages is sound, since genetic psychology favours the view that all the important types of intelligent action are present germinally at about the third year of life, and subsequent development involves, not new forms but increasingly complex examples of functions already present in embryo. It is maintained that the point scale method is definitely superior to other varieties for testing psychopathic subjects and delinquents, and that it is more amenable to statistical treatment; but neither of these claims has been justified by experience.

MENTAL GROWTH

Much discussion has centred round two fundamental topics in the theory of mental measurement, namely the rate and limits of mental growth, and the constancy or variability of an individual's mental ratio. There is much conflicting evidence on both these points. In the first rush of enthusiasm the earlier workers believed that the mental ratio of a child was fixed and definite and would cling to him for the rest of his days. Subsequent research has thrown some doubt on this conclusion. Dr Doll for instance as the result of repeated examination of the same feeble-minded persons over a series of years concluded that the mental ratio was so fluctuating as to be worthless for prognosis. Professor Terman who, as we saw above, believed that the ratio was constant has recently taken up a much more cautious attitude. He points out that the mental ratio is subject to a serious mathematical disqualification on the ground that its probable error is relatively very large, as is also that of a mental age. The mental ratio for psychopathic subjects does not, according to his later view, always remain constant and for normals its constancy is only approximate or rather expresses a tendency.

Dr Wallin examined over a hundred children who failed to make satisfactory progress in a special school for subnormal cases. He tested them at intervals varying from half a year to six years, and found that the mental ratios in several cases differed by several units. He concluded that " it is frequently impossible to determine for years whether a young mental subnormal is feeble-minded or not." He made use both of Binet's earlier and later scales and of the Stanford revision, obtaining similar results with each of them; and inferred that the differences in the mental ratio, however measured, are too large to be ignored, and, in individual cases surprisingly large.

More recently he compared the Stanford revision with certain group tests and concluded that the inconsistencies as to mental age are so glaring that mental tests give no reliable means of grading pupils for the purpose of instruction.[8]

Investigations on normal children have so far led to a contrary view. Pupils from eight to sixteen years of age were re-tested by the Stanford revision at different periods, 43 at intervals of four years, 127 after two years and 298 after a year. For the year's interval the difference of mental ratio ranged from 7·2 to 4·2. For all the intervals combined only 8·5 per cent. of the cases shewed a difference of more than ten points and 89 per cent. had a difference of eight points or less. The duller pupils seemed on the whole to lose a small amount and the brighter to gain.[9]

A careful re-examination of elementary school children up to the age of fourteen by the same tests each time shewed a similar state of affairs.[10] The fluctuations that were observed were attributed to the method of marking, which assigns so many months to each test passed. It was observed that practice in the same tests once a year appeared to have little effect, since the children are never told whether their answers are correct, and the same wrong answer is, on the whole, apt to be given in successive years. There were 371 children examined (169 boys and 202 girls) and some of them were re-tested at the end of the first, second and third years after the initial test and 42 at yearly intervals of four years. The following table shews the changes in mental ratio observed.

Interval	1 year	2 years	3 years
No. of cases . . .	204	110	57
Median change . .	+ ·2	− ·6	0

The middle 50 per cent. of the change for the three years was between the limits of −5·1 and 6·0 points. The next table shews the changes for those examined four times :

	1st test	2nd test	3rd test	4th test
Average mental ratio	98·7	102·2	102·4	99·7
Change	...	+3·5	+ ·2	−2·7

The correlation coefficient between the marks of the first and fourth test was ·84.[11]

Similar conclusions were reached by Professor Rugg and Miss Colloton [12] after reviewing all the previous work on re-testing of about 1500 cases, and themselves testing and re-testing at intervals of about a year more than 130 individuals by the Stanford scale. They came to the conclusion that confidence could be placed in the approximate constancy of the mental ratio. The average difference found by all previous investigators for intervals ranging from six months to five years was, according to their calculations, five units. The typical positive differences (taking only the middle 50 per cent. of cases into account) were less than six points and the typical negative differences three points. They found also that the coefficient of correlation between the first and second of their own tests was ·84.

By the use of his revised scale on different groups of defective children between the ages of six and a half and fourteen and a half, Dr Burt demonstrated that the mental ratios varied but little ; on the whole there appeared to be a drift towards diminution. He annually examined the same set of 34 individuals in mentally defective schools for six successive years. The average ratios dropped from 63·7 to 57·1 and in all but eight cases the ratio was smaller at the end of five years than at the beginning. Another test, made in two successive years on 72 children in a school for defectives, shewed that 2 had remained constant, 17 had declined, but 53 had definitely advanced. In one case the advance was sufficiently great to enable the child to reach a mental ratio of 90, which is high enough to be considered normal. This instance is not typical, for seldom do such children advance one mental year per annum. Burt states that, although the rule is not established, the weight of evidence seems to shew that with subnormal children " low mental ratios tend to become yet lower with the lapse of time."

A similar conclusion has been reached by independent observers [13] with regard to border-line cases, i.e. children in ordinary schools who are referred for special examination as to their mental condition. By examining about 60 such children with the Stanford-Binet tests at different intervals, ranging from one to four years, it was found that half of them shewed a loss in mental ratio on the second occasion, the average drop being 6·3 points. The tendency to decline was most marked in those whose initial ratios were between 60 and 80.

It seems, then, that there are cases of deferred maturity, where development is not arrested but postponed. Such cases are also found in children in ordinary schools ; so that in London a second scholarship examination is held for those who ' bloom late.' There are also individuals of an opposite kind whose mental deficiency may be deferred till a later date, but such instances are very rare indeed.

The differences stated by different observers as to the constancy of the mental ratio and with regard to its change are sometimes the result of using different tests or different versions of the same scale. Again a pupil very frequently scatters his successes over different parts of the scale which makes comparison with other pupils unsafe, unless the device of the London revision is adopted of making the intervals between all parts of the scale approximately equal, and this is only partially possible. Sometimes, too, and this is a point of technique which only very experienced investigators can avoid, the examination is not carried out over a sufficiently wide range of the scale, since a pupil may fail in all the tests of a particular year in the scale and succeed later.

The fact that the mental ratio appears, on the whole, approximately constant has led to the assumption, which is apparently justified by experiment, that intellectual growth as measured by the Binet scale is not uniform from year to year but steadily decreases with age. It can be shewn mathematically that if the rate of growth were the only factor determining the constant mental ratio then the curve of growth would be logarithmic, the formula being $y = \log x$ where y represents the degree of maturity and x the chronological age. The curves of growth of all individuals might be of this form all parallel to one another but of different heights. A consideration of the logarithmic curve shews that for all practical purposes the curve very soon becomes asymptotic to the line of time. In other words, mental growth ceases for practical purposes at a fairly early age. Professor Terman used a mental age of 16 for all adults in finding their mental ratios, this being the age at which growth in intelligence is supposed practically to cease. Using the point-scale method Messrs Yerkes and Wood concluded that the rate of intellectual development diminishes from the fifth year onwards; between the years 16 and 18 there is a slight, irregular increase, which ceases almost entirely at 18 years. Later observers have suggested a surprising limit of 13 or 14 years which was based on the results obtained with the American army tests. Burt, however, as the result of more careful measurements adheres to the age of 16 as the limit. Dr Ballard,[14] by the use of graded ' absurdity tests ' in which marks were given for detecting and explaining absurd statements, shewed that in two large secondary schools the maximum marks were obtained at the age of 15 years. By extending his investigations so as to include about two thousand individuals, and pooling the results, he concluded that the rate of growth of intelligence gradually slows down, does not improve much after twelve, and is almost imperceptible at 16. A year of mental age is consequently not a fixed unit, but gradually diminishes as we ascend the scale of life. It should be observed that although the growth is very small after 16 yet, as it still continues, there may be a measurable amount in a decade.

These conclusions should be compared with the results of a research by means of a group test given to English grammar school girls and boys and University students.[15] There were 227 boys and 37 girls examined, 87 University men and 97 women ; and in addition, for purposes of comparison, 8 men and 18 women with degrees in Honours and 6 University Professors and lecturers. The written examination consisted of tests of synonyms, analogies, mixed sentences, completions and reasoning, one mark being assigned to each correct answer. In order to make the marking mechanical, alternative answers were printed and the subjects had simply to underline the correct answers. The table below shews the results (omitting decimal points) for all the subjects, the maximum possible mark being 189.

Age	11-12	12-13	13-14	14-15	15-16	16-17	16-17	17-18	17-18	22½	23
Sex	B	B	B	B	B	G	B	G	B	M	W
Marks	84	91	100	109	112	116	125	129	131	130	127

The Honours students and lecturers gained the following marks :

Age			22 y. 2 m.	22 y. 7 m.	Professors, etc.
Sex	.	.	W	M	...
Marks	.	.	131	142	175

The correlation of the marks of the various groups of boys and girls with the teachers' estimates was from ·62 to ·78. It will be observed that the marks steadily rise till about 130 but are not appreciably higher for the University students than for the older schools pupils. There is an increase up to about 17 years and little or no increase thereafter, whence the investigator concluded that "Intelligence, apart from experience, ceases to grow, except among men of exceptionally high ability." It must be remembered that the same total score in such a group test can be made from widely different scores in the individual tests, and consequently only doubtful value can be placed upon a single figure expressing the general result in terms of a mental ratio. Thus, in the reasoning test alone, the marks at 17 years of age were two and a half times those obtained at the age 11–12 years, and this was slightly increased amongst the University students ; so that a mental ratio based on reasoning tests only would shew a different result.   It is instructive to compare the figures just given with those obtained by the same group test given to all the six hundred boys in Rugby School.[16] As in the former case, the boys had simply to underline the correct reply.   In a previous test at the same school, on a smaller group, the results had been found to correlate with the masters' independent estimates of intelligence to the extent of ·83.   The head master stated that from his knowledge of the boys the results were a good indication of a boy's industry and " teachable ability."   The maximum possible mark this time was 200 and the following tables, as before, give the marks to the nearest whole number ; but for purposes of comparison with the previous table the numbers must be proportionately reduced.

Upper School	*Classical Side* *School Forms*					*Modern Side* *School Forms*				
Age (y. and m.)	17·8	17·11	16·4	16·2	15·6	17·8	17·4	17·1	16·6	16·5
Marks . .	163½	160	157	142	155	160½	150	137	146	136

Middle School	*Upper*						*Lower*				
Age	15·9	16·0	15·8	15·4	15·1	14·11	15·3	14·11	14·8	14·5	14·5	14·6
Marks	141	144	128½	131½	130	132½	114	120½	120	122	114½	109½

Lower School—Age 13·11.   Average mark 106.[17]

The head master thinks that the above figures " seem to disprove the contention that there is very little change in a boy's intelligence between 16 and 18."

The experimental facts concerning the growth of intelligence and the constancy of the mental ratio may be interpreted as being the result of two possible causes, either that the growth curves of all individuals, as previously stated, whilst shewing diminishing rates with time are parallel at all stages of growth, or that the curves of different individuals diverge from each other with time. Both these assumptions have been challenged.[18] The results obtained by the use of the various point-scale methods of measuring ability have been shewn to yield curves of growth approximating to the form of a straight line up to the age of 14 years. This would imply that up to this age the rate of growth is uniform. Further, the weight of the evidence yielded by such scales appears to incline towards the view that not only is growth in maturity uniform but that the lines of growth of all individuals are parallel. It would be rash, however, to assume that the results of the point-scale method are interchangeable with those of the Binet scale, or that either can be compared with those of dissimilar group tests ; and further after the age of fourteen there are decided indications that the rate of growth as tested by the various point scales does slacken down, even though its subsequent form is linear.

Objection has been taken to the attempt to measure the rate of mental growth by any limited series of tests on two grounds, namely that not sufficient mental functions are explored and also that there is less chance of shewing improvement at the later ages ; since the number of suitable tests is insufficient and it is more difficult to make an advance from a higher score than from a lower. In order to avoid one of these difficulties a large battery of scholastic and mental tests of very diverse kinds was fired at over a hundred and sixty children from 9 to 15 years of age ; the tests being given annually for two or three years.[19] The median gains in the whole series of tests measured in units of standard deviation were calculated ; and it seemed as if such gains were roughly constant for each age, indicating that the rate of mental growth does not vary between these ages. The number of cases examined is too small to justify a positive conclusion, but the method of employing a very large number of tests and re-testing the same individuals annually by exactly similar tests is a sound one.

ABILITY AND ATTAINMENTS

From what has been said it is clear that success in the Binet-Simon tests is not dependent on ability or maturity alone. Indeed, ability and maturity *in vacuo* are empty conceptions, and the attempt to measure native intelligence or ' mother wit ' apart from the material on which it is exercised is seductive but impracticable. Among the hosts of influences which determine the score obtained in the tests by any individual the chief is undoubtedly educational opportunity ; in fact, many of the tests are direct measures of school work. Hence those who appear most retarded mentally are still more retarded educationally ; feeble intelligence results in still feebler scholastic acquirements.

Using the method of partial correlations Dr Burt calculated that of the mental age of a child found by the London version of the tests " one-ninth is attributable to age, one-third to intellectual development, and over half to school attainments. School attainment is thus the preponderant contributor to the Binet-Simon tests." When the effects of age and intelligence are discounted the tests, contrary to a widespread belief, shew little correlation with ability in arithmetic but a decided correlation with linguistic subjects, especially composition. From this, it would be reasonable to conclude that the best single indicator of a child's intelligence would be found in his ability in composition.

The connection between scholastic attainments and the ability to do well in mental tests has been confirmed by an investigation of certain selected groups of metropolitan children.[20] Mental ratios were found by means of the Stanford-revision tests, and educational ratios, which are the counterpart of these, by means of very simple standardised tests of reading, adding, subtracting and spelling. The tests were given to children in special schools for physically defective children, to canal-boat children and to gipsies. Amongst over 150 physically defective boys and girls, mainly between six and twelve years of age, the mental ratio was 86·7 and educational ratio 86·9. When a comparison was made between the average attendance at school of more than eighty of these children the correlation coefficients between the percentage of attendances and the mental and educational ratios respectively were found to be the same, namely ·31. Thus the effect of physical defects is to reduce the mental ratio because it decreases the amount of schooling.

The canal-boat children attend school either little or not at all, but as far as health, cleanliness, morality, feeding and clothing are concerned their parents compare favourably with town dwellers of the same class. The average mental ratio for 76 of such children was found to be 69·6 which is only slightly higher than that found by Dr Burt for mentally defectives. But these children are by no means of the defective class. The clue to their poor performance in the tests lies in the fact that they are handicapped severely by their lack of educational opportunity, for the very youngest amongst them test normally. A startling fact was disclosed by comparing the children in the same family, namely that an increase of age is found to be associated with a decrease of mental ratio, shewing that the ability to cope with the tests depends on a scholastic frame of mind. Similar conclusions were suggested by the examination of gipsy children whose attendance at school is irregular but more frequent than that of the canal-boat children. The mental ratio of sixty of the gipsies was 75·4 whilst their educational ratio was 77·4 ; the correlation coefficient between average attendance and these ratios was ·37. As with the canal-boat children there was found a decrease of mental ratio with an increase of age, but not to the same extent since they have more schooling.

Both Binet and Terman, agreeing in this respect with others, found that children of superior social status have a higher mental ratio than those of a lower status. Thus, in the Stanford investigation the children were grouped into three classes, superior, average and inferior and it was found that the average ratio for the superior social group was 107 and for the inferior 93, which is " equivalent to a difference of one year in mental age with seven-year olds, and to a difference of two years with fourteen-year olds." Professor Terman attributes the difference, not however on very cogent grounds, to a superiority in heredity, i.e. to a better intellectual strain.

Further evidence was obtained by Burt in two schools in a London borough, one ' superior ' the other ' poor ', at opposite ends of the social scale as compared with the general average of all schools in the borough. The children of the superior school turned out to be nearly a year ahead of the average in mental age and the poor school were more than a year behind. From the known fact of the influence of school attainments on the Binet scale it is not surprising to learn that the preeminence of the superior school was more marked during the earlier years, sinking after the age of ten to about half its previous magnitude.

Messrs Duff and Thomson roughly classified the occupations of the parents of over 13,400 Northumberland children over eleven and under thirteen years of age, so as to shew differences of social standing, of skill and responsibility. They found that the average mental ratio was highest amongst the children of professional classes, namely 112·2, managers 110, and higher commercial classes 109·3 ; and lowest amongst the children of miners and quarrymen, namely 97·6, agriculturists, 97·6 and low grade labourers, 96·0. These results are hardly comparable with the former since they were

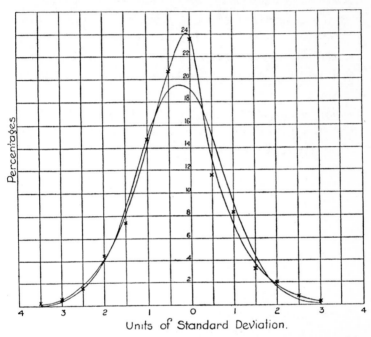

Units of Standard Deviation.

Diagram of Distribution of Intelligence drawn from numbers obtained by Burt. The upper curve shews the actual distribution, the lower curve the theoretical percentages for a normally distributed group.

obtained by means of the Northumberland group tests, whose correlation with the Stanford revision is however high, i.e. ·8. A rough classification into brain workers and hand workers shewed that the children of the former had an average ratio of 106·6 and the latter 98·6 ; the average of all the children being 99·6.[21]

A curious and illuminating fact has been brought to light

by the investigations in London schools, which seems to be in favour of the view that the differences in mental ratio, due to social status, are not the effects of nature but of nurture. The order of difficulty of the various tests differs both for children of differing social grades and also for the sexes. There is a distinct parallelism between tests which are easier for girls and for those which are easier for children of a better social class. One ground for the similarity lies in the partial similarity of environment, for girls are more supervised, sheltered and detained at home than boys, so that their external conditions tend to approximate to those of children in general of a higher social grade. It should be stated, however, that the variations in the order of the tests for differences of social status and sex are not very great in number or degree.

THE DISTRIBUTION OF INTELLIGENCE

Professor Terman had found that for over 900 unselected school children between the ages of 5 and 14 years the distribution of intelligence, as measured by his revised scale, was very symmetrical. The actual figures were as follows from which it will be seen that the frequency of the different grades decreases gradually in both directions from the median grade.

Mental ratio	56-65,	66-75,	76-85,	86-95,	96-105,	106-115,	116-125,	126-135,	136-145
Percentage	·33%,	2·3,	8·6,	20·1,	33·9,	23·1,	9·0,	2·3,	·55

The symmetry of this table should be compared with that of the following figures for the distribution of ability obtained by examining over 2700 children by the Northumberland group test.

Mental ratio	up to 60,	61-70,	71-80,	81-90,	91-100,	101-10,	111-20,	121-30,	131-40,	140 and over
Percentage	·3,	2·4,	8·8,	15·2,	23·9,	22·4,	15·2,	8·6,	2·9,	·3

Burt has treated the question of the distribution of intelligence at the ordinary elementary school age for London children very thoroughly. He combined the results of the percentages obtained at the different ages into a single frequency diagram and compared this with the results which would have been obtained if intelligence were distributed in accordance with the 'normal curve' of frequency. His figures for ordinary children have been used to construct the diagram given in the text, where the normal curve is superimposed for purposes of comparison. He says that the figures, if they do not corroborate, do not in any way contradict the hypothesis that ability is distributed in close conformity with the normal curve of frequency. The asymmetry can be readily accounted for, by the absence of adequate tests for brighter children of the older ages.

GROUP TESTS

The tests originating with Binet are intended to be given by the examiner to individual subjects and to be accompanied by a report on the manner in which such subjects deal with the single tests. Up to the year 1917 such individual tests held the field, although sporadic attempts at testing groups of persons simultaneously by written tests had been made. In 1917 a committee of American psychologists met to produce a group examination in order to classify recruits for the army.[22] They examined the previous tests of both individual and collective varieties. A complete group test, the work of Mr A. S. Otis a member of the committee, existed in manuscript and was similar in form to that finally adopted for the army tests. It must always be remembered that a group test gives no indication of the numerous minute, but extremely valuable, indications of mentality which an individual test offers the examiner. Further it is dangerous to apply a group test, outside very narrow limits, to other uses than that for which it has been prepared. Certain criteria determined the choice of the test adopted by the committee and these may be classified as psychological and administrative. There are four psychological criteria and every group test should be constructed strictly in accordance with them. The tests should have a high degree of validity as a measure of intelligence, being compared in this respect with independent estimates obtained either from those who know the persons, or from individual tests. The range of difficulty must be wide enough to test higher and lower levels of intelligence so that " if 50 per cent. of the group tested, or even 20 per cent., make zero scores, the test is unsatisfactory as a measure of a wide range of intelligence." Moreover the test ought to be as completely independent of schooling and educational advantages as possible ; a criterion hard to seek. It may be that some of the conclusions drawn as to the limits of the growth of intelligence partly rest on the fact that an examination attitude is cultivated in educational establishments which the adult, released from their toils, finds irksome and difficult to settle into again. Finally the material used should arouse the interest of the examinees.

All the other criteria are purely administrative and are aimed at examining and correcting as rapidly as possible, eliminating personal bias in correcting answers, avoiding coaching and demanding a minimum of writing in recording answers. Many enthusiastic testers appear to forget that these are all purely matters of convenience and have no psychological significance.

The committee selected a number of tests believed to have a high degree of validity as indicators of intelligence and gave them to selected groups. On the basis of these trials ten were chosen and given to a large variety of subjects in

the army, colleges, institutions for feeble-minded and so on.
Each test consisted of separate items the number of which
was so fixed that five per cent. of individuals or less in any
average group would be able to finish the entire series in the
time allowed. This was in order to give the superior persons
a fair chance ; the inferiors were catered for by one or two
sample items correctly answered and printed at the beginning
of each test so as to act as shock absorbers, and all the items
were set out in increasing order of difficulty. The tests were
checked by comparing their results with those obtained from
subjects who had previously been examined by individual
tests, and by teachers' estimates and officers' ratings. Professor Thorndike checked the validity, reliability and significance of the tests by statistical methods. As a result of all
this sifting eight tests were finally chosen and received the
name of army *alpha* group tests. Another group test known as
army *beta* group test was constructed for illiterates who
could not read English and was " in effect, although not in
strictness test for test, alpha translated into pictorial form."
The tests were given to nearly one and three-quarter million
men, but as the scoring and interpretation was entirely in
terms of military needs it is dangerous to generalise the
results. Even in their own sphere it was stated that " there
are convincing evidences that some men are not fairly measured
by either alpha or beta tests and that the provision of careful
individual examination " is necessary in such cases. The
reliability coefficient was ·95 and the correlation coefficient
with Stanford-Binet tests was from ·8 to ·9 for adults; for
American school children the coefficient of the alpha tests
compared with teachers' estimates turned out to be from
·67 to ·82. An application of these tests to seventy English
grammar school boys in the fourth and fifth forms [23] yielded
a coefficient of ·48 when compared with their ranks in school
subjects. When compared with the marks obtained in the

U

school certificate examination of a University the correlation was ·60.

Group tests have been widely employed in many countries for educational purposes to gauge differences in average intelligence in different schools and areas ; and in England have been most frequently used to pick out children from the elementary schools capable of profiting by a secondary education. In almost every case they have been employed as a supplement to the ordinary scholastic examination and are not intended to replace the latter. Where the children in small country schools are deprived of the educational advantages enjoyed by urban children, group tests are most valuable in redressing the balance. Professor G. H. Thomson has designed a useful test with this object in view known as the Northumberland mental test.[24] He prepared several tests including some examples used in the *alpha* series and devised certain new ones. These were tried on about fourteen hundred school children from $10\frac{1}{2}$ to $13\frac{1}{2}$ years of age in different parts of the country and thereby the unsuitable tests were discarded. Six types of suitable examples survived. The test lasts for one hour, and speed is eliminated as practically all children tested can finish all they can do in an hour. A couple of typical examples are shewn worked out in the printed tests, and, on the day before the test is set, a ten-minute practice-test is given as a safeguard against stupor pædagogicus. It has been found that pupils thoroughly enjoy the tests, so that in this respect as in the others, the criteria above enumerated were satisfied. In the preliminary investigations it appeared that the rural districts gave results which were more than a year behind those of a large city ; consequently when the tests are to be used in any area it is as well to use scores derived from the results in the same area. Generalisation in group tests is always hazardous and as far as possible the scores of each group should be used to measure the individuals within the group. A group of fifty children whose mental ratio was determined both by the Stanford-Binet tests and by the Northumberland tests yielded a correlation coefficient of about ·8.

A large number of other group tests have been devised and used, but as no psychological principles are involved in their construction or use other than those considered above, it is unnecessary to enter into details in this book. The student will find a bright account of a number of such tests in *Group Tests of Intelligence* by Dr Ballard.[25] It is interesting to observe that, in the attempt to make the tests suitable for educational prognosis, the testers have long since exhausted their ingenuity and have been compelled to fall back on well-worn scholastic material such as reading, arithmetic and general information. Although most of the standardised examiners despise their predecessors they appear to be unable to act without their material. Strenuous attempts have been made in America to devise group tests suitable for testing candidates for college. Professor Thorndike has constructed a group test of a composite form involving many of the *alpha* type together with absurdity tests, reasoning tests and others, and also scholastic tests, the whole taking two and a half hours. This battery was fired off at two hundred and fifty women students of average age $18\frac{1}{2}$ years on entering college and again each year in succession till they graduated.[26] As part of their normal procedure these unfortunate students were pestered thirty times with various college examinations during their undergraduate course ; yet the college is described as one " for the liberal arts." There were one hundred and fifty who survived. The correlation coefficients for the survivors between the marks in the academic examinations and the tests are shewn below.

Year . . .	1	2	3	4
Pearson Coefficient	.56	.43	.36	.38

It is usually accepted by experimenters, although no proof is forthcoming that such tests to be considered satisfactory should have a correlation coefficient with ordinary examinations marks lying between the limits of ·40 and ·60.

The mean correlation coefficient of the academic marks alone for the four years was ·68, and this figure may therefore be taken to be the highest which could be expected with the tests, since one sample of academic achievement could not, save by chance, agree more closely with a measure of intellectual ability than with another sample of itself. The decrease in the amount of correlation in the successive years was explained by the fact that the group became more homogeneous academically owing to the elimination of those who could not tolerate the examinations. The conclusion reached by the investigator was that although the tests can forecast a student's success in college as accurately as school records or college entrance examinations, yet they cannot be used alone to predict academic success but supply useful supplementary information in doubtful cases. One is left wondering whether the predictive power does not rest entirely on those portions of the test which are of a scholastic nature.

From time to time attempts have been made to compare the various kinds of group tests with one another. One such comparison was recently made with five group scales including the Northumberland variety which were given to about three hundred English children between the ages of 10 to 14 years in elementary schools and a girls' boarding school.[27] The average coefficient of correlation of all the five scales with the examination marks in ordinary school subjects turned out to be ·46, whilst an independent comparison with the teachers' estimates of the intelligence of the pupils yielded an average correlation coefficient of ·30. The different scales correlated among themselves produced high coefficients ranging from ·88 to ·70, and the experimenter inferred that the various scales measure much the same thing.

Possibly they may since many group tests are constructed more or less after the manner of alpha tests, with variations, but the assumption rests on precarious grounds. A coefficient of correlation obtained from large numbers may obscure individual differences. Thus two different group tests were given by the same person to 120 school children [28] and the correlation coefficient by the rank difference method was ·64 ; but six pupils changed rank more than 60 places whilst the median change of rank from one test to the other was 18 places. It was observed that " if these 120 pupils had been divided on the basis of the intelligence scores of one test into 4 class sections of ordinary size, 52 per cent. of them would have been in the wrong section according to the other test." As two forms of the same test usually yield very high correlation coefficients, sometimes well over ·9 the investigator doubted whether the group tests " though called general intelligence tests are really measuring the same element in the pupils' endowment."

Examples of individual and group tests are given at the end of the chapter. There are a large variety of other tests including performance tests involving no use of language, but the manipulation of pictures, models, etc. In addition there are vocational and scholastic tests. The last are of great educational significance but illustrate no additional general psychological principles and so are not dealt with here.[29]

SOME OBJECTIONS

In addition to the various criticisms that have been incidentally made up to this point there are some fundamental objections to mental tests which must now be briefly considered. A game can only be played properly when the players agree, explicitly or tacitly, to abide by the same rules, which agreement gives a certain ' set ' of mind. In giving a mental test the experimenter takes for granted that the person will assume this attitude of ' make-believe.' But a bright child may resent this attitude and refuse to adopt it, when an incorrect answer from the examiner's point of view may only mean that the child has adopted some other supposition. The universe of discourse within which the examiner expects his reply may not be the universe which the child is exploring. It may also happen that bright children regard the questions as ridiculous (which they often are) and the procedure as silly (which it sometimes is) and so refuse to play this particular game. Group tests cannot take into account this incalculable factor and it is always assumed that the ability to make the examiner's assumptions is an essential part of intelligence. In the latest published group test [30] the following examples, chosen at random, occur : " What do we tell people the truth to save them from being ? *Angry ? Excited ? Deceived ? Unhappy ?* " A child who told his parents an untruth might make them angry, excited and unhappy without deceiving them. Which of these four replies is an unfortunate youthful casuist to select ? " Stamps are put on—*tables ? letters ? pictures ? trees ?* " Everybody knows that tables are sometimes stamped in public places, pictures in library books nearly always are spoilt in that way and I have seen trees stamped in forests to indicate the route. Which is the correct reply to choose ?

Experimenters always claim that they get into friendly and intimate relations with the pupils when giving individual tests, but it may well be doubted whether this is possible in the time necessary to administer the Binet tests. Moreover the necessity of adhering, more or less, to rigid formulæ, which is the condition for making comparative observations, militates against the exploration of a child's powers and leads to examination stupor. This was well brought out by the Danish psychologist, W. Rasmussen [31] who tried the tests on his own daughters and found that they were far too easy for children brought up in freedom in a highly cultivated home. He treated the whole thing as a game and got replies which he regarded rightly as signs of intelligence though they would have been rejected by a mental tester as not in accordance with the standard answers. There is for instance a test in the eighth year series in which a child is asked to count backwards from 20 to 1 and he gave this to one of his daughters of 5 years 8 months. When she got into difficulties at the number 13 he heard her begin to count *forward* under her breath and he considered this ' an excellent proof of intelligence, the method of procedure being improvised on the spur of the moment, entirely on her own initiative.' But no mental tester would pass this as he would consider it not playing the game, so the child who does it is considered to that extent to lack intelligence.

A very acute objection against the tests was urged by the late Professor J. A. Green.[32] He pointed out that intelligence is correlative to the universe in which it works, it does not work *in vacuo:* thus a dog may be a very intelligent animal within its own universe of action. As the universe expands so the intelligence grows ; hence, when a man does no better than a boy in a given set of tests this does not mean that they have the same intelligence, since if we wish to give a test to both it must obviously be within the universe of the boy's capacity otherwise we should have no means of comparison. This may be put more generally thus : if we have two individuals A and B we have two universes to consider a and b. If the mental efficiency of A in universe a is x and that of B in b is y we cannot compare the efficiency of A and B until we know the relative complexity of the two universes.

WHAT IS INTELLIGENCE ?

Having traced the development of mental tests and considered the more important variations and refinements of
method, the question arises as to what it is that the tests
measure. The answer to this apparently straightforward
question is by no means obvious. It has been widely assumed
that the ability to do well in mental tests is a sign of a high
degree of intelligence and, in fact, the tests are frequently
called intelligence tests. This name begs the question as it
rests on the belief that the nature of intelligence is known,
whereas in fact the most diverse views are held on the subject
amongst competent psychologists. So divergent are the
opinions that some authorities have been compelled to take
up the position that the sole ability measured by the tests is
the power to deal with mental tests.

In a symposium on the definition of Intelligence, to which
the contributors were the leading American psychologists
who had taken an important part in developing the tests, the
disagreement was very pronounced.[33] One contributor went
so far as to affirm that so little is known about the nature of
intelligence that discussion about it is almost worthless.
Another, who has devised tests of his own and employed them
widely affirmed that he was not interested in what intelligence
is ; all that he required to know was what such tests will do
in solving practical problems of grading in schools and other
institutions. Intelligence would thus be a hypothetical concept
or working hypothesis which is helpful in practical work and
about which it is not essential to have absolutely clear ideas.
Such a view has something to commend it from the practical
standpoint, for it is frequently possible to make practical use
of a concept even though its ultimate nature is not known,
just as it is feasible to use and to measure energy from an

electricity department though neither the nature of energy nor electricity can be defined by the user. There is nothing, therefore, in this theoretical difficulty which would militate against the attempt to measure intelligence by the tests.

The simplest criterion suggested in the symposium was included in the epigrammatic definition that " Intelligence is the capacity to acquire capacity." Indeed it would be strange were it not so ; for whatever view may be taken of the nature of intelligence our only means of gauging it is by its performances. For intelligence, properly considered, is concerned with problems, suppositions or propositions, i.e. with meanings sought or discovered. An individual possesses intelligence in so far as he is able to adapt his actions and thought to the meanings, obvious or implied, in his physical or social environment. Mental tests rest on the assumption that the persons examined have had the normal opportunities of learning. A certain amount of knowledge is always presupposed, and those are not far out who assume that a properly constructed examination in school acquirements, is, whatever else it may be, a test of intelligence. At all events, as we have had reason to see, the mental tests so far produced depend on school attainments much more than on any other factor. There is also a growing body of opinion, amply confirmed by practical experience in mental testing, that it is impossible to divorce intelligence from emotional and volitional characteristics.

Psychological analysis has long since destroyed the belief in such conceptions as simple desire, unalloyed feelings, pure reason and similar notions ; and it is now generally held that all normal mental states must be viewed from three aspects, the cognitive, affective and conative. We should suspect, then, that the notion of pure intelligence is a pure abstraction. Several of the contributors to the symposium, mainly on the ground of practical considerations, took this view. Thus it was urged that such qualities as mental balance, control, steady purpose, etc. are all implicated in the idea of intelligence ; and these are mainly conative activities. Again, a person's emotional attitude, his degree of energy and perseverance undoubtedly affect his intelligence. It is difficult to believe that a mental test, given by a stranger and lasting less than an hour, can provide adequate scope for the display of such emotional and moral traits. The more profound and deliberate type of intelligence must surely escape such perfunctory treatment. In all mental testing emotional and volitional data should be taken into account by consulting teachers who have had prolonged intercourse with the individuals tested. Some of these difficulties had been foreseen by Binet and Simon during the period when they were constructing their metrical scale of intelligence. They pointed out correctly that to succeed in school work demands will, character, docility, regular habits and especially continuity of effort. But they were of the opinion that these qualities are hardly called into play in the tests and that, therefore, intelligence could be sharply distinguished from scholastic ability. In this view they were undoubtedly mistaken, and although Binet described intelligence as being displayed by suitable adaptation to the environment and was aware that scholastic attainments influenced the tests, he failed to see that the dominating part of the environment of a child was the school and scholastic tradition.

It was pointed out above that the assumption that mental tests measure General Intelligence or Ability was open to challenge, and some have gone so far as to maintain that to talk of Intelligence is merely to hypostatise a general name. In a word, whilst there are intelligent acts there is no reason to assume that there is a real entity called General Intelligence, but that this is simply a name for the average of all such acts. Much discussion has centred round this point and the matter is by no means settled. According to the ' *non-focal* ' view of the nature of intelligence, ability to perform any test depends on a complex of heterogeneous factors ; and if ability in any two performances is positively correlated the result is due to the degree in which the elementary factors happen to coincide in the two cases. On the ' *multifocal* ' theory ability to cope with a test depends on the particular mental level to which it appeals, such as sensory, ideational, etc. and two performances will be positively correlated when they call into action powers at the same level of consciousness. Finally there is the ' *unifocal* ' theory according to which one common factor called General Ability is always brought into play in performing any mental test ; and the amount of correlation between two performances, in so far as it does not depend on similarity of content or form in the tests, depends on the extent to which the common factor is involved.[34]

Professor Spearman, who is responsible for the unifocal view bases his belief in the existence of the common factor on the results of experiments in correlating various psychophysical or mental tests. A variety of different tests calling into activity sensory, motor, associative, volitional and other functions are given to groups of individuals and the coefficients of correlation between every pair of tests are calculated. Sets of mental or scholastic tests are dealt with in the same fashion. It is found in these cases that the measures of correlation are as a rule positive and frequently high, and whilst they are sometimes low they are only very rarely negative. These coefficients are also found to have a relationship to each other called the hierarchical order, that is, they may be arranged in rows and columns so that each is greater than any other to the right of it in the same row or, below it in the same column ; and the magnitudes follow a definite rule. The theory in question is sometimes known as that of ' Two Factors ' for it is thought that the performances of any individual in any intellectual activity, such as a mental test, depend on a general factor entering into them all in various degrees, and a specific factor peculiar to each test ; and further that there are no group factors involved, unless the tests are very similar. The nature of the argument which is believed to necessitate the existence of the general factor has been stated lucidly in the following manner. Suppose we consider a series of psycho-physical functions which we may call A, B, C, D, E, and " Let us for illustration assume that these are specific mani-festations of one common process, more or less essential to them all and therefore connected with them in various degrees ; then if A correlate with C, D, etc. in progressively diminishing degrees in that order, any other function of the same series such as B will also correlate with C, D, etc. in progressively diminishing degree in the same order ; and similarly if the correlation of C with A be higher than C with B then the correlation of D with A will also be higher than that of D with B ; so of E and similarly through the series in either direction. The system of correlations between each possible pair in such a series is called a hierarchy." *

Another equivalent method of defining a hierarchy is given by the equation

$$\frac{r_{ap}}{r_{aq}} = \frac{r_{bp}}{r_{bq}}$$

where r_{ap} is the coefficient of correlation between any two tests or functions a and p ; and similarly of the others. If the tests a, b, p, q are not obviously similar it is argued that the relationship expressed by the equation can only hold if there is some general intellective factor common to all the performances, and no group factors. It follows, as a corollary from the equation, that in any table of correlations arranged as a hierarchy every column has a perfect correlation with

* Burt. I have substituted letters for words to make the argument clearer.

every other one. Professor Spearman has demonstrated that all the work which had been done in the direction of correlating the results of tests for many years by different investigators satisfies this condition. The general factor is supposed to be due to a common fund of intellectual energy so that " every intellectual act appears to involve both the specific activity of a particular system of cortical neurones and also the general energy of the whole cortex." Now the conception of mental energy assumed in this statement is of very doubtful validity ; and if any analogy with energy in the physical sense of the term is implied it is definitely erroneous. Physiology, at any rate, knows of no fund of nervous energy for as Dr Adrian has said " speaking from a purely physiological point of view, it seems to me that the less we say about nervous and mental energy the better." Nor has psychology any use for such an energy fund as our study of fatigue in the next chapter will shew.

Experimental evidence shews that the tests which have the highest correlation with all other tests are those which depend most on voluntary attention ; and further that when the same tests are repeated till they become mechanical, so that little attention is required, the degree of correlation tends to diminish. On both these grounds it is inferred that the general factor is the power to concentrate attention. Thus we are almost driven to the conclusion that mental tests measure volition rather than intelligence, and lest we should hesitate to take the last step Dr Webb has asserted that his investigations on Character and Intelligence demand a second general factor other than general ability, namely persistence of motives or steadiness of purpose. Luckily, however, Dr Maxwell Garnett has prevented us from confounding the intellect with the will by the discovery, made with the aid of original mathematical devices, of another group factor called ' cleverness ' which is found whenever the tests are sufficiently similar.

Much confusion has been introduced into these experimental and statistical matters by the neglect of general consideration and the confusion of the subjective with the objective standpoints. It is sometimes forgotten that the numerical results of mental tests are concerned only with the objective side of experience and that the subjective aspect is a more or less happy inference from the data so obtained. Historically, the failure to distinguish carefully between the active subject on the one hand and the objects of his activity on the other led to the exploded doctrine of the structure of the mind as a congeries of separate faculties. But if we keep steadily before us the fact that there is only one ultimate mode of psychical activity to wit, attention, we are led to look in the direction of the objective aspect of consciousness for an explanation of the varieties of mental powers. Nobody has stated the correct position more succinctly than Professor J. Ward who says: [35] " At first sight it looks rather as if the kind of activity might vary while the object remained the same ; that, e.g., having perceived an object, we later on remembered or desired it. It would then be most natural to refer these several activities to corresponding faculties of perception, memory and desire. . . . Nevertheless, a more thorough analysis shews that when the supposed faculty is different the object is never entirely and in all respects the same. Thus, in perception, e.g., we deal with ' impressions ' or primary presentations, and in memory and imagination with ' ideas ' or secondary presentations. In desire the *want* of the object gives it an entirely different setting, adding a new characteristic, that of *value* or *worth*."

The fact that mathematical analysis of the results of the correlation of mental tests shews that the activity of attention is a factor common to all performances, is an interesting but unnecessary confirmation of this psychological analysis ; and indeed what else could anybody expect ? Dr Maxwell

Garnett's group factor of 'cleverness,' is, we are told, closely allied to wit or humour and cheerfulness and not merely cognitive. It leans, in other words, to the affective side of subjective processes. Now we have frequently seen that to describe the facts of experience we require not less than three sets of descriptive terms, cognitive, affective and conative. These attitudes are observable in varying degree in every psychical state; yet one of them may on occasion be reduced to a bare minimum. Such diminution is hardly likely to occur to the conative factor under the conditions of mental testing, and it would be equally difficult to effect a reduction in the process of cognition unless the tasks were absolutely mechanical. On the other hand the affective element may well decrease indefinitely during the process of the tests, as when the person ceases to be interested but has not yet become bored. We ought, therefore, to have anticipated that the results of mental testing would display a general conative factor and a group affective factor; and further we should be led to expect the existence of another general factor, corresponding to the cognitive side of consciousness and evident in all performances. The student may confidently anticipate that when some future investigator searches statistically in the proper quarter he will discover a general factor consisting of clearness of apprehension mingled with sound judgment as an essential feature in the conception of intelligence.

Before this consummation has been reached, however, Professor G. H. Thomson has delivered an attack on the methods used to prove the theory of the Two Factors.[36] He made artificial experiments by means of dice throws and card drawings so as to obtain correlations due to group factors selected at random. His method was to assign chance numbers obtained in these ways to certain letters of the alphabet thus getting a series of values for 'imitation mental tests.' When the correlations between these numbers was worked out and arranged in rows and columns all the criteria of the hierarchical order were found to be satisfied. The hierarchical order can consequently be produced without the necessity of invoking a general factor, but simply by the arrangement of group factors allocated by chance throws of dice and drawings from a pack of cards. In this way " it was found that in every case a very considerable degree of perfection of hierarchical order was produced, quite as high as that found in the correlation data of experimental psychology." A hierarchy amongst correlation coefficients may consequently be a chance phenomenon due to taking a sample instead of the whole population, and does not require any theory of a general factor to account for it. Professor Thomson, accordingly, proposes to substitute a ' sampling theory of ability ' according to which there are a group of abilities involved in carrying out any test, such factors being a sample of the whole number of elemental abilities which the subject possesses. In order to account for intellectual ability he uses the analogy of a game, where the chance of winning, other things being equal, depends on good team work, that is a group acting together as a unit. But no amount of mathematical analysis can eliminate the general factor of attention without eliminating consciousness.

In the experimental investigations into the meaning of intelligence so far considered the correlations between different tests have been measured by taking the results of initial trials of various abilities. There is a serious objection to this procedure owing to the great variability displayed by the same individual in the preliminary attempts to accomplish any task. Suppose it were desired to find out whether skill in cricket goes with excellence in tennis. It would be palpably absurd to take the results of the first few games or, indeed, to take any results until the individuals had found their level of ability. For the same reason it is better to continue the tests time after time until the person reaches his limit of capacity in each particular test. Professor Hollingworth [37] accordingly tested a group of subjects with half a dozen tests, instances of which were given over two hundred times until the limit of skill was reached as was shewn by the fact that a large number of subsequent trials produced no further improvement. The results of each test were correlated with all the others at various stages of the practice from the first to the last trial. It was found that the value of the correlations became markedly greater the longer the practice was continued; the average correlation coefficients of each test with all the others increasing from ·065 to ·490. There was some indication in these investigations that the coefficients of correlation cease to increase when the practice level is reached, and thereafter begin to decline. As long as practice improves performance, i.e. until the plateau is reached, there is a decided increase; but any drop from the plateau, such as may be brought about by slackened effort, leads to a decrease in the value of the correlation.

Professor Hollingworth thinks that the results favour the theory of general ability; for if this exists evidence should be sought in the ultimate capacity of the individuals. The earlier tests would be vitiated by chance variability, momentary attitudes, strangeness, etc. and being subject to these errors would not be true measures of ability. When each individual has reached the limit of his efficiency a fair sample is obtained and, then only, those who excel in one test also excel in the others. These conclusions are not well established since the number of individuals examined was very small, but the method is useful and, though the results have received a certain confirmation, further research in this direction would yield valuable results.

X

SAMPLES OF INDIVIDUAL TESTS

Dr Burt considers that for normal children the Binet-Simon tests yield the most accurate measurements at the ages of 6, 7 and 8 years.   The following are therefore given as samples of the London Revision in average order of difficulty.

Age VI

(Children aged 5 to 6 should do half the following in addition to previous tests.)

1 Knows (without counting) number of fingers on right hand, left hand, both hands.
2 Counts 13 pennies.
3 Copies a large diamond shape (2½ × 1½ inches) recognisably.
4 Copies legibly from script : " See little Paul."
5 Names days of week without error in 10 seconds.
6 Names without error 4 coins, 1s., 1d., 6d., ½d.
7 A visiting - card (2½ × 3½ inches) is cut in two diagonally. The triangles are placed so that the hypotenuses are at right angles.   The child fits them together properly.
8 Defines by stating their use 3 out of 5 of the following : horse, chair, mother, table, fork.
9 Repeats 5 numbers (1 trial correct out of 3) 52947......63852......97318.
10 Describes items in 2 out of 3 prescribed pictures.
11 Repeats after the examiner the following : " We are going for a walk ; will you give me that pretty bonnet ? "
12 Shews his (a) right hand ; (b) left ear.

Age VII

(Children aged 6 to 7 should do half the following.)

1 Recognises missing features (3 out of 4) ;   (a) man's head—mouth missing ;   (b) woman's head—eye missing ;   (c) woman's head—nose missing ;   (d) woman with missing arms.
2 Adds without error 3 pennies and 3 half pence (in 15 secs.).
3 States difference between (2 out of 3 in 2 mts.) : (a) fly—butterfly ;   (b) wood—glass ;   (c) paper—cardboard.
4 Writes legibly from dictation : " The pretty little girls."

Age VIII

(Children aged 7 to 8 should do half the following.)

1 Reads, without assistance, a prescribed passage enumerating 20 items and recalls 2 items out of the 20.
2 Answers the following questions (2 out of 3) :   What would you do—(a) if missed train...... ;   (b) if broke something belonging to somebody else...... ;   (c) if struck accidentally by boy or girl ?

3 Counts backwards from 20 to 1 (in about 30 secs. with only one mistake).

4 Gives full date. Day of week. . . . Day of month. . . . (3 days' error allowed) . . . . month . . . . . year.

5 Gives change for 2d. out of 1s. (from the following ¼d., ½d., 1d., 6d., 2s., 2s. 6d., 10s., £1).

6 Repeats 6 numbers (1 trial correct out of 3) : 250364 . . . . . . 853916 . . . . . . 471582.

SAMPLES OF GROUP TESTS

The following are samples from the *alpha* tests, the first and last item being selected in every case.   In all the tests except the first, one or more items are solved as a guide.

Test 1   Directions (12 items).

(*a*) Look at the circles (5 circles of 1 cm. diameter side by side are drawn).

(*a*) Make a cross in the first circle and also a figure 1 in the third.

(*b*) Look at 12 (the figures 1 to 9 printed in bold type). If 7 is more than 5, then cross out the number 6 unless 6 is more than 8 in which case draw a line *under* the number.

Test 2   Arithmetical problems (20 items).

(*a*) How many are 30 men and 7 men ?

(*b*) A commission house which had already supplied 1897 barrels of apples to a cantonment delivered the remainder of its stock to 29 mess halls. Of this remainder each mess hall received 54 barrels. What was the total number of barrels supplied ?

Test 3   Practical judgment (16 items).

Make a cross before the best answer.

(*a*) Cats are useful animals, because
— they catch mice,
— they are gentle,
— they are afraid of dogs.

(*b*) Why is it colder nearer the poles than nearer the equator ? because
— the poles are always farther from the sun.
— the sunshine falls obliquely at the poles.
— there is more ice at the poles.

Test 4   Synonyms and Antonyms (40 items).

If two words of a pair mean the same or nearly the same, draw a line under *same*.   If they mean the opposite or nearly the opposite, draw a line under *opposite*. If you cannot be sure, guess.

(*a*) wet—dry   same—opposite.
(*b*) encomium—eulogy   same—opposite.

Test 5   Disarranged sentences (24 items).

> Below are some mixed sentences. Some of the sentences are false and some true. Think what each *would* say if the words were straightened out, but don't write them yourself. If what it *would* say is true, draw a line under the word " true " ; if what it *would* say is false, draw a line under the word " false." If you cannot be sure, guess.

> (*a*) lions strong are   true—false.

> (*b*) repeated call human for courtesies associations
> true—false.

Test 6   Number Completion Series (20 items).

> Look at each row of numbers below, and write the two numbers that should come next.

> (*a*) 3   4   5   6   7   8 . . . . . .
> (*b*) 3   6   8   16   18   36 . . . . . .

Test 7   Analogies (40 items).

> In each line, below, the first two words are related to each other in some way. What you are to do is to see what the relation is between the first two words, and underline the word in heavy type that is related in the same way to the third word.

> (*a*) gun—shoots : : knife — RUN   CUTS   HAT   BIRD

> (*b*) cold—ice : : heat — LIGHTNING   WARM   STEAM   COAT

Test 8   General Information (40 items).

> In each of the sentences below you have four choices for the last word. Only one of them is correct. Draw a line under one of these four words which makes the truest sentence. If you cannot be sure, guess.

> (*a*) *America* was discovered by Drake   Hudson   Columbus   Balboa

> (*b*) *Scrooge* appears in Vanity Fair, The Christmas Carol, Romola, Henry IV

The following are samples of novel tests used in the *Northumberland* tests. They are selected from the easier or shorter examples.

> *Extra word.*

1 The pupil is required to underline the *extra* word.

> Example : wood, cork, stone, boat, bladder—stone because the others float.

> grapes, wool, oranges, apple, banana

Schema.

2 The following schema is explained and two relationships are solved as a guide.

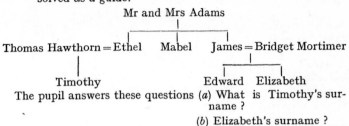

Mr and Mrs Adams

Thomas Hawthorn = Ethel   Mabel   James = Bridget Mortimer

Timothy   Edward   Elizabeth

The pupil answers these questions (*a*) What is Timothy's surname ?
(*b*) Elizabeth's surname ?
(*c*) Who is Timothy's uncle ?

Middle word.

3 The pupil has to arrange *mentally* the five words in each line
in their proper order and underline the middle word.

Example : minute   second   year   <u>hour</u>   week
elephant   sheep   <u>mouse</u>   cow   puppy

Hindustani Test.

4 The sentences below are in a foreign language and their meanings are given in English. In each English sentence a word
is underlined and you have to underline the word which
corresponds to it in the foreign sentence.

1. Kuch malai   some <u>cream.</u>
2. Kuch puri leoge   <u>will</u> you take some cake ?
3. Misri leoge   will you take <u>sugar ?</u>

This example is worked out fully and two more difficult examples
are set.

CHAPTER XII

MENTAL FATIGUE

The Forms of Fatigue—Influence of the Environment—Psychological
Factors—Symptoms of Fatigue—Sex Differences in Fatigue—
Methods of Measuring Fatigue—Fatigue and Rhythm

THE FORMS OF FATIGUE

DURING the last quarter of a century a considerable amount of
experimental research has been directed to the study of the
problems of fatigue, but the nature of mental fatigue has
remained obscure and the methods suggested for measuring
it are consequently very diverse.   The origin of the difficulties
lies in the failure to distinguish between various forms of
fatigue, coupled with search in the wrong directions.   Physiological or muscular fatigue was the first form to be investigated, and the methods and results have been too readily
applied to the case of mental fatigue.   From the point of view
of education it is desirable to understand the processes that
have been employed : for if a sound method of detecting and
measuring mental fatigue can be found it will play an important part in determining the distribution of the subjects in the
curriculum, the length of school periods and the time devoted
to work and recreation.   Within the last decade a beginning
has been made in the investigation of industrial fatigue, and
the conclusions reached, especially those for improving the
environmental conditions of work are applicable to schools
and will be briefly described later on.

Biologically, fatigue has been regarded as a defensive

function intended to ward off exhaustion. In accordance with this conception it has been defined as " a subjective impression with an objective impotence." But this assumed parallelism, between the feeling of fatigue and lack of power to work, rests on no solid foundation. It is possible to have the subjective feeling without diminished capacity and *vice versa*. Dr Rivers has recorded an instructive example from his own experience. He made a record each night of the contractions of a small group of muscles : one such reading was taken after a very fatiguing day, when he was so tired, that " it was only by a great effort that I brought myself to carry out my usual task." To his great surprise he produced a curve " very much larger than usual." [1] A similar phenomenon was observed by Miss M. Smith who carried out prolonged experiments on fatigue, produced by deprivation of sleep. As a result of her experiences over three years she states that the subjective feelings bear no relation to the objective demonstration of fatigue. " Subjectively I had no criterion whatever for the stage when the objective records shewed continuous deterioration nor yet for the return to the normal." [2] It is, in fact, as difficult to give a biological significance to subjective fatigue as to the emotion of fear. As in the latter case the feeling may injuriously affect the activity necessary to safeguard the welfare of the organism, so in the former the feeling is no true index of the state of physiological fatigue, and so does not subserve well-being.

We may distinguish three forms of fatigue which, however, are closely interwoven, (a) objective fatigue as shewn by abnormalities in activity or output of work, (b) subjective fatigue or a feeling of inability, resting partially on certain bodily sensations and (c) physiological fatigue, which is a state of a particular organ or organs. Diminished power of activity, it must be remembered, is a relative state depending partly on the difficulty of the task, as is shewn by the observation that a muscle, for instance, may be completely fatigued for lifting a particular weight, but nevertheless capable of lifting freely a lighter weight ; and relative also to the interest taken in the task.   The physiological state has no necessary conscious concomitant, but is inferred from chemical and physiological evidence.   Further, we must distinguish between lassitude and fatigue, the former being weariness due to monotony, lack of interest, etc. in which neither physiological fatigue nor subjective fatigue is necessarily present, yet there is diminished capacity for the task to be performed.

It seems hardly necessary to support this last statement by experimental data but nevertheless such evidence is forthcoming.   Certain individuals performed three simple tasks two mainly mental, namely adding figures in their heads, and adding figures by means of a comptometer, and a third physical, i.e. pulling at regular intervals against a spring. They worked for two and a half hours both in the morning and the afternoon, with an hour's interval for lunch, over a period of six weeks.   On certain days they confined themselves each to one of the three tasks, whilst on other days they had spells at each task in turn.   The amount of work done was in every case greater on the days of varied work than on the unvaried days, being from 4 to 24 per cent. in excess.   Also the accuracy of the work, as measured by the number of the errors in the first two tasks, was greater by more than 25 per cent. on the days of varied work.   It is consequently uneconomical to maintain the same form of activity throughout a long spell of work, and a considerable increase of quantity and improvement in quality results from variety.   Introspective records shewed that the results were due to the boredom and monotony of an unchanging task.

Subjective fatigue is a very complex state, consisting not only of fatigue sensations referred to different organs, but also of a feeling of inertia shewn in a disinclination to begin new

work.   There is also, hypersensitivity to noises, sometimes
accompanied by visual hallucinations : and what is more
important still, a heightened emotional excitability which,
by causing a feeling of exaltation, may result in an increased
power of work.   As previously stated, the subjective feelings
are no guide to objective fatigue : very bad work being sometimes accompanied by a conviction that it is remarkably
good.   There is some evidence to shew that temperamental
differences take a predominant part in determining the subjective differences to fatigue for the same kind of work.

The physiological state of fatigue may be briefly described,
but it is mainly with the other varieties that we shall be concerned since from the educational standpoint they are the most
important.   Whilst it would be rash to assume that the
incidence and development of mental fatigue follow the same
course as physiological fatigue, the relation of mind to body
makes a study of the latter a necessary part of the former.
In this study there are two factors to be considered, an energy
factor and a toxic factor.

During muscular contraction the tissues give out heat and
perform work as the result of the breaking down of glycogen,
an animal starch, stored in the muscles themselves and also
in the liver, as in a reservoir, from which supplies may be
drawn at need, as for instance after excessive labour.   The
glycogen is first broken down chemically into sugar, and then
into lactic acid, and by this means chemical energy is converted
into mechanical tension.[3]   When the muscles are again in a
state of rest the chemical process is reversed, so that the
greater part of the lactic acid is reconverted into glycogen, a
substance of higher potential energy.   The adrenal endocrine
gland aids this effect, for the internal secretion which it pours
into the blood defers the onset of fatigue in muscle and assists
in its recovery.   After a muscle has been fatigued the injection
of adrenalin into the blood will rapidly restore it to its resting

condition. This, it does, by liberating sugar from the stored supply in the liver. Excessive doses of adrenalin may produce an excess of sugar so that glycosuria results. Similar effects are produced by hard labour as in athletic contests and in examinations, after which some students shew temporary glycosuria. In order that the above chemical change may be reversible under normal conditions a supply of oxygen is necessary. If oxygen is not available the lactic acid accumulates and fatigue ensues, so that it is the accumulation of products of lower potential energy, and not primarily the exhaustion of supplies which is the immediate precursor of physiological fatigue. As a result of the recovery process the muscular system regains chemical energy. Although these facts have been established for the case of muscles excised from the body it is evident that good ventilation, by securing a proper supply of available oxygen, is an important condition in counteracting the effects of physiological fatigue.

In the living body the efficient performance of work depends not only on the state of the muscular apparatus, but also on the integrity of the central nervous system which initiates and distributes impulses to action, and on the conducting peripheral nerves which convey the impulses to the muscles. Now the conducting nerve fibres are practically unfatiguable ; thus the sciatic nerve has been shewn capable of conducting nervous impulses after continuous stimulation for ten hours, whilst the central nervous system, on the other hand, is more readily fatiguable. The parts of the nervous system most easily fatigued are the end-organs which are the nervous structures at the point of union of muscle and nerve, and the synapses or points of junction where adjacent nerve fibres meet. So that what really happens when the muscular system fails to respond to an effort of the will is a blocking of the nervous impulses at the synapses and the end-organs. There is also a central inhibition produced by the activity itself. For, when a muscle is voluntarily contracted, impulses are sent up the nerve fibres to the centres in the central nervous system the effect of which is to inhibit the impulses which normally travel down other fibres and produce further contractions in that muscle. Consequently, although a tired man refers his feelings of fatigue to sensations in his muscles, it is probable that by no voluntary effort can the muscles be completely fatigued ; for they are guarded, as it were, by the failure of the nervous impulses to find an open path to stimulate them. It is as though an electric tram were ready to start but could not establish proper contact with the overhead wires, or the connection at some junction had broken down.

But the muscular system may cease to respond for another reason. When a muscle with its attached nerve is isolated from the body and the nerve is stimulated for a long period, the ensuing contractions sooner or later progressively decline in amplitude and the time of each contraction progressively increases. If, however, the muscle is washed by a stream of salt water it recovers. The blood acts as a flushing agent in the living body so that the movements are not damped down. Moreover if an extract of fatigued muscle is injected into the body of another animal the latter shews signs of fatigue. These observations would appear to shew that in addition to lactic acid certain poisonous metabolites are produced by muscular activity. Fatigue of the muscle system, therefore, is not to be compared with the failure of fuel in a steam engine, or with the running down of a clock-weight, but rather with the clogging of wheels in some mechanism by dirt.

It is necessary to warn the student against a too-ready application of the results of physiological fatigue established by means of experiments on excised muscles. For the functioning of any organ of the body is controlled and regulated by impulses generated by the cells of other organs. Thus the source of impulses which gave rise to muscular activity is to be sought in other parts of the body, notably the nervous system. And it is hazardous to assume that an electrical stimulus can be a complete substitute for the normal impulse arising from such other cells. An impulse originating in living cells can exercise control over the functions of other cells. For example, there is a group of cells in the heart known as ' the pacemaker ' because of their influence on the rhythm of that organ ; and certain nerve cells possess the same power. It is by the influence of these structures that the organs of the body are caused to work harmoniously together.[4] The importance of this co-ordination of the activities of the living body will appear in the sequel.

There is some reason to suppose that an antitoxin is formed in the living body which counteracts the effects of the poisons referred to above. For a person is able, by practice, to acquire a relative immunity to some particular form of fatiguing process, as shewn by the delay in the onset of the symptoms of fatigue and their diminished duration. Not the least of the valuable results of disciplined study beyond the point at which the pupils would cease of their own accord, is the acquired habit of immunity to mental fatigue thereby induced. Any system of work in schools, which permits pupils below the age of 16 to cease applying themselves to a particular subject when they think they have had enough of it, is detrimental to their future resisting powers. Nobody seems to have called attention to this danger in the Dalton and similar plans of work for young scholars.

INFLUENCE OF THE ENVIRONMENT

Valuable information concerning the environmental causes of industrial fatigue has been accumulated [5] and some of the results have a direct bearing on schoolroom conditions, so that the student of education should be familiar with them.

In industry the degree of fatigue developed depends largely on the methods of work adopted, being much less in the case of the steadier and more systematic worker. Unduly long hours of work have been shewn to produce absolutely less output ; thus a reduction in hours from 66·7 to 55·5 per week of heavy labour resulted in an average hourly increase of output in the ratio of 100 to 137, and an increase of total output in the ratio of 100 to 119. Output is always low on Monday and at the end of the week. The former is known as the " Monday effect " and is due to the difficulty of settling down to work after the excitement or change of the week-end, and the partial loss of the effects of habituation. The present author has been assured that the men in a College eight always row worse on Monday than on other days of the week. The latter is due to the effects of fatigue which are cumulative during the week. There is also a seasonal variation, so that in some kinds of heavy work which involve high temperatures the output is greatest in Winter and least in Summer. Work done under artificial illumination even of the best kind causes production to fall, and when natural lighting is resumed some time is necessary before the output again becomes normal. Ventilation has a decided effect on output. Good ventilation prevents disease by removing dust and germs, stimulates muscular and mental activity by its physiological action, and is a psychological stimulus in that it reproduces to some extent the invigorating conditions of outside air. Dr Hill has shewn that these results of good ventilation depend on the *physical* rather than on the *chemical* properties of the air. A current of dry air cools the skin and stimulates the nerve endings. The blood instead of flushing the surface vessels is deflected to the visceral organs ; and the cool skin stimulates deeper breathing and increases the circulation so as to improve the health generally. Moreover the absorptive power of the air is increased when it is in motion, thus removing moisture exhaled from the lungs and evaporated from the skin : whilst stagnant air combined with moist heat causes the mucous lining of the throat to become turgid, providing a suitable culture medium for disease germs of influenza and consumption. Thus, to decrease fatigue and danger of disease, the air in a well-ventilated schoolroom should be cool, dry, diverse in temperature in different parts, and in motion produced by a cross draught.

PSYCHOLOGICAL FACTORS

We have seen that the structure of the nervous system acts as a screen to ward off the danger of excessive muscular fatigue by blocking the paths of the nervous impulses. The chief line of defence, however, against all the forms of fatigue, especially subjective or mental fatigue is psychological. It is impossible to over-estimate the importance of psychological factors in dealing with problems of fatigue ; and the neglect of them has vitiated the interpretation of experimental results. For every form of mental excitement influences the capacity for activity so that the bare knowledge that a piece of work is about to begin or end may have a decided effect on the amount a person is able to accomplish.[6] When the capacity for a particular sort of work is diminishing, as shewn by lessened output, a strong mental incentive may counteract this effect. Amongst such incentives are the desire to do well or to get finished, or to secure a reward ; whilst more important than all of them is an interest in the work itself or in some of its concomitants. The most convincing proof that the factors we are considering are purely psychological is to be found in the influence of suggestion on the ability to accomplish a task. It has been demonstrated, for instance, that when a person has been lifting weights, by means of an ergograph, until he can no longer raise a given mass, the mere suggestion that a portion of the weight has been removed, although nothing has really happened, will enable him to continue lifting. And the contrary effect has also been observed; when it is suggested that a mass has been added the person is unable to move the weight even though in actual fact a portion has been removed. Also there may be a lessened output of a particular variety of work when no fatigue is present and when capacity is not diminished, simply as a result of mind-wandering due to extraneous incentives or impulses to some other kind of activity. In fine, the quantity of specific work a person is able to accomplish seems to be a function of the intensities of the various sorts of stimuli to activity, the most important being the amount of interest he has in the task.

The above considerations must be borne in mind in considering the value of the various methods that have been used or suggested for estimating fatigue. Professor Muscio has recently called in question the possibility of finding any test of fatigue on the ground that, before the application of such a test, we must know independently what degree of fatigue is present. A similar objection has been taken to any attempt to measure Intelligence by mental tests since we require to know the grade of a person's Intelligence in order to be sure that the test itself has any diagnostic value. Moreover, as it is impossible to observe a person's capacity directly, it must be inferred from the quantity and quality of his output; but we have seen reason to think that the relation between them is frequently obscured by lack of interest, etc. Often, too, as was pointed out above, output is relatively good when the subject is undoubtedly fatigued but is stimulated by some strong incentive; so that the relation between fatigue and poor output is not a constant one, but merely expresses a general tendency. With these considerations in mind, Professor Muscio defined fatigue as " a condition caused by activity, in which the output produced by that activity tends to be relatively poor ; and the degree of fatigue tends to vary directly with the poorness of output." Although general and local fatigue are probably comparatively distinct, little harm will be done if the definition is modified so as to include in it the output which is produced not only by the activity itself, but by activities of a similar nature and difficulty.

One other difficulty remains which has been brought to light by the experiments, previously mentioned, on fatigue due to loss of sleep. As estimated by the quality of the output a state of fatigue displays two phases ; an immediate passing condition when the person is stimulated to do better work, followed by a later prolonged state characterised by general loss of accuracy, weakened inhibition, and loss of retentiveness. It is possible, however, that the more accurate work accomplished in the first phase was due to interest in the result of the experiments with its accompanying sub-conscious excitement.

These are, certain definite psychological and psycho-physical influences, first pointed out by Kraepelin, which serve to mask the measurable effects of fatigue as estimated by the quantity of output. Such are (a) practice or habit, including also familiarisation or feeling at home with the work, (b) warming-up or getting up steam, by which is meant the process of getting habituated, (c) swing, or the mood for the activity, the effect of which as also of the previous influence may be interfered with by a pause, (d) spurts, which frequently occur at the beginning or end of a period of activity owing to some mental incentive. Finally, and more fundamental than all of these is (e) rhythm of work which, owing to its importance, will be considered in detail later in the chapter.

SYMPTOMS OF FATIGUE

The growth of experimental science tends to be inimical to observations of a general nature, since it is recognised that in order to collect scientific facts the observer needs a technical training. It might be expected that the sympathetic observations of teachers would be serviceable in discovering the prominent signs of mental fatigue. Galton, with his indefatigable zeal and passion for collecting data of every conceivable kind, circulated a *questionnaire* and received replies from over a hundred teachers regarding the symptoms of fatigue both in themselves and their pupils.[7] The object of his questions was to discover the signs and incipient effects of mental fatigue with the ultimate purpose of finding out the causes of nervous breakdown. Whilst his suggestions for investigation in other directions such as sensory acuity, mental imagery, and anthropometry have been acted on by others and have borne fruit, it is strange that his researches in this direction have been allowed to lapse completely. The inquiry established the following instructive facts.

The commonest sign of incipient mental fatigue in school children is restlessness which is shewn in a variety of ways, such as sudden muscular movements, twitchings of fingers, grimaces, tendency to nervous laughter and general lack of motor co-ordination, leading to bad writing and, in extreme cases, to disordered speech. Sometimes there are disturbances of circulation shewn by cold feet and pallor or flushing of the face, with congested eyes. The rhythm of breathing is modified—by an acceleration of the number of respiratory movements and a reduction of their amplitude. Irritability also arises in consequence of which children become cross. When the fatigue is more pronounced it is indicated by headaches and accompanied by sleeplessness, talking in sleep and some-

Y

times somnambulism.   As far as the senses are concerned, the observation of teachers shews that both hearing and vision are affected ; especially the latter.   There may be a heightened susceptibility to sounds or the contrary, a diminution of sensibility.   Vision is often disturbed partly as a result of excessive eye strain, but as the following case attested by Galton shews there are more deeply rooted causes in the nervous system.   A lady teacher during a prolonged period of continuous study was subject to attacks of colour-blindness which disappeared with rest.   During such attacks she confused orange with ivy green, and blue with dingy yellow.   After a year's cessation from work she recovered, but was still prone to temporary periods of colour-blindness during mental fatigue.

The mental effects of overstrain, produced by excessive fatigue, have been well summarised by Dr C. S. Myers who describes the mental disorders directly induced by overwork which also affect the bodily processes.   " The failure of the higher intellectual processes results, on the psychical side, in a loss of control over the unpleasant conflicting experiences of the past, the memories of which, through such higher control have hitherto—it may be unconsciously—been inhibited or repressed from consciousness.   Fatigue impairs this inhibition, and bygone conflicts, together with repressed unsatisfied impulses and cravings, are now free to surge forth from the unconscious to which they have been previously banished. Thus the mind becomes tormented with the emotional experiences of the past. . . .   Neither over the worries of the past, nor over those of the present, has the self any adequate mastery ; and it has no longer the power to view them in the proper perspective.   They are like restive horses which have escaped from control and bolt away, bearing their driver along with them.   The emotional experiences thus engendered are accompanied by over-stimulation of certain organs of internal secretion, exhaustion of which reacts in turn harmfully on the organism. A shortage of psychical as well as of physical, reserve forces arises." [8]

We may summarise the symptoms described in this section in a single formula by saying that mental fatigue is indicated by a loss of physiological balance and disturbed rhythm.

SEX DIFFERENCES IN FATIGUE

One of the most important factors in the consideration of the question as to whether there should be any differentiation of the school curriculum for boys and girls respectively is their relative susceptibility to physical and mental fatigue. Dr Adami who has reviewed the anatomical and physiological evidence has shewn that after the onset of adolescence, which occurs shortly after the beginning of the secondary school period of the pupil's school career, girls are more susceptible to nervous strain and nearer to the fatigue point. Data on the subject are scarce and somewhat obscure, but the experience of teachers seems to leave no doubt that, on the whole, girls are more liable to overstrain and worry than the majority of boys.

There is some evidence also that during the secondary school age girls are more variable than boys with regard to tests of fatigue, especially at puberty. A coefficient of variation may be obtained by dividing the average of a group of subjects by their mean deviation and in this way the variabilities for different ages may be compared. By means of a fatigue test the following coefficients were found : [9]

Ages	6	7	8	9	10	11	12	13	14	15	16	17
Boys	·41	·43	·34	·30	·34	·32	·33	·42	·35	·35	·30	·43
Girls	·33	·33	·30	·38	·37	·30	·48	·40	·51	·50	·48	·32

In comparing boys with girls it is necessary to remember

that as regards anatomical age, determined by such things as the growth of teeth, hair, etc., girls are six months in advance of boys at the age of 5 and two and a half years at the age of 15. This means that " the girl is proportionately almost adult while the boy is still adolescent and the initial periods of strain fall at different periods." Apart from differences of stature and weight in the sexes at corresponding ages there is a physiological difference which is very important from the point of view of fatigue. Up to the age of puberty the composition of the blood is the same in boys and girls, but thereafter the specific gravity is lower in women than in men and remains so until about the age of 45 to 50. This state of affairs is due to the fact that man's blood contains relatively less water and more red corpuscles. Consequently the proportion of hæmoglobin is less in the adolescent girl and remains so, and this indicates a lessened capacity for absorbing oxygen and for metabolic rehabilitation. Women are, therefore, nearer the threshold of anæmia than men and general experience bears out this observation. During the years of secondary education, boys are not only physically stronger but have greater reserves of strength.

Again, the essential organs of sex act as endocrine glands elaborating and discharging into the blood stream certain secretions, called hormones, which are carried to other parts of the body and exert a selective influence on those tissues and organs concerned in the production of secondary sexual characters which are peculiar to the sexes. Moreover, other endocrine glands, such as the thyroid in the neck and the adrenals on the kidneys are brought into mutual functional relationship with the sex organs by means of the blood stream. Such connection appears to be of significance in regard to the quantity of calcium in the body ; and calcium salts are thought to play a part in maintaining the blood pressure and in controlling the excitability of the muscles. Although the evidence is by no means strong, it is believed that there are differences in the drain of calcium from the blood which shew themselves at the time of puberty for " in the female the calcium metabolism becomes unstable, whereas in the male it remains relatively constant." Defective calcium metabolism is the cause of softening of the bones which leads to spinal curvature and postural defects which, it is well known, are commoner amongst girls than boys.

The internal secretions produced by the endocrine glands produce an effect on the organism very similar to that caused by drugs, namely variations in the pulse and blood pressure, in organic tone, in deferring the onset of fatigue and generally in exciting or depressing the bodily functions. It will be noticed that such bodily changes are characteristic of emotional expression and, as some of the hormones are different in the sexes, it would be reasonable to expect a difference in emotional functioning and mood accompanied by different susceptibility to emotional and nervous strain. Owing to these considerations, and also to the fact that boys are less industrious and conscientious than girls, presenting a more obstinate resistance to the pressure of overwork by the cultivation of a spirit of healthy idleness, it comes about that girls, especially at the period of adolescence, are nearer to the fatigue point. If a girl is given too severe mental work she breaks down under strain ; whilst the boy in similar circumstances, with less conscientiousness, gives up the work ; in this way acquiring an immunity to scholastic fatigue.

METHODS OF MEASURING FATIGUE

It is now time to consider the more important of the various methods which have been employed or suggested to measure fatiguability. These may be divided into *Active* methods, in which the person examined has to exert voluntary activity, muscular or mental ; and *Passive*, in which certain non-voluntary phenomena supposed to be indicative of a state of fatigue are tested. Amongst the latter, tests of sensory acuity were frequently employed in the earliest attempts to measure fatigue. There was a twofold reason for this choice. Experimental psychology had been largely concerned with measurements of sensation, and when a fatigue test was required the investigators naturally turned to the subject they were most familiar with. They also made the obvious assumption that the effects of fatigue would be most readily displayed in a diminution of sensory acuity, for they held the view, though not consciously formulated, that there was a fund of energy at the disposal of the subject, which, having been more or less used up by physical or mental work left a smaller amount at the disposal of the senses.

Now there is a serious objection to such a view of the nature of fatigue, which has been well stated by Dr E. D. Adrian.[10] He points out that the term energy is employed in two different senses, biological and physical, as when we speak of a man of energy or the energy of a moving body. " In both phrases we are using ' energy ' to mean the capacity to do work, but in the first case work means biological or ' purposive ' activity, and in the second it means physical work, the product of a force into a distance. . . . If we speak of ' mental energy ' (to take the extreme case), we may mean something analogous to physical energy, but it is obvious that it must be defined in quite different terms. Mental work, and mental forces and resistances may have a clear enough meaning for us, but it is a meaning which involves ideas of life and purpose. Mental energy may perhaps be regarded as the product of the force into the resistance overcome (though both are imponderables) but because there is an analogy there is no reason to suppose that this mental energy will follow any of the generalisations which have been observed for the energy changes in material systems." In particular we have no right to assume that when there is a state of mental fatigue brought about by mental activity there must be a corresponding decline in the amount of " energy " available for sensory activity. Independent observation or experimental evidence is necessary in order to verify such a hypothesis.

A considerable volume of work has been performed in this connection on the sense of touch. If two compass points are placed simultaneously on any part of the skin it is found that they must be separated by a certain minimum distance called the spatial threshold, which varies on different parts of the body, before the person can discriminate the two touches. At distances below the threshold the double touch appears single. It was believed that fatigue would make the discrimination of the points more difficult. The only consistent results which emerged from this æsthesiometric method were that the threshold of tactile acuity was raised after formal gymnastic exercises whilst games lowered it. In other words gymnastics are work whilst games are play. But there is no convincing evidence that variations of the threshold are proportional to variations in fatigue.

Sensibility to pain has been measured by means of an algesimeter, an instrument for exerting a pressure of known intensity on the surface of the skin by means of a blunt point attached to a spring. Some observers have found that mental fatigue raises the threshold of pain, others state that it is lowered.

Tests of the acuity of vision and of hearing have likewise been employed, and it has been asserted that the limiting range of sight and hearing diminishes in the evening after a day's work. The results are more consistent for auditory than for visual acuity, but in neither case very convincing.

Measurements of the variation in blood pressure before and

after mental effort have also yielded no very consistent results, but there is some evidence of a decrease of systolic pressure after work, accompanied by a change in respiration. All such methods shew great individual differences and are seriously affected by factors other than fatigue, such as emotion or sickness; and unless the results of passive methods can be shewn, by independent evidence, to be positively correlated with those of the active methods their value remains problematical.

Although the speed of a reaction is not wholly dependent on the will of the subject we may regard reaction-time experiments as forming a sort of transition from passive to active methods. In simple reaction-time experiments the person responds to a single sensory stimulus such as a letter, word or colour, or a simple shock, by pressing a key or uttering a word; and the time necessary to make the reaction is recorded automatically —usually by an electric device, the reacting movement making or breaking a circuit. It might be supposed that the muscular response would be slower in a state of fatigue, but the results are variable; for the subject sometimes has a smaller reaction-time after a period of intensive work, or at the end of a day's labour. For complex reaction-time experiments the subject responds to some stimulus such as a light or a sound, by choosing between two or more reactions; or he may be required to react to some definite stimulus but to refrain from reacting to others. Here, too, we often get apparently paradoxical results for the reaction may be made more quickly when the person is presumably in a state of fatigue after work. It is evident that either the reaction-time is not regularly prolonged owing to fatigue, or that the experimental results have been wrongly interpreted; and the latter alternative is probably the correct one as will be seen later. There are some results, however, which shew that reaction-times are slower at the end of a week's work, which has been interpreted to mean that the effects of fatigue are cumulative. A most ingenious and interesting reaction-time experiment was suggested by Galton which can be used with even the youngest of school children, being in fact an enjoyable game. The teacher and the pupils hold hands in a ring, the latter with eyes closed. At a time noted on a watch the teacher squeezes the right hand of the adjacent pupil who passes it on to the next pupil, and so on, until the squeeze goes the round and reaches the teacher again, when the time is noted; or, preferably, several circuits may be made continuously at one time. If the total time taken is divided by the number of pupils in the circuit and by the number of circuits we arrive at the average reaction-time for each pupil. Galton must have played this delightful game himself for he has stated that the squeeze usually takes one second to pass through each dozen or fifteen pupils.

Tests of muscular strength as shewn by the ergograph, an instrument in which the contractions of the finger muscles are registered, the rest of the hand and the arm being clamped in a fixed position; or by the dynamometer in which a spring is pressed in the hand and its movements recorded on a dial are the active methods most widely used in the past. With these are allied such tests as the rapidity of tapping a Morse key, or the accuracy of movement as shewn by dart-throwing, or the number of repetitions required to learn a set of non-sense syllables, etc. The ergograph has been applied to the measurement of mental fatigue in school children, as it was thought that concentrated attention would produce loss of muscular power in accordance with the hypothesis previously mentioned. It was hoped, at one time, to be able to measure the relative fatiguability of different school subjects by the ergographic method. The instrument was also employed to demonstrate the influence of alcohol, coffee, tea, etc., on fatigue. In using an ergograph variations occur both in the number and the height of the contractions, leading to the belief that there is both a central and peripheral factor in fatigue. All such conclusions are vitiated by the effect of the psychological factors which, as stated before, produce irregular and contradictory readings.

It is evident that in order to measure mental fatigue the most suitable means are active methods in which mental activity is indicated by the quantity and quality of the mental work which is done. Various simple mental operations have been used for this purpose, such as the performance of simple additions or multiplications, in which the amount of work is estimated by the number of examples done correctly in a given time, and the quality by the number and nature of the errors. Of a similar nature are those tests consisting of dictations or arithmetical problems of similar length and difficulty performed before and after a period of mental work. By analysing the nature of the mistakes in dictation, such as those due to the transposition or omission of letters and so forth, some attempt has been made to estimate the quality of the work.

Individual differences are of very great significance and psychological disturbing conditions render difficult the interpretation of the results. Nevertheless it has been stated, by some observers, that the spontaneous appearance of fixed habits due to the home environment of the children can be detected in the mistakes that are made, and that fatigue is thus indicated by the loss of higher control over later formed school habits. On the other hand the onset of fatigue is frequently masked by the action of previously acquired stable habits ; so that diminution of speed or accuracy in the tests is not invariably shewn when fatigue is obviously present.

Other methods of an active kind have been suggested and used, such as the filling in of blank spaces left in a printed text, the reproduction of a series of numbers read to the subject at a uniform rate and so forth, A very useful test which would repay further investigation is that of associated words, employed by Miss M. Smith. It demands a double mental effort, namely the recognition of relationships between successive words and the retention of the right sequence. A list of forty words is used each having some connection with its successor as for instance, sheep, grass, plain, beautiful, Apollo, Greece, candle, etc. The list is read to the subject at the rate of one word in two seconds, after which, being given the first word, the whole series has to be reproduced. Failure to give the correct word in ten seconds counts as an error, whilst a wrong word corrected in ten seconds is half an error. The effect of a state of fatigue is greatly to increase the number of errors, since attention is difficult to sustain. But lack of attention may be due to causes other than fatigue, such as lack of interest and this, as before, renders doubtful the interpretation of results in all such methods.

A review of the various devices that have been employed makes it clear that any trustworthy method of estimating mental fatigue must conform to certain essential conditions. The active method should be followed and the tests must be mental and not physical or sensory. Psychological factors must be allowed for or balanced by means of control experiments performed on subjects who are not fatigued. The nature of the work by which fatigue is measured ought to be similar to the kind of work which has produced the fatigue. Attempts to draw conclusions from the amount of work done in the tests must be abandoned, which implies that the calculations should be made on some other basis than that of quantity. Finally the interest of the persons examined must be maintained at a maximum by securing their active co-operation.

Some of these conditions are satisfied by the following investigation of mental fatigue in school children.[11] Different classes of boys and girls were examined by preliminary tests consisting of arithmetical problems graded according to their ages. Every class was divided on the basis of the marks gained by the individual pupils into two equal teams A and B ; each pupil in team A being matched against one of team B who had secured the same number of marks, so that the teams were of equal ability. In what follows we shall ignore the class of infants seeing that they were only six and a half years of age. The equivalent groups worked identical problem tests in the first morning period and the last afternoon period of the school day, respectively, with the following results :

| | Average age | | | Average mark | Coefficient of variability [12] |
	Years	Months			
Boys	10	7	Morning group A	47·8	30
		.	Afternoon ,, B	44·6	33
Boys	12	9	Morning group A	19·4	8·2
			Afternoon ,, B	18·9	9·0
Girls	11	0	Morning group A	10·2	14
			Afternoon ,, B	9·6	20

If we confine our attention to the marks gained by each team it will be seen that the morning groups were superior to the afternoon groups to the extent of 6 to 7 per cent. for the younger children and 3 per cent. for the older. Mr Winch, who performed the experiment, followed in the footsteps of all his predecessors and based his conclusions regarding fatigue on the capacity and accuracy of the pupils as shewn by their marks. He inferred in this way that mental work of an arithmetical kind appears to be less affected by the fatigue engendered by the school day as the children increase in age and that for the older pupils the fatigue effects are negligible.

But inferences of a totally different kind are suggested by the figures if properly interpreted. The relative variabilities of the different groups are shewn in the last column of the above table, and if the experimenter had used these numbers he would have had a very different tale to tell. For it has been shewn repeatedly that the quantity of the work done is no true index of the state of fatigue. We must look for the effects of fatigue in the direction of steadiness of work rather than of quantity. Regarded from this angle both afternoon groups of boys are more variable by about 10 per cent. than their corresponding morning groups, whilst the afternoon team of girls has become quite ragged, being over 40 per cent. more variable than their morning competitors.

FATIGUE AND RHYTHM

Enough has now been said to shew the fallacy of attempting to estimate fatigue by the amount of work that a subject is able to accomplish. For, although a fatigued person may feel impotent to continue the fatiguing work, we have ample reason to believe that by an effort of will he can conquer this, and so defeat the purpose of any test. But although he can accomplish the task, and do it even accurately, he cannot command his voluntary attention. Mental fatigue is displayed by a diminution of the power of *steady* attention to which the subject is liable as the result of mental work; and physical fatigue is shewn in the same manner. If experimenters had devoted their researches to this aspect of fatigue instead of attempting to estimate capacity or accuracy it is probable that a suitable fatigue test would long since have been discovered. Isolated observations have been made from time to time which indicate that this is the very kernel of the problem of fatigue. Thus, in Miss Smith's prolonged and careful study of the fatigue state, one of the experiments consisted in marking dots with a pencil accurately in the centres of a large number of small irregularly disposed circles on a moving sheet of paper.[13] Attention was so disturbed owing to fatigue that " the loss of control as evidenced by the inability to restrain the hand from making unaimed extra dots is very marked and is as characteristic of the fatigue state as the loss of efficiency shewn by the ineffective aiming." Further evidence is provided by a study of the windmill illusion. If one gazes at a windmill from the side, at a little distance away, the movements of the arms appear to change direction from time to time owing to disturbances of attention. By setting up a small windmill in a laboratory it was found that in normal circumstances, trying by an effort of will to maintain the windmill revolving in one direction as long as possible, there were on the average seven apparent changes of direction per minute. During prolonged fatigued states the number of changes of direction increased greatly, mounting up to between thirteen to forty for several days. That is to say voluntary attention in states of fatigue is subject to large uncontrollable fluctuations as long as the fatigue effects persist.

The author of this book undertook the task of investigating such disturbance of attention in school children by the following method. Printed texts, of suitable difficulty, were used in which there were no divisions between the words or sentences, no paragraphs and no punctuation ; so that the appearance of the text was simply a continuous series of letters. The subjects were schoolboys whose average age was 14 years and who were the brightest class in a Central School. Instructions were carefully given by the head master who told the boys that this was a competition for accuracy in which two teams would compete against each other. All the boys were exceptionally keen throughout the whole experiment, and on every occasion asked which team was winning. At the beginning of every test the importance of accuracy was emphasised and they were told that they would be heavily penalised, in marks, for inaccurate work. They were instructed to divide the text by short vertical lines between each word

and to place a cross above the line to indicate a full stop.   A
five-minute test, by a stop-watch, was given on each occasion
and at the end of each minute a signal was made, when the
subjects drew a horizontal line under the last word they had
done.   In this manner a record was obtained of the number
of words marked off during each of the five minutes.   One
mark was given for each word correctly marked and two marks
for each full stop correctly placed ; whilst one mark was
deducted for each incorrect word,[14] and two marks for each
stop wrongly inserted or omitted.   In order to habituate the
boys to the procedure, and to give as much preliminary practice
as possible, a five-minute test was given to the whole class on
three successive occasions, each separated by one day ; two
in the morning shortly after school began and one in the
afternoon during the last school period.   A final practice test
was given a fortnight later so as to ensure that any unconscious
habituation should have its full effect ; a sort of incubation
period.   On the basis of these four tests the class was divided
into two groups A and B of equal ability.   There were 13 in
each group.   Four boys who had disobeyed instructions were
eliminated ; two of them were the brightest boys in the class,
who in their eagerness to make a good score, had rushed the
work, doing a lot but doing it badly !   The class was told
that any other boy who disobeyed instructions would be
thrown out of the teams, and this was effective.   To stimulate
them to competition still further the total marks gained by
each team were stated on each occasion.

The experiment proper began one week later on a Thursday,
as it was assumed that scholastic fatigue would be better
displayed near the end of the week.   Group A was given a
five-minute test (1) shortly after the school assembled in the
morning, and group B was given the same test during the last
lesson of the afternoon.   On the following day (Friday)
group B was given test (2) in the morning and group A took

it in the afternoon. The number of marks gained per minute by each boy was found ; thence the mean variation and the coefficient of variability for the five-minute test were calculated for each boy. The following table exhibits the average of the results for each group at the different periods.

			Average mark per minute.	Average coefficient of variability.	
Thurs.	a.m.	Group A	34·1	11·9	Test (1)
	p.m.	Group B	34·0	14·0	
Fri.	a.m.	Group B	32·0	16·0	Test (2)
	p.m.	Group A	30·4	17·2	

A study of these figures shews that the variability of the individuals of the afternoon group exceeds that of the morning workers, both when the average amount of work done is practically the same (Thursday) and also when the quantity of work done is less (Friday). The figures suggest that the effects of fatigue are cumulative at the end of the school week. One great advantage of this test over all others is that the subject's conscious effort or interest does not directly affect the measurable results. For the subject is trying to gain marks, whilst the experimenter is not immediately concerned with these, but with the variability of the marks during a short period. Here, then, is the direction in which future investigation must search for the effects of fatigue. Mental fatigue does not necessarily diminish the amount of the work done ; whereas the uncontrollable fluctuations in voluntary attention have here been shewn to produce measurable effects in subjects whose interest was maintained at a very high pitch by the spirit of competition.

Bearing in mind the clue we now have for detecting fatigue it is interesting to see that where published results give detailed figures, for short periods of work, the view here presented is confirmed though the authors themselves are often unaware of the implications of their data. In a recent experiment in which eight college students performed arithmetical additions for a continuous period of 10 hours, with a break of about half an hour for lunch, the number of examples correctly done in each of the first and last 10-minute periods is set forth in the succeeding table.[15]

	1	2	3	4	5	6	7	8	9	10
First 10 minutes	45	37	36	43	34	36	38	40	37	38
Last 10 minutes	42	34	38	33	45	34	37	39	35	42

Now the mean number correct in the first 10-minute period is 38·4 and in the last 37·9, a difference of just over one per cent., which apparently yields no indication of fatigue. But there *must* be fatigue after such an effort and the figures for the variability coefficients clearly shew it, being 6·7 and 8·7 respectively, an increase of thirty per cent.

A striking confirmation of the theory that the real effects of fatigue are to be sought in increased variability has recently been obtained by a new method of measuring fatigue of the eyes.[16] A series of printed words were exhibited on two vertical planes at distances of about 9 inches and 45 inches respectively from the eye. The person tested had to accommodate his eye rapidly to read the words first on the one plane and then on the other, backwards and forwards, alternately. By an ingenious electrical device it was possible to measure the time required by the internal and external muscles of the eye to bring the words into focus at each distance, i.e., the time of the act of fixation and accommodation. A large number of readings was taken, and the percentage of correct perceptions at each distance and the average accommodation time were found. The ratio of the former of these quantities to the latter is called the fixation-accommodation coefficient. A set of readings was taken for each person examined, and the coefficient was calculated. Then he was placed under conditions where the illumination could be controlled and

z

measured, and he engaged in reading for some time, either in a very dim light which put a very severe burden on the eyes, or in normal illumination, or in light of some intermediate intensity. At the end of a measured period, varying from one to two and a half hours, the coefficient was again found by means of tests exactly similar to the original ones. In this way it was quite easy to determine the variation in the combined accuracy of discrimination and rapidity of accommodation brought about by the fatigued state of the eye, induced by prolonged reading.

A comparison of the coefficients antecedent and subsequent to the reading revealed wide variations in the susceptibility of different persons to fatiguing conditions. Whilst the coefficients of some subjects were found to diminish markedly, as a result of the strain of reading, as might be expected, others were highly resistant to fatigue, and their coefficients increased owing to a heightened ocular capacity, so that words which could not be distinguished in the preliminary tests could be clearly seen in the final tests, owing possibly to the formation of antitoxins to fatigue. These cases were the extremes, for intermediate grades occur. There is one remarkable characteristic in which the extreme grades differ from one another, which is exactly similar to that found by the author of this book in the investigation previously described. When the mean deviations of each of the series in the preliminary and final tests were compared, it was found that those whose ocular capacity diminished, as the result of fatigue, exhibited a more pronounced increase in variability. This implies that their muscular co-ordinations are less under their voluntary control; so that the effect of fatigue is " to increase the variableness of the muscular adjustments in the less resistant types."

There is little doubt that experiments on reaction-times, sensory acuity, muscular power, and all the other devices named for measuring fatigue would have shewn the same peculiarity if it had been sought after. Galton, with remarkable insight, anticipated that the phenomenon would occur in reaction-time observations but nobody appreciated the pregnant hint. In describing the experiment for infants mentioned above he said, "We should expect to find *uniformity* in successive experiments when the pupils are fresh ; *irregularity* and prevalent delay when they are tired " (italics mine). This means that the regular rhythm of the action would break down during a state of fatigue.

General biology lends strong support to the theory that variability is of the very essence of fatigue by its demonstration that all life is rhythmic. Alternating periods of full activity and complete rest are of normal occurrence in living tissues. Such a rhythm has been observed in the capillary blood vessels of muscles and skin, in the glomerular vessels of the kidneys, and has also been noticed in voluntary muscle. Similar fluctuations are observable in the hot and cold sensations derived by stimulating the heat and cold spots on the surface of the body. Thus nerves, muscles and glands are subject to the principle of rhythmic action. Professor Herring has put forward a novel theory to explain such fluctuations based on the view that when any organ is active only a portion of the tissue units come into play.[17] In moderate activity of any organ the groups of units which are in action constantly change so that all the units are employed in rotation " individual units coming into action and going out of action in orderly sequence." This prevents undue fatigue of the separate units, permits varying degrees of graded activity of the organ, as a whole, and maintains a reserve which can be brought into play when necessity arises. From the simplest to the most complex forms of organisms we may observe this characteristic property. The protoplasm itself in plant cells moves in a definite cyclic flow and the cilia of animal cells pulsate rhythmically. Passing to the higher physiological processes such as heart beat, respiration, etc., we find that these too are essentially rhythmical, and there are more embracing rhythms of the whole organisms such as regular nocturnal sleep. By far the most instructive examples of this all-pervading rhythm are, from our point of view, presented by the nervous system, especially in reflex actions.[18] Thus the flexion-reflex of the dog's hind leg which consists of a flexion at knee, hip and ankle is produced by any nocuous stimulus applied to the leg. It may also be excited by electrical stimulation of the skin of the limb, and in that case the undulatory movements proceed in the region of about ten per second, independently of the rate of delivery of the electrical shocks and even when the stimulus is a constant current. Similar results are observable in the well-known scratch-reflex of the spinal dog,[19] which consists of a rhythmic alternation of flexion and extension at hip, knee and ankle. The reflex is brought about by a stimulus applied to any part of a large saddle-shaped region of the skin over the shoulder and back, when the impulse travels along the spinal cord and the peculiar scratching movement of the leg takes place. Professor Sherrington whose work in this sphere is classical noticed that the rhythm of the scratching movement, as far as its rate is concerned, is independent of the rhythm of the stimulus. A large variety of different stimuli are capable of evoking the reaction, yet, " under all these various modes of excitation (heat-beam, constant current, double and single induced currents, high frequency currents, and mechanical stimuli) the rhythm of the flexor response remains . . . almost the same." And further " no mode or intensity of stimulation to which I have had recourse converts rhythmic clonic beat into a maintained steady contraction." More striking still, when the reflex is in progress as the result of stimulation of the skin at one point, stimulation at some other point also producing the reflex " does not break the rhythm of the reflex or complicate it in any way."

There is obviously something peculiar to the organism itself, due it is believed to some feature of the conduction at the synapses in the neurones of the spinal cord, which renders reflex actions autonomic in their rhythm.

Again continuous stimulation of a certain part of the ' face area ' of the cerebral cortex provokes a rhythmic alternating opening and closing of the jaws, as in eating. So that nervous rhythmical activity is not limited to actions carried out by the lower centres but is observable when the initiation of the impulse has its seat in the brain.

When fatigue begins to set in for a reflex action, owing to prolonged excitation, the rhythm slows down becoming more sluggish and finally the action becomes less steady and less accurately adjusted : " it becomes tremulous and the tremor becomes progressively more marked and irregular."

Closely associated with this characteristic of the central nervous system is the fact, noted in an earlier chapter, that certain specific rhythms of activity and pause provide the most effective means of training in habit-formation. Finally, passing to mental activity itself we see the same characteristic. "There is no such thing," says Professor James,[20] "as voluntary attention sustained for more than a few seconds at a time. What is called sustained voluntary attention is a repetition of successive efforts which bring back the topic to the mind. The topic once brought back, if a congenial one, develops ; and if its development is interesting it engages the attention passively for a short time. . . . This passive interest may be short or long. As soon as it flags, the attention is diverted by some irrelevant thing, and then a voluntary effort may bring it back to the topic again ; and so on, under favourable conditions, for hours at a time." Until, in fact, fatigue sets in when

358 EDUCATIONAL PSYCHOLOGY

such repeated voluntary effort becomes more and more difficult to sustain.

Since living process is essentially rhythmical anything which baulks the rhythm is bound to interfere with action and make it more difficult. Fatigue, by upsetting the rhythm, acts as a drag on physical and mental activity. Conversely any device for maintaining steady rhythmical action tends to ward off fatigue, as is well shewn by the effect of music in enabling soldiers to march long distances in heavy kit. All forms of labour, mental or physical are carried on with greater ease when a rhythm adapted to the particular sort of work is established and maintained, and without it the toil is apt to become a burden. Mental fatigue strikes at the very core of mental activity by impeding the regular pulsation of voluntary attention. So it comes to pass that when for any reason the rhythm of attention is thwarted, and uncontrollable fluctuations occur, a feeling of subjective fatigue supervenes though the capacity for work may shew no sign of diminution, whilst on the other hand diminished capacity in the absence of disturbed attention yields no such feeling.

REFERENCES

CHAPTER I

1. *Introductory Lectures on Psycho-Analysis.* Allen & Unwin (1922), p. 249.
This is easily the best as it certainly is the most persuasive book on the subject, but it is scientifically weak.

2. *The Interpretation of Dreams,* trans. by Brill. Allen & Unwin (1920). Ch. 7, p. 425.

3. *Op. cit.,* p. 425.

4. *Essay.* Bk. 2, Ch. 21, par. 20.

5. *Outlines of Psychology.* Höffding. Macmillan (1896). Ch. 4.
Much can still be learnt from this useful treatise.

6. *History of Association Psychology,* by Warren. Constable (1921).
Gives much biographical information. The author is in sympathy with Associationism.

7. *Op. cit.* Warren, p. 32. This figure was borrowed by James in his chapter on *Habit* and passed into general psychology.

8. Autobiography, by J. S. Mill. 2nd ed. Longmans (1873), p. 108.

9. Locke's *Essay.* Bk. 2, Ch. 33.

10. *The Senses and the Intellect.* (1868.) Ch. 2. For Professor Semon's views see *The Mneme.* Allen & Unwin (1921).

11. See *Psychology, from the standpoint of a behaviourist.* Watson, Lippincott Co. (1919). This is an excellent book on *Physiology.* Provided that he does not think he is reading Psychology the student will learn much from it concerning the physical basis of mind.

12. *The Analysis of Mind.* B. Russell. Allen & Unwin (1921), Lecture 4. A clear exposition of the notion of Causality.

13. *An Outline of Psychology.* Methuen (1923). Chs. 8, 15, 17, more especially pp. 259–63 and p. 396 ff.

14. *Education and World Citizenship.* Maxwell Garnett. Cambridge University Press (1921). Ch. 12.
See my Review of this, *Brit. Journ. of Psy.,* vol. 12, p. 188 ff.
The part of this book dealing with the relations of schools and colleges should be read by every student of Education.

15. *Psychological Principles.* J. Ward. Cambridge University Press (1918). Ch. 4, par. 7.
Consult also his *Naturalism and Agnosticism.* A. & C. Black (1899). The importance of subjective selection is clearly brought out.

16. *Principles of Psychology.* Macmillan. Vol. 1, ch. 9.
The title of this chapter itself constituted a new departure.

17. *Growth of Mind.* Koffka. Kegan Paul : and Harcourt, Brace & Co. (1924).
The theory is expounded from the educational standpoint. See my review of this in *Brit. Journ. of Psy.*, vol. 16, p. 56.
18. *Groundwork of Psychology* (1905). Ch. 11.
19. Inheritance of Acquired Characters. Detlefsen. *Physiological Reviews* (Baltimore). Vol. 5, No. 2 (1925).
A good summary of the present position.
20. *Heredity.* Chapters 1, 7, 14.
His verdict on the Inheritance of Acquired Characters is "not proven."
21. *Op. cit.* Ch. 17, par. 4.
Remarks very acute ; but he was unacquainted with more modern work.
22. Quoted in Ward's *Principles*, p. 420, note.
23. *Biometrika.* Vol. 3. On the Inheritance of Mental and Moral Characters in Man.
24. *Francis Galton Laboratory Memoirs*, I (1907). The Inheritance of Ability. Schuster and Elderton.
Also, *Biometrika.* Vol. 14 (1923). Summary of Present Position with regard to the Inheritance of Intelligence. Elderton.
25. The measure used in the text is the mean square contingency coefficient.
26. *An Introduction to the Study of Heredity.* Macbride. Home University Library (1924). Ch. 4, gives all the favourable evidence.
27. Watson. *Op. cit.*
28. *Brit. Med. Journ.*, Aug. 11th, 1923, p. 256. An account of the International Physiological Congress (Edinburgh), where Pavlov communicated his results. An account in English of Pavlov's recent work is to be published.
Note.—The most penetrating brief account of Heredity on the biological side, will be found in a small book by E. Rabaud, *L'Hérédité.* Armand Colin, Paris (1921). Especially good in dealing with Mendelian Inheritance.
The little that is known about Mendelian characters in Man is well summarised in *Die Rehoboter Bastards* by E. Fischer, published by G. Fischer (Jena, 1913).

CHAPTER II

1. *Montessori and her Inspirers.* R. F. Fynne. Longmans (1924).
2. *Problems of Philosophy.* Ch. 7. Home Univ. Library.
3. The fraction ⅔ means that the person can read only at 6 metres letters which are read by the normal eye at 9 metres : and so on.
4. *Cambridge Anthropometry.* Arts. by J. Venn, in *Journ. of Anthropological Institute*, vol. 18 (1888), and *Nature* (March 1890).
5. All the data are to be found in the various reports issued by County and Boro' Education Authorities, and are summarised in the

Annual Reports of the Chief Medical Officer. Board of Education—H.M. Stationery Office.

6. Ce que voient les yeux d'enfant. E. Cramausel. *Journ. de Psychologie* (1924).

7. Is myopia inherited or acquired ? Ruckmich. *Journ. of Ed. Psy.* Vol. 4 (1913).

8. Reliability of school tests of auditory acuity. Peterson and Kuderman. *Journ. of Ed. Psy.* Vol. 15 (1924).

9. Les acuités sensorielle. Foucault. *Journ. de Psychologie* (1924).

10. Inertia of eye and brain. Cattell. *Brain.* Vol. 8 (1885).

11. The relative legibility of the small letters. Sanford. *Amer. Journ of Psy.* Vol. 1 (1888). Relative legibility of different faces of printing types. Roethlein. Same journal. Vol. 23 (1912).

The latter art. is much the most important so far. New evidence will soon be forthcoming.

12. Power of the eye to sustain clear seeing under different conditions of lighting. Ferree and Rand. *Journ. of Ed. Psy.* Vol. 8 (1917). Effect of Intensity of illumination on Acuity. Same authors. *Amer. Journ. of Psy.* Vol. 34 (1923).

13. Table of logarithms, by Babbage. London (1827).

14. *Psychology and Pedagogy of Reading.* Huey. Macmillan (1910). The best introduction to the subject. Summarises all the preceding work and deals with the question of types, etc., for school books.

See *Report of British Association on Influence of school books on eyesight.* 2nd ed. To be obtained from the Secretary. Gives useful information about type and spacing for school books.

CHAPTER III

1. *Principles of Psychology.* Vol. I, ch. 11.

2. The whole notion of mental activity is admirably presented in Ward's *Psychological Principles.* Ch. 3.

3. See 'Obliviscence and Reminiscence.' *Monograph Supplement of Brit. Journ. of Psy.* (1913). Pp. 70 ff. and 82.

4. A Revision of Imageless Thought. *Psychological Review.* Vol. 22 (1915).

5. The notion that a remembered fact must, of necessity, be a sensorial image, visual, auditory, verbal, etc., though supported by nearly all psychologists is a mere assumption with no convincing evidence in its favour. Feelings are often confused with images.

6. This lecture is printed in full with all the diagrams in *Brit. Journ. of Psychology.* Vol. 15 (1924). Art. on " A study in preperception."

7. *Text-book of Experimental Psychology.* Myers. Camb. Univ. Press (1911), p. 141.

Lewes' account of Preperception is given in *Problems of Life and Mind. Third Series. Problem 2nd* (1879). James borrowed freely from this, including the terminology.

CHAPTER IV

1. *Inquiries into Human Faculty.* F. Galton. Everyman Series. First published in 1883. Can still be read with profit.

2. Distribution and functions of Mental Imagery. Betts. *Teachers' College* publications, Columbia Univ. (1909).

3. *Experimental Psychology of the Thought Processes.* Titchener. Macmillan (1909), p. 7.

4. *Critical Examination of Psycho-Analysis.* Wohlgemuth. Allen & Unwin (1923), p. 25.

5. Nature of the Mental Image. *Psy. Review.* Vol. 15 (1908).

6. Galton. *Op. cit.* Section on Mental Imagery.

7. The intellectual respectability of muscular skill. Pear. *Brit. Journ. of Psy.* Vol. 12 (1921).

8. *L'Etude experimentale de l'Intelligence.* Binet. Schleicher Frères. Paris (1903). One of the best books on the sympathetic study of individual differences in children.

9. Mental Ass. in School Children. Rusk. *Brit. Journ of Psy.* Vol. 3.

10. Recherches Comparatives sur la mémoire des formes. Piéron, *L'Année Psychologique.* 21st year (1920).

11. A marked case of mimetic ideation. Colvin. *Psy. Review.* Vol. 17 (1910).

12. Piéron. *Op. cit.*, p. 147. The article contains a very acute analysis of mental imagery.

13. Imagery in Imaginative Literature. Peers. *Journ. of Exp. Pedagogy.* Vol. 2 (1913–14).

14. Conditions which arouse mental images in thought. C. Fox. *Brit. Journ. of Psy.* Vol. 6. Also Bartlett on Functions of Images. Same journal. Vol. 11. Comstock, Relevancy of Imagery, etc., *Amer. Journ. of Psy.* Vol. 32 (1921).

15. Titchener. *Op. cit.*, p. 19.

16. On meaning. Pillsbury. *Psychological Review.* Vol. 15 (1908).

17. The phenomenon of meaning. Ogden. *Am. Journ. of Psy.* Vol. 34 (1923).

18. Titchener. *Op. cit.* Gives an admirable summary of this work.

19. *Family life of Heine.* Translated by Leland. Heinemann (1896), p. 149.

20. Forster's *Life of Dickens.* Book 9, Ch. 1.

21. *Memories of Whistler.* Way. Lane (1912).

22. A qualitative investigation of the Effect of Mode of Presentation, etc. O'Brien. *Amer. Journ. of Psy.* Vol. 32 (1921). The following papers may, with advantage, be consulted. On the nature of images. G. Dawes Hicks. *Brit. Journ. of Psy.* Vol. 15 (1924). The view taken is very similar to that suggested in this book; though it is arrived at on general grounds. Factors in the Mental Process of School Children. Carey. *Brit. Journ. of Psy.* Vol. 7.

A revision of imageless thought. Woodworth. *Psy. Review*. Vol. 22 —one of the best articles on the topic.

On meaning. A Symposium. *Psy. Review*. Vol. 15.

An objective interpretation of meaning. Kantor. *Am. Journ. of Psy*. Vol. 32.

Meaning and Imagery. Moore. *Psy. Review*. Vol. 24.

A useful book on some points of this Chapter is *The Meaning of Meaning*. Ogden and Richards. *Int. Lib. Psych*. (1923).

For Eidetic Imagery. Allport. *Brit. Journ. of Psy*. Vol. 15 (1924). Note especially the looseness of the whole investigation and its unscientific nature.

Note.—Whenever an author thinks that an image is a faint copy of a sensation the rest of his remarks on the subject may be ignored.

CHAPTER V

1. *The Republic*. Bk. 7, 518 E. Jowett's translation.

A similar view to Plato's is held by Dewey, who says : " All virtues and vices are habits which incorporate objective forces. They are interactions of elements contributed by the make-up of an individual with elements supplied by the out-door world. They can be studied objectively as physiological functions, and can be modified by change of either personal or social elements." *Human Nature and Conduct*. Allen & Unwin (1922), sect. 1. The author thinks that the study of habit is the key to social psychology and develops this view philosophically.

2. *Story of My Life*. Hodder & Stoughton (1903). Ch. 3.

3. Groves. *Dictionary of Music*. Art. Handel.

4. *Memoirs* of Benvenuto Cellini, by himself. Bk. 1, sect. 7.

5. *Adolescence*. Vol. II (1904), p. 484.

6. *An Outline of Psychology*. Methuen. Ch. 6 (1923).

7. *The Great Society*. G. Wallas. Macmillan.

8. Dewey. *Op. cit*. Sect. 1.

9. Bryan and Harter. Studies in the physiology and psychology of the telegraphic language. *Psy. Review*. Vols. 4 and 6 (1897–1899).

These are still the most exact and complete studies of the habit curves, and repay careful reading.

10. The significance of learning curves. Peterson. *Journ. of Exp. Psy*. Vol. 2 (1917).

The curves in the text were obtained by combining the results of 23 students' attempts to learn to toss 2 balls with one hand catching one whilst the other was in the air. Each practice period was continued until the total number of successful catches reached 200. The practice was continued daily until for 5 days in succession they made no errors (misses). This is open to the objection that each practice period does not give the same amount of practice. The art. is suggestive.

11. Artificial syllables of 3 letters, such as wov, nim, etc.

These must be constructed in accordance with a very rigid plan (see Myers, *Text-book of Exp. Psy.*) so as to eliminate meaning as far as possible. Otherwise all work with them is wasted time.

12. G. Wallas. *Op. cit.* Ch. 5.

13. Experiments in Learning, etc. Smith and McDougall. *Brit. Journ. of Psy.* Vol. 10 (1919–20).

14. Dewey. *Op. cit.*, p. 71.

15. *Principles of Psychology.* Vol. I, ch. 16, p. 663.

16. James. *Op. cit.* Vol. I, ch. 4, p. 108.

17. Smith and McDougall. *Op. cit.*

18. On this whole section admirable accounts are given in two books in the *Int. Lib. Psych.*, namely, Köhler's *Mentality of Apes* (1925), and Koffka's *Growth of Mind* (1924).

19. McDougall. *Social Psychology.* 13th ed., p. 102.

20. Köhler. *Op. cit.*, p. 225.

21. *Manual.* 3rd ed., p. 395.

22. McDougall. *Op. cit.* Ch. 4.

23. Called *association by similars* because the chimes at different times are similar.

24. *Groundwork of Psychology.* (1905.) Ch. 11.

25. Dewey, *op. cit.*, makes the remark, " To understand the existence of organised ways or habits we surely need to go to physics, chemistry and physiology rather than psychology." The whole tenor of our chapter shews that this is a mistake, but it is true enough of the objective manifestations of a habit.

26. The learning curve equation. Thurstone. *Psychological Bulletin.* Vol. 14 (1917), p. 64. See a criticism of this in *Psy. Review.* Vol. 25 (1918), p. 81, by Blair.

27. Hence when $n=0$ the time taken to perform a new task is *not* infinite : p tells us what previous experience, before the experiment begins, has contributed to its successful performance.

28. The equation of the learning function. Meyer and Eppright. *Amer. Journ. of Psy.* Vol. 34 (1923).

29. A translation of Ebbinghaus' original paper is given in *Memory.* Columbia Teachers' College (1913).

30. For children there is slight evidence to shew that the decay is slow at first and more rapid later on.

Note.—Most of the extensive literature on Habit is tarred by the physiological brush. The following articles by Piéron are strongly recommended, Sur les phénomènes de mémoire, etc., *L'Année Psychologique* (1913) : Recherches Comparatives sur la mémoire, *L'Année Psy.* (1920).

CHAPTER VI

1. Butler's *Unconscious Memory*. Fifield (1910). Ch. 6 contains a translation of Hering's famous lecture on Retentiveness called ' On Memory.' See also Butler's *Life and Habit*. Fifield.
Consult also Rignano on *Biological Memory*. Int. Lib. Psych. (1925).
2. *Matière et Mémoire*. Bergson. F. Alcan. Paris (1908). Ch. 2.
3. Some experiments in learning and retention. Smith and McDougall. *Brit. Journ. of Psy.* Vol. 10 (1919–20). A very suggestive article containing useful experiments and methods.
4. Memory and the direction of associations. Wohlgemüth. *Brit. Journ. of Psy.* Vol. 5.
5. Ward's *Psychological Principles*. Ch. 4, par. 7.
6. The relation of length of material to time taken for learning, etc. D. O. Lyon. *Journ. of Educ. Psy.* Vol. 5 (1914). An important contribution to the subject with an account of heroic experiments extending over 4 years.
7. 'Obliviscence and Reminiscence.' *Monograph Supplement.* Vol. I. *Brit. Journ. of Psy.* (1913).
8. A study in logical memory. S. D. Austin. *Amer. Journ. of Psy.* Vol. 32 (1921). This art. really deals with memory and not with habit which is the bane of articles on the subject.
9. Should poems be learnt by school children as ' wholes ' or in ' parts.' Winch. *Brit. Journ. of Psy.* Vol. 15 (1924).
This art. is vitiated by the antiquated methods used by the children in the schools.
10. *Introd. Lectures on Psycho-Analysis*. Eng. tr. Allen & Unwin (1922). Ch. 4. Also Freud's *Psycho-pathology of Everyday life*. Fisher & Unwin (1920).
11. *Instinct and the Unconscious*. Camb. Univ. Press (1920), Appendix I.
12. Influence of Feeling on Memory. Wohlgemüth. *Brit. Journ. of Psy.* Vol. 13 (1923). Also, Influence of Subjective Preference on Memory. C. Fox. Same vol. of *Brit. Journ. of Psy.*
13. *Text-book of Exp. Psy.* Camb. Univ. Press. Ch. 13, p. 165 (1911).
14. Mach. *Science of Mechanics*. Ch. 4, sect. 4.
15. *Mental Physiology*. 6th ed. (1881), ch. 10.
16. *Psychology for Teachers*. Arnold (1906), p. 70.
17. *Principles*. Vol. I, ch. 16.
An interesting theory of forgetting has been put forward by A. Lynch in his *Principles of Psychology*, G. Bell & Sons (1923). Pt. III, ch. 2. By learning considerable extracts of poetry by heart and testing himself at long intervals he found that he could remember the ' inspirational ' parts but not the parts which merely served to connect these, i.e. the ' padding.' In this way he thinks it is possible to analyse a work of art æsthetically, on the ground that " the essential characteristic expression of a passage is retained, and the accidental forgotten." If this is so, it is a striking confirmation of the influence of interest on memory dealt with in the text.

CHAPTER VII

For the earliest experiments the following books give good summaries.

Educational Psychology. Thorndike. Kegan Paul (1913). Vol. II, ch. 12.

The Learning Process. Colvin. Macmillan (1911). Chs. 14, 15.

The Educative Process. Bagley. Macmillan (1914). Ch. 13.

1. Plato's *Republic*. Bk. VII, 526 B and 527 C. The first extract is Jowett's translation amended, and the second has been retranslated as he does not give the exact meaning.

2. See Locke's *Educational Writings*. Ed. by Adamson. Camb. Univ. Press, and an art. by Phillips in *Brit. Journ. of Psy.* Vol. 13, p. 1.

3. *Essays on a Liberal Education*. Macmillan (1867). Ch. 2. Art. by H. Sidgwick. The book is a series of arts. giving the point of view of the best thinkers of the period.

4. *Schools Inquiry Commission* (1868). Vol. 5, p. 677.

5. Same Commission, vol. 5, p. 726. Also see the evidence given by other women witnesses ; and Adamson's *Short History of Ed.* Camb. Univ. Press, p. 323.

6. *Essays on a Liberal Education*. Art. by Wilson, p. 267.

7. *Principles*. Vol. I (1890), ch. 16, p. 666, *note*.

8. Memory and Formal Training. *Brit. Journ. of Psy.* Vol. 4 (1911).

It is difficult to understand why the doctrine was called " formal training." Its more modern name of ' transfer of training ' is unintelligible—what we are looking for are the *effects* or *consequences* of training. The best name of all would be *generalised* training.

9. Transfer of Training in relation to Intelligence. Brooks. Critique of methods of estimating and measuring transfer of training. Gates. Both in *Journ. of Ed. Psy.* Vol. 15 (1924).

10. Methods and Results of a class experiment in learning. Dearborn and Brewer. *Journ. of Ed. Psy.* Vol. 9 (1918).

11. A comparison of two types of learning. *Journ. of Ed. Psy.* Vol. 9 (1918).

12. Mental Discipline in High School Studies. *Journ. of Ed. Psy.* Vol. 15 (1924).

13. General v. group factors in mental activities. Thomson. *Psy. Review*. Vol. 27 (1920).

14. Ward's *Psychological Principles*. Ch. 3, par. 1.

15. *Mentality of Apes*. Köhler. Int. Lib. Psych. (1925). Ch. 8. An excellent book on the topic of this chapter. Who would have expected apes to solve the problem !

16. *British Med. Journ.* Aug. 1923, p. 256.

17. *Republic*. Bk. VII, 531 E.

18. Russell. *Mysticism and Logic*. Longmans (1921). Ch. 4. On the study of mathematics. The whole book should be read.

19. *Cambridge Review*. April 24th, 1925. Neill, p. 338.

There is a vast literature on the topic of the chapter, but a good deal of it is worthless owing to primitive mental atomism, or crude associationism which now masquerades under a new name, to wit 'mental factors'; but the more it changes its designation the more it remains the same. The various volumes of the *Journ. of Ed. Psy.* will provide copious references.

CHAPTER VIII

1. *The Psychology of Suggestion.* B. Sidis. Appleton (1911).

2. *Instinct and the Unconscious.* Rivers. (1920).

3. *La Suggestibilité.* Binet, Schleicher Frères. Paris (1900). A very useful book with interesting experiments and dealing with suggestibility in the normal life. See also, De la suggestibilité naturelle, *Rev. Psychol.*, 38 (1894), pp. 337–47. Binet et Henri.

4. *The Master and his Boys.* S. S. Harris. Warren & Son, Ltd. Winchester (1925), p. 18 ff.

The whole book is worthy of very careful study. The quotation given in the text deals incidentally with 'sneaking,' a topic which is admirably dealt with by Simpson in *An Adventure in Education.* Sidgwick & Jackson, 1917.

5. *Mental and Scholastic Tests.* P. S. King (1921), p. 195.

6. *Life of Lord Rayleigh* by his son. Arnold (1924).

7. An Experimental Study of Sensory Suggestion. Edwards. *Amer. Journ. of Psy.* Vol. 26 (1915).

8. Individual and Sex Differences in Suggestibility. Brown. *Univ. of California Publications in Psy.* Vol. 2, No. 6 (1916).

9. Trotter. *Instincts of the Herd in Peace and War,* quoted by Hart in *Psy. of Insanity.* Camb. Univ. Press, p. 105.

10. Quoted in Mill's *Logic.* Bk. II, ch. 3, par. 3.

11. The influence of the form of a question. Muscio. *Brit. Journ. of Psy.* Vol. 8 (1915–17).

12. *Suggestion in Education.* Keatinge. Black (1907).

13. Keatinge. *Op. cit.,* p. 125.

There is not much of value concerning suggestibility in the *normal state,* collected together in any one volume or article. But the following contain useful points not referred to above. Suggestion and Mental Analysis. Brown. Univ. of London Press (1922). Suggestibility with and without prestige in children. Aveling and Hargreave. *Brit. Journ. of Psy.* Vol. 12 (1921–22).

The opinion of Professor Hill quoted in the text is to be found in *Youth and the Race,* ed. by Marchant. Kegan Paul (1923), p. 269.

CHAPTER IX

1. *Studies in Word-Association.* Jung. Transl. by Eder. Heinemann. *Analytic Psychology.* Jung. Baillière Tindall & Cox (1917).

Psychological Types. Jung. Int. Lib. Psych., also deals with points in this chapter.

2. A study of assoc. in children.   Rand and Rosanoff.   *Psy. Review*, 20 (1913).

An investigation into the rate of assoc.   Anderson.   *Journ. of Ed. Psy.* (1917).

Mental Assoc. in Children.   Rusk.   *Brit. Journ. of Psy.*   Vol. 3.

3. The Relation of Complex and Sentiment.   *Brit. Journ. of Psy.* Vol. 5.

4. *A Neglected Complex.*   Bousfield.   Kegan Paul (1924).

5. *Introductory Lectures on Psycho-Analysis.*   Freud.   Allen & Unwin, 1922, ch. 6, p. 90.

6. *The Neurotic Constitution.*   Adler.   Kegan Paul (1921).   *Individual Psychology.*   Adler.   Int. Lib. Psych. (1924).

7. *Childhood's Fears.*   Morton.   Duckworth (1925).

A study by a head master illustrated by cases of his own pupils. He calls the complex ' inferiority—fear-complex.'

8. *Neurotic Constitution.*   Introd. p. xii.

9. *Instinct and the Unconscious* (1920).   Rivers.   Ch. 2.

10. Rivers.   *Op. cit.*

11. A study in feeling and emotion, etc.   Flügel.   *Brit. Journ. of Psy.*   Vol. 15 (1925).

12. *Introd. Lectures on Psycho-Analysis*, p. 298.   Freud has another Principle called the Reality Principle.   See his *Collected Papers*, vol. 2 (1924).

13. *Principles of Psychology.*   James.   Vol. 2, p. 550.

14. *Three Contributions to the Theory of Sex.*   Freud.   Nervous and Mental Disease Publishing Co.   Washington.   2nd ed. (1920).

15. *Youth and the Race.*   Edited by Marchant.   Kegan Paul (1923).   This consists of the evidence given before the National Birth Rate Commission.

16. *The Neurotic Constitution*, p. 31 ff.

17. *Three Contributions, etc.*, p. 62.

18. *Op. cit.*, p. 55.

19. *A Critical examination of Psycho-Analysis.*   Allen & Unwin. Ch. 7.

A clever examination of the subject.   Should be read by everybody who has been infected by the doctrines.   The principles are examined in a light and witty style but very acutely.

20. *Papers on Psycho-Analysis.*   E. Jones.   Baillière Tindall & Cox (1913).   See the chapter on Psycho-analysis and Education which is simply a rehash of Freud's views.

21. *Child Psychology.*   Rasmussen.   Gyldendal.   See vol. 2.   The Kindergarten Child.

22. See Wohlgemuth, *op. cit.*, ch. 7, for parts of this analysis.

23. Rivers.   *Op. cit.*   Chs. 15 and 16.

24. Bousfield.   *Op. cit.*   Ch. 3.

25. *Youth and the Race.*   Dr Sibly's evidence, p. 183.   Dr Rivers also gave evidence and referred, apparently with approval to the doctrine of infantile sexuality, adding that he knew nothing about it from his own experience.

26. *Op. cit.*   Evidence of Tansley.   In some ways the most striking evidence in the book ; gives an account of how he trained his own

children in sex matters. He has the advantage of being a distinguished biologist himself and could therefore do things outside the range of other parents.

27. *Op. cit.* Evidence of the head master of Charterhouse.

Note.—I have not referred to the minor psycho-analysts since they simply deal with unsavoury detail and add nothing to our knowledge.

CHAPTER X

1. Russell. *Mysticism and Logic.* Longmans. Ch. 4.

2. Adamson. *Short history of Ed.* Ch. 1.

3. Croce. *The Essence of Æsthetic.* Heinemann (1921), transl. by Ainslie.

4. Bréal. *Semantics,* trans. by Cust. Heinemann (1900). *The King's English.* Clarendon Press. *The Meaning of Meaning.* Ogden and Richards. Int. Lib. Psych. (1923). Chs. 9 and 10.

Seeing that the use of language is the most distinctive human characteristic it is a matter of wonder that Semantics is not more widely studied by psychologists.

5. A happy translation of the Ger. Einfühlung.

6. Preface to 2nd ed. *Lyrical Ballads* (1800).

7. Poems of Coleridge, ed. by E. H. Coleridge. Oxford Press (1912), p. 503.

8. *Analytical Psychology.* Jung. (1917). Chs. 11 and 14. Also *Psychological Types.* Int. Lib. Psych. (1924).

9. *British Journ. of Psy.* Vols. 2 and 3. Arts. by Bullough. Vol. 7. Art. by Myers and Valentine, Vol. 13, art. by Myers.

10. *Florentinische Nächte.* Page after page of Ch. 1 is a detailed series of romantic pictures induced by music.

11. *L'Art.* Rodin. Ch. 2. Grasset. Paris (1924).

12. *Op. cit.*

13. Psychical Distance, etc. Bullough. *Brit. Journ. of Psy.* Vol. 5.

14. *The Play Way.* Caldwell Cook. Heinemann.

15. See the chapter on Mental Imagery.

16. *The Gentle Art of Making Enemies* by Whistler.

17. As Lamborn in the *Rudiments of Criticism.* Clarendon Press (1916). Ch. 9. This is the sole objection to an otherwise suggestive and admirable book.

18. *Victorian Poetry.* J. Drinkwater. Hodder & Stoughton (1923). Pt. 2, ch. 3.

19. Indiv. Diffs. in listening to music. *Brit. Journ. of Psy.* Vol. 13 (1922).

20. *The Music of Life.* C. T. Smith. P. S. King & Son (1919).

21. Published by the Gramophone Co., 363 Oxford St., W.

22. Lamborn. *Op. cit.* See also Perse Playbooks. Heffer (Cambridge).

23. See chapter on Mental Imagery.

24. 22 men and 15 women.

2 A

25. The Nature of Rhythmic experience. Isaacs. *Psy. Review.*
Vol. 27 (1920).

26. See the *Play Way.*

27. *Rhythm, Music and Education.* Dalcroze. Chatto & Windus
(1921). Also an art. in *Psyche.* Vol. 5, p. 121.

Reference may also be made to Some exps. on Æsthetics. Feasey,
Brit. Journ. of Psy., Vol. 12, and an art. by Wheeler in Vol. 13.

On the subject of Rhythm in nature see *Life.* Shipley. Camb.
Univ. Press. Ch. 12.

An excellent account of æsthetic theory is to be found in *The
Beautiful,* by H. R. Marshall. Macmillan (1924). More recently the
field has been covered by Richards in *Principles of Literary Criticism.*
Int. Lib. Psych. (1925).

CHAPTER XI

The study of mental tests should begin with the various articles in
L'Année Psychologique. See especially

A propos de la mesure de l'intelligence. Binet (1905).

Méthodes nouvelles pour faire le diagnostic différentiel, etc. Binet
and Simon (1905).

Le développement de l'int. chez les enfants. Binet and Simon (1908).

Nouvelles recherches sur la mesure du niveau intellectuel, etc.
Binet (1911).

L'echelle métrique de l'intelligence, etc. Saffiotti (1912). Deals
with a novel method of marking the tests.

1. *Montessori and her Inspirers.* Fynne. Longmans (1924).

2. *Education as a Science.* Bain, 5th ed., 1885, p. 16.

3. The term ' mental ratio ' is preferable to Intelligence Quotient
(I.Q.), since the latter presupposes that the tests measure Intelligence.

4. *Measurement of Intelligence.* Terman. Harrap (1916).

5. Both published by P. S. King & Son (London). Useful biblio-
graphies are given.

6. Comparative Variability of different ages. Henmon and Living-
stone. *Journ. of Ed. Psy.* Vol. 13 (1922).

7. A point scale for measuring mental ability. Yerkes and Foster.
Warwick and York (Baltimore), 1923.

8. Results of re-tests by means of the Binet Scale. Wallin. *Journ.
of Ed. Psy.* Vol. 12 (1921). Same journal. Vol. 14 (1923), p. 231.

9. Additional re-tests by Stanford Revision. Garrison. *Journ. of
Ed. Psy.* Vol. 13 (1922).

10. Constancy of the Intelligence Quotient. Gray and Marsden.
Brit. Journ. of Psy. Vols. 13 and 15 (1923 and 1925).

11. I have omitted dec. points in this and later cases owing to their
doubtful value. See Notes on Interpretation of Correlation Measures.
Hamilton. *Forum of Ed.* Vol. 2 (1924).

12. Constancy of the Stanford-Binet I.Q., etc. *Journ. of Ed. Psy.*
Vol. 12 (1921).

13. *Journ. of Ed. Psy.* Art. by Henmon and Burns. Vol. 14 (1923),
p. 247.

14. The limit of the growth of int. Ballard. *Brit. Journ. of Psy.* Vol. 12.

15. Investigation of group int. tests. Dobson. *Brit. Journ. of Psy.* Vol. 15 (1924).

16. *Psychological Tests of Educable Capacity.* H.M. Stationery Office. (London) 1924. Gives a bibliography.

17. I have tried the same group test on 28 Cambridge graduates and the average mark was 161.

18. Interpretation and Application of I.Q. Freeman. *Journ. of Ed. Psy.* Vol. 12. Growth of Int. and the I.Q. Same vol. Art. by Peterson.

19. Rate of Mental Growth. Brooks. *Journ. of Ed. Psy.* Vol. 12.

20. *Mental and Scholastic tests among retarded children.* Gordon. Board of Ed. pamphlet. No. 44. H.M. Stationery Office.

21. Social and Geog. Distribution of Int., etc. Duff and Thomson. *Brit. Journ. of Psy.* Vol. 14 (1923).

22. *Mental Tests in the American Army* by Yoakum and Yerkes. Sidgwick & Jackson (1920).

23. An application of American Army tests. Bowie. *Brit. Journ. of Psy.* Vol. 13 (1923).

24. The Northumberland Mental Tests. Thomson. *Brit. Journ. of Psy.* Vol. 12 (1921).

25. Pub. by Hodder & Stoughton, 1922.

26. Mental tests for Selection of Univ. students. Rogers. *Brit. Journ. of Psy.* Vol. 15 (1925).

27. Comparison of certain Int. Scales. Wilson. *Brit. Journ. of Psy.* Vol. 15 (1924). The other tests were Terman's, Otis, National and Simplex.

28. Reliability of Rankings by Group tests, etc. Geyer. *Journ. of Ed. Psy.* Vol. 13 (1922).

29. Some of the best will be found in Burt's Mental and Scholastic tests.

30. *A measure of int.* Spearman. Methuen (1925).

31. *Child psychology.* Rasmussen. Vol. 2. Gyldendal.

32. *Psy. Tests of Educable Capacity*, p. 229.

33. Int. and its Measurement. *Journ. of Ed. Psy.* Vol. 12 (1921).

34. The following arts. in *Brit. Journ. of Psy.*:
Some exp. results in correlation of Mental Abilities. Brown. Vol. 3. Exp. tests of General Intelligence. Burt. Vol. 3. General Ability. Hart and Spearman. Vol. 5.

35. *Psychological Principles* (1918). Ch. 3.

36. General v. group factors in mental abilities. Thomson. *Psy. Review* (1920). *Essentials of Mental Measurement.* Brown and Thomson. Camb. Univ. Press (1921). Manifold theories of the Two Factors. Spearman. *Psy. Review* (1920). General Int. objectively determined. Spearman. *Am. Journ. of Psy.* (1904).

37. Correlation of Abilities, etc. Hollingworth. *Journ. of Ed. Psy.* Vol. 4 (1913).
Influence of Practice on correlation of abilities. Strickland. Same journal. Vol. 9 (1918).

The following should also be consulted :
Education and World Citizenship. Maxwell Garnett. Camb. Univ.
Press. *Proceedings* of VIIth International Congress of Psychology
(1924). Camb. Univ. Press. Communications on *Nature of Intelligence,* and *Conception of Nervous and Mental Energy.*

CHAPTER XII

1. *Influence of Alcohol on Fatigue.* Rivers. Arnold (1908).
2. A contribution to the Study of Fatigue. Smith. *Brit. Journ.
of Psy.* Vol. 8.
One of the best contributions to the subject in all respects. Deals
especially well with subjective fatigue.
3. Chemical Dynamics of Muscle. F. G. Hopkins. *John Hopkins'
Hospital Bulletin.* Vol. 32 (1921).
4. See a letter by Sir J. Mackenzie. *Times,* London, Feb. 11th, 1925.
5. By the Industrial Fatigue Research Board. The results are
published in a series of Reports by H.M. Stationery Office, London.
6. Rivers. *Op. cit.*
7. *Journ. of Anthropological Institute.* Vol. 18 (1889). Art. by
Galton.
8. *Mind and Work.* C. S. Myers. Univ. of London Press (1920),
p. 164.
9. Researches on Physical and Mental Development of School
Children. Gilbert. *Studies from Yale Psychological Laboratory.*
Vol. 2 (1894).
10. VIIth International Congress of Psychology. *Proceedings.*
Camb. Univ. Press. (1924), p. 158. Paper by Adrian. See also a
paper by C. S. Myers in the same Proceedings.
11. *Brit. Journ. of Psy.* Winch. Vol. 4 (1911).
12. This coefficient was calculated thus $\frac{m.\ v.}{Av} \times 100$.
Not all the coefficients are given by Winch as he, like others, failed
to appreciate their great significance.
13. Smith. *Op. cit.*
14. The tests were all chosen from suitable portions of Macaulay's
History, Ch. 3. Note that a boy really loses 3 marks for an incorrect
word, as by making a wrong stroke he misses 2 words and in addition
a mark is deducted.
15. Fatigue and work curve from a 10-hour day in addition. Reed.
Journ. of Educ. Psy. (1924). The author was unaware of the deduction
which could be made from his figures.
16. A method of measuring fatigue of the eyes. R. E. Wager.
Journ. of Educ. Psy. Vol. 13 (1922).
This is a sound art. viewing the subject from the right standpoint.
17. *Brit. Med. Journ.* Aug. 4th, 1923. P. 203.
18. *Integrative Action of the Nervous System.* Sherrington. Constable (1911). Lect. 2.

19. A dog whose spinal cord is transected in the neck so as to eliminate the action of the higher nervous centres.

20. *Principles of Psychology.* Vol. I, p. 420.

Although there is a large literature on Fatigue much of it is confused owing to the fact that the authors have been searching for the wrong effects.

The following may be consulted:

Experimental Pedagogy. Claparède. Arnold. Ch. 5. Gives all the earlier work up to 1910.

Fatigue and Efficiency. Goldmark. Ch. 2. Russell Sage Foundation. New York (1912). Gives earlier physiological work.

Fatigue. Mosso. Allen & Unwin (1915). Very readable. The first use of the ergograph.

Any good textbook on physiology will give more modern work.

Differentiation of the Curriculum, etc. Appendix 5. H.M. Stationery Office (1923). Gives sex differences.

Is a Fatigue Test Possible? Muscio. *Brit. Journ. of Psy.* Vol. 12 (1921–22). A good theoretical art. on the definition and measurement of fatigue. He reaches the conclusion that no single test is possible. Our discussion has shewn that almost any test is suitable provided that the correct calculations are made.

INDEX

This Index does not include the Notes on pages 359 to 373

PRINTED IN GREAT BRITAIN BY
THE EDINBURGH PRESS, 9 AND 11 YOUNG STREET, EDINBURGH